Lung Cancer

Editors

DANIEL MORGENSZTERN
ROY S. HERBST

HEMATOLOGY/ONCOLOGY CLINICS OF NORTH AMERICA

www.hemonc.theclinics.com

Consulting Editors
GEORGE P. CANELLOS
H. FRANKLIN BUNN

February 2017 • Volume 31 • Number 1

ELSEVIER

1600 John F. Kennedy Boulevard • Suite 1800 • Philadelphia, Pennsylvania, 19103-2899

http://www.theclinics.com

HEMATOLOGY/ONCOLOGY CLINICS OF NORTH AMERICA Volume 31, Number 1
February 2017 ISSN 0889-8588, ISBN 13: 978-0-323-49650-6

Editor: Stacy Eastman
Developmental Editor: Kristen Helm

Hematology/Oncology Clinics (ISSN 0889-8588) is published bimonthly by Elsevier Inc., 360 Park Avenue South, New York, NY 10010-1710. Months of issue are February, April, June, August, October, and December. Business and Editorial Offices: 1600 John F. Kennedy Blvd., Ste. 1800, Philadelphia, PA 19103—2899. Customer Service Office: 3251 Riverport Lane, Maryland Heights, MO 63043. Periodicals postage paid at New York, NY and at additional mailing offices. Subscription prices are $397.00 per year (domestic individuals), $742.00 per year (domestic institutions), $100.00 per year (domestic students/residents), $453.00 per year (Canadian individuals), $919.00 per year (Canadian institutions) $536.00 per year (international individuals), $919.00 per year (international institutions), and $255.00 per year (international and Canadian students/residents). International air speed delivery is included in all Clinics subscription prices. All prices are subject to change without notice. **POSTMASTER:** Send address changes to Hematology/Oncology Clinics of North America, Elsevier Health Sciences Division, Subscription Customer Service, 3251 Riverport Lane, Maryland Heights, MO 63043. Customer Service (orders, claims, online, change of address): Elsevier Health Sciences Division, Subscription **Customer Service, 3251 Riverport Lane, Maryland Heights, MO 63043. Tel: 1-800-654-2452 (U.S. and Canada); 314-447-8871 (outside U.S. and Canada). Fax: 314-447-8029. E-mail: journalscustomerservice-usa@elsevier.com (for print support); journalsonlinesupport-usa@elsevier.com (for online support).**

Reprints. For copies of 100 or more, of articles in this publication, please contact the Commercial Reprints Department, Elsevier Inc., 360 Park Avenue South, New York, New York 10010-1710; Tel.: 212-633-3874, Fax: 212-633-3820, E-mail: reprints@elsevier.com.

Hematology/Oncology Clinics of North America is covered in MEDLINE/PubMed (Index Medicus), EMBASE/ Excerpta Medica, and BIOSIS.

Contributors

CONSULTING EDITORS

GEORGE P. CANELLOS, MD
William Rosenberg Professor of Medicine, Department of Medical Oncology, Dana-Farber Cancer Institute, Boston, Massachusetts

H. FRANKLIN BUNN, MD
Professor of Medicine, Division of Hematology, Brigham and Women's Hospital, Harvard Medical School, Boston, Massachusetts

EDITORS

DANIEL MORGENSZTERN, MD
Associate Professor of Medicine; Director, Thoracic Oncology Program, Division of Oncology, Washington University School of Medicine, Washington University, St Louis, Missouri

ROY S. HERBST, MD, PhD
Ensign Professor of Medicine, Chief of Medical Oncology, Associate Director for Translational Research, Yale School of Medicine, Yale Cancer Center, Smilow Cancer Hospital at Yale-New Haven, New Haven, Connecticut

AUTHORS

KATHRYN C. ARBOUR, MD
Department of Medicine, Memorial Sloan Kettering Cancer Center, New York, New York

JODY C. CHUANG, MD, PhD
Post-doctoral Fellow, Divisions of Hematology and Oncology, Department of Medicine, Stanford Hospital and Clinics, Stanford, California

MEGAN DALY, MD
Assistant Professor of Radiation Oncology, University of California Davis Medical Center, Sacramento, California

SIDDHARTHA DEVARAKONDA, MD
Fellow, Division of Oncology, Washington University School of Medicine, St Louis, Missouri

LINGLING DU, MD
Fellow, Division of Oncology, Washington University School of Medicine, St Louis, Missouri

GREG DURM, MD
Assistant Professor of Clinical Medicine, Division of Hematology/Oncology, Indiana University Simon Cancer Center, Indianapolis, Indiana

RAMASWAMY GOVINDAN, MD
Professor of Medicine; Anheuser Busch Chair in Medical Oncology; Director, Section of Medical Oncology, Division of Oncology, Alvin J Siteman Cancer Center, Washington University School of Medicine, St Louis, Missouri

NASSER HANNA, MD
Professor of Medicine, Division of Hematology/Oncology, Indiana University Simon Cancer Center, Indianapolis, Indiana

REBECCA S. HEIST, MD, MPH
Assistant Professor of Medicine, Harvard Medical School; Department of Thoracic Oncology, Massachusetts General Hospital, Boston, Massachusetts

ROY S. HERBST, MD, PhD
Ensign Professor of Medicine, Chief of Medical Oncology, Associate Director for Translational Research, Yale School of Medicine, Yale Cancer Center, Smilow Cancer Hospital at Yale-New Haven, New Haven, Connecticut

HATIM HUSAIN, MD
Division of Hematology and Oncology, Moores Cancer Center, University of California, San Diego, La Jolla, California

GREGORY P. KALEMKERIAN, MD
Professor, Division of Hematology/Oncology, Department of Internal Medicine, University of Michigan, Ann Arbor, Michigan

KAREN KELLY, MD
Professor of Medicine, University of California Davis Medical Center, Sacramento, California

YING LIANG, MD, PhD
Associate Professor, First Division, Department of Medical Oncology, Sun Yat-sen University Cancer Center, State Key Laboratory of Oncology in South China, Collaborative Innovation Center for Cancer Medicine, Guangzhou, Guangdong, China

ASHIQ MASOOD, MD
Assistant Professor of Medicine, Division of Oncology, Alvin J Siteman Cancer Center, Washington University School of Medicine, St Louis, Missouri

SOHAM MORE
Division of Hematology and Oncology, Moores Cancer Center, University of California, San Diego, La Jolla, California

DANIEL MORGENSZTERN, MD
Associate Professor of Medicine; Director, Thoracic Oncology Program, Division of Oncology, Washington University School of Medicine, Washington University, St Louis, Missouri

AYESHA MURTUZA, MD
Division of Hematology and Oncology, Moores Cancer Center, University of California, San Diego, La Jolla, California

SUCHITA PAKKALA, MD
Assistant Professor, Interim Section Chief of Hematology/Oncology at Emory Midtown, Department of Hematology and Medical Oncology, Winship Cancer Institute, Emory University School of Medicine, Atlanta, Georgia

SOO J. PARK, MD
Division of Hematology and Oncology, Moores Cancer Center, University of California, San Diego, La Jolla, California

SURESH S. RAMALINGAM, MD
Professor, Department of Hematology and Medical Oncology; Deputy Director, Winship Cancer Institute, Emory University School of Medicine, Atlanta, Georgia

GREGORY J. RIELY, MD, PhD
Department of Medicine, Memorial Sloan Kettering Cancer Center, Weill Cornell Medical College, New York, New York

BRYAN J. SCHNEIDER, MD
Associate Professor, Division of Hematology/Oncology, Department of Internal Medicine, University of Michigan, Ann Arbor, Michigan

KIT TAM, MD
Hematology Oncology Fellow, University of California Davis Medical Center, Sacramento, California

PAMELA VILLALOBOS, MD
Post-doctoral Fellow, Department of Translational Molecular Pathology, The University of Texas MD Anderson Cancer Center, Houston, Texas

HEATHER A. WAKELEE, MD
Associate Professor, Division of Oncology, Department of Medicine, Stanford Cancer Institute, Stanford University, Stanford, California

SAIAMA N. WAQAR, MBBS, MSCI
Assistant Professor of Medicine, Section of Medical Oncology, Washington University School of Medicine, St Louis, Missouri

IGNACIO I. WISTUBA, MD
Professor and Chair, Department of Translational Molecular Pathology, The University of Texas MD Anderson Cancer Center, Houston, Texas

BRIAN D. WOODWARD
Division of Hematology and Oncology, Moores Cancer Center, University of California, San Diego, La Jolla, California

Contents

Preface: Evolving Treatment Options for Lung Cancer   xiii

Daniel Morgensztern and Roy S. Herbst

**Next-Generation Sequencing of Lung Cancers: Lessons Learned and
Future Directions**   1

Siddhartha Devarakonda, Ashiq Masood, and Ramaswamy Govindan

> Targeted therapies and immune checkpoint inhibitors have significantly improved outcomes in a sizable fraction of patients with metastatic non–small cell lung cancer. Nevertheless, a majority of patients with lung cancer continue to have poor outcomes. The ability to comprehensively characterize the genomic alterations in various subtypes of lung cancer has the potential to transform cancer care by facilitating the identification of novel treatment strategies. The objective of this review is to summarize key findings from recent studies that have sequenced a large number of lung cancer samples and discuss the diagnostic, prognostic, and therapeutic relevance of these findings.

Lung Cancer Biomarkers   13

Pamela Villalobos and Ignacio I. Wistuba

> The molecular characterization of lung cancer has changed the classification and treatment of these tumors, becoming an essential component of pathologic diagnosis and oncologic therapy decisions. Through the recognition of novel biomarkers, such as epidermal growth factor receptor mutations and anaplastic lymphoma kinase translocations, it is possible to identify subsets of patients who benefit from targeted molecular therapies. The success of targeted anticancer therapies and new immunotherapy approaches has created a new paradigm of personalized therapy and has led to accelerated development of new drugs for lung cancer treatment. This article focuses on clinically relevant cancer biomarkers as targets for therapy and potential new targets for drug development.

Neoadjuvant and Adjuvant Therapy for Non–Small Cell Lung Cancer   31

Jody C. Chuang, Ying Liang, and Heather A. Wakelee

> The use of 4 cycles of cisplatin-based adjuvant chemotherapy is now the standard of care for patients with resected stage II and IIIA non–small cell lung cancer. Neoadjuvant chemotherapy lacks the same level of data as adjuvant treatment, but meta-analyses of this approach support its use. Selection of patients who are most likely to benefit from chemotherapy remain elusive. Ongoing adjuvant trials are exploring biomarkers, molecularly targeted agents, postoperative radiation therapy, and immunotherapy.

Treatment of Locally Advanced Non–Small Cell Lung Cancer   45

Kit Tam, Megan Daly, and Karen Kelly

> Locally advanced non–small cell lung cancer is a heterogeneous disease with typically poor outcomes. Select patients may benefit from the integration of surgery, whereas patients with bulky, multistation, or contralateral (N3) mediastinal involvement are managed with definitive chemoradiation. Attempts to improve outcomes through induction, consolidation, or maintenance chemotherapy or radiation dose escalation have not demonstrated a survival benefit. Current research efforts focus on the integration of novel systemic agents that exploit tumor-specific driver mutations, augment anti-tumor immune response, or enhance radiation sensitivity.

First-Line Systemic Therapy for Non–Small Cell Lung Cancer   59

Rebecca S. Heist

> Major advances in the treatment of metastatic non–small cell lung cancer have led to significant incremental improvements in patient outcomes. Platinum-based combination therapy remains the cornerstone of first-line therapy. The addition of biologic agents, such as bevacizumab or necitumumab, in selected populations has shown benefit over chemotherapy alone. The advent of maintenance therapy has also improved overall survival outcomes in selected populations of patients. Ongoing studies will further refine optimal treatment in the first-line setting and further advance first-line treatment options.

Second-Line Chemotherapy and Beyond for Non–Small Cell Lung Cancer   71

Greg Durm and Nasser Hanna

> The landscape for the second- and third-line treatment of advanced non–small cell lung cancer has changed dramatically over the last two decades. Immunotherapeutic agents have become a preferred choice following progression on platinum-based first-line chemotherapy. However, there remains a role for cytotoxic chemotherapy and pemetrexed and docetaxel (with or without ramucirumab) are approved for single-agent use in the second-line setting. With the discovery of new genetic alterations and the development of novel targeted drugs, the treatment of advanced non–small cell lung cancer following progression on first-line therapy continues to become more complicated as new treatment algorithms evolve.

Epidermal Growth Factor Receptor Mutated Advanced Non–Small Cell Lung Cancer: A Changing Treatment Paradigm   83

Suchita Pakkala and Suresh S. Ramalingam

> Activating mutations in the epidermal growth factor receptor (EGFR) are present in approximately 15% of US patients with lung adenocarcinoma. EGFR tyrosine kinase inhibitors are associated with high response rate and progression-free survival for patients with non–small cell lung cancer with this genotype. Gefitinib, erlotinib, and afatinib are the EGFR tyrosine kinase inhibitors that are presently in clinical use. Understanding resistance mechanisms has led to the identification of a secondary mutational

target, T790M, in more than half of patients, for which osimertinib has been approved. This article reviews the current treatments, resistance mechanisms, and strategies to overcome resistance.

Diagnosis and Treatment of Anaplastic Lymphoma Kinase–Positive Non–Small Cell Lung Cancer   **101**

Kathryn C. Arbour and Gregory J. Riely

Anaplastic lymphoma kinase (*ALK*) gene rearrangements occur in a small portion of patients with non–small cell lung cancer (NSCLC). These gene rearrangements lead to constitutive activation of the ALK kinase and subsequent ALK-driven tumor formation. Patients with tumors harboring such rearrangements are highly sensitive to ALK inhibitors, such as crizotinib, ceritinib, and alectinib. Resistance to these kinase inhibitors occurs through several mechanisms, resulting in ongoing clinical challenges. This review summarizes the biology of ALK-positive lung cancer, methods for diagnosing ALK-positive NSCLC, current FDA-approved ALK inhibitors, mechanisms of resistance to ALK inhibition, and potential strategies to combat resistance.

New Targets in Non–Small Cell Lung Cancer   **113**

Soo J. Park, Soham More, Ayesha Murtuza, Brian D. Woodward, and Hatim Husain

With the implementation of genomic technologies into clinical practice, patients have seen meaningful benefits with targeted therapy for oncogene-addicted cancer, and we have identified new molecular dependencies in non–small cell lung cancer. The clinical success of tyrosine kinase inhibitors against epidermal growth factor receptor and anaplastic lymphoma kinase activation has shifted treatment options toward the separation of subsets of lung cancer and the administration of genotype-directed therapy. Drug development is underway for a host of new molecular targets. This review highlights treatment options, including clinical trials for ROS1 rearrangement, RET fusions, NTRK1 fusions, MET exon skipping, BRAF mutations, and KRAS mutations.

Immunotherapy in Lung Cancer   **131**

Lingling Du, Roy S. Herbst, and Daniel Morgensztern

The treatment of patients with good performance status and advanced stage non–small cell lung cancer has been based on the use of first-line platinum-based doublet and second-line docetaxel. Immunotherapy represents a new therapeutic approach with the potential for prolonged benefit. Although the vaccines studied have not shown benefit in patients with non–small cell lung cancer, immune checkpoint inhibitors against the PD-1/PD-L1 axis showed increased overall survival compared with docetaxel in randomized clinical trials, which led to the approval of nivolumab and pembrolizumab. Because only a minority of patients benefit from this class of drugs, there has been an intense search for biomarkers.

Advances in Small Cell Lung Cancer   143

Gregory P. Kalemkerian and Bryan J. Schneider

Small cell lung cancer (SCLC) is an aggressive neuroendocrine tumor characterized by early metastatic spread and responsiveness to initial therapy. The incidence of SCLC has been declining in the United States in parallel with the decreasing prevalence of cigarette smoking. Limited stage disease is potentially curable with chemoradiotherapy followed by cranial irradiation. Extensive stage disease is incurable, but systemic chemotherapy can improve quality of life and prolong survival. Nearly all patients relapse with chemoresistant disease. Molecularly targeted therapy has failed to yield convincing clinical benefits. Nevertheless, many biologically rational strategies, including immune checkpoint inhibition, show promise in ongoing clinical trials.

Systemic Treatment of Brain Metastases   157

Saiama N. Waqar, Daniel Morgensztern, and Ramaswamy Govindan

Lung cancer continues to be the leading cause of cancer-related mortality in the United States. Brain metastases are a significant problem in patients with lung cancer and have conventionally been treated with whole-brain radiation. This article reviews the data for systemic chemotherapy to treat brain metastasis from lung cancer and examines the activity of small molecule tyrosine kinase inhibitors for the targeted therapy for brain metastases from *EGFR*-mutant and *ALK*-rearranged non–small cell lung cancer. Future directions for evaluating the role of immunotherapy in treating brain metastasis are also discussed.

Index   177

HEMATOLOGY/ONCOLOGY CLINICS OF NORTH AMERICA

FORTHCOMING ISSUES

April 2017
T-Cell Lymphoma
Eric D. Jacobsen, *Editor*

June 2017
Upper Gastrointestinal Malignancies
Manish A. Shah, *Editor*

August 2017
The Treatment of Myeloid Malignancies
with Kinase Inhibitors
Ann Mullally, *Editor*

RECENT ISSUES

December 2016
Aggressive B- Cell Lymphoma
Laurie Sehn, *Editor*

October 2016
Direct Oral Anticoagulants in Clinical
Practice
Jean Marie Connors, *Editor*

August 2016
Imaging of Neurologic Complications in
Hematological Disorders
Sangam Kanekar, *Editor*

ISSUES OF RELATED INTEREST

Surgical Oncology Clinics of North America, July 2016 (Vol. 25, No. 3)
Lung Cancer
Mark J. Krasna, *Editor*
Available at: http://www.surgonc.theclinics.com/

Thoracic Surgery Clinics, May 2015 (Vol. 25, No. 2)
Lung Cancer Screening
Gaetano Rocco, *Editor*
Available at: http://www.thoracic.theclinics.com/

THE CLINICS ARE AVAILABLE ONLINE!
Access your subscription at:
www.theclinics.com

Preface

Evolving Treatment Options for Lung Cancer

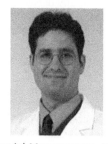 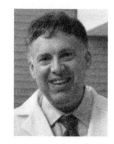

Daniel Morgensztern, MD   Roy S. Herbst, MD, PhD
Editors

Lung cancer is the leading cause of cancer mortality worldwide. Despite the poor outcomes, particularly for patients with advanced stage, there has been remarkable progress in the biology and treatment of lung cancer over the last 15 years. In this issue of *Hematology/Oncology Clinics of North America*, we have assembled a team of experts to review the management of lung cancer, including the current standards and future directions.

The issue begins with a review of lung cancer genomics by Drs Devarakonda, Masood, and Govindan, who summarized the key findings from the most important studies using next-generation sequencing. Subsequently, Drs Villalobos and Wistuba review the lung cancer biomarkers, a major component of the pathologic diagnosis and therapy decisions, with a detailed description of the histologic subtypes, genomic biomarkers, and immunotherapy.

The following articles describe the standard therapy for non–small cell lung cancer (NSCLC). Drs Chuang, Liang, and Wakelee review the role for neoadjuvant and adjuvant therapy, including the recently completed and ongoing studies with targeted therapy. Drs Tam, Daly, and Kelly describe the standard of care for patients with locally advanced NSCLC, including the chemotherapy choices, radiation therapy techniques, complications, and surveillance. Dr Heist reviews the standard treatment options for the initial treatment of patients with stage IV NSCLC, including the chemotherapy backbone, maintenance therapy, and the role of monoclonal antibodies against vascular endothelial growth factor and epidermal growth factor receptor (EGFR). Second-line therapy and beyond is reviewed by Drs Durm and Hanna, who describe the data supporting the use of docetaxel, pemetrexed, the combination of docetaxel plus ramucirumab, and erlotinib in patients with *EGFR* unknown or wild type.

The development of targeted therapy has provided a remarkable benefit for patients harboring specific genetic alterations. Drs Pakkala and Ramalingam review the treatment of patients with *EGFR* mutation, including the initial studies, mechanisms of

Hematol Oncol Clin N Am 31 (2017) xiii–xiv
http://dx.doi.org/10.1016/j.hoc.2016.09.001
0889-8588/17/© 2016 Published by Elsevier Inc.

resistance, and use of third-generation drugs. Drs Arbour and Riely provide the standard therapy for treatment with *ALK*-positive tumors, including the role of first- and second-generation drugs, mechanisms of resistance, and the important issue of central nervous system disease. Drs Park, Murtuza, Husain, and colleagues review the biology, current and emerging data on multiple targets, including *ROS1*, *RET*, and *NTRK1* fusions, BRAF V600E, KRAS, and c-MET exon 14 skipping mutations.

The use of immune checkpoint inhibitors has revolutionized the therapy of NSCLC, with two drugs already approved for patients with previously treated tumors. Drs Du, Herbst, and Morgensztern describe the current data with vaccines and immune checkpoint inhibitors, including the recently completed randomized clinical trials comparing antibodies against PD-1 or PD-L1 to docetaxel and the predictors for benefit from immunotherapy.

Progress in the treatment for patients with small cell lung cancer (SCLC) has been slow with no major changes in the standard of care for the last 15 years and no proven benefit from targeted therapies. Nevertheless, there have been encouraging results over the last two years. Drs Kalemkerian and Schneider provide a detailed review on the management of SCLC, including the choices of chemotherapy, role for thoracic and prophylactic cranial irradiation, and the emerging therapies, such as immune checkpoint inhibitors and rovalpituzumab tesirine (Rova-T), an antibody drug conjugate against DLL-3.

Brain metastases represent a significant problem for patients with both NSCLC and SCLC. Drs Waqar, Morgensztern, and Govindan review the standard of care for patients with brain metastases, including the roles for radiation therapy, chemotherapy, targeted therapy, and the emerging data with immune checkpoint inhibitors.

We thank the authors for their outstanding contributions and hope that readers enjoy this very thoughtful and updated review on the management of lung cancer.

Daniel Morgensztern, MD
Thoracic Oncology Program
Washington University
660 South Euclid Avenue, Box 8056
St Louis, MO 63110, USA

Roy S. Herbst, MD, PhD
Yale School of Medicine
Yale Cancer Center
Smilow Cancer Hospital at Yale-New Haven
New Haven, CT 06519, USA

E-mail addresses:
dmorgens@wustl.edu (D. Morgensztern)
Roy.herbst@yale.edu (R.S. Herbst)

Next-Generation Sequencing of Lung Cancers

Lessons Learned and Future Directions

Siddhartha Devarakonda, MD[a], Ashiq Masood, MD[b],
Ramaswamy Govindan, MD[c],*

KEYWORDS

- Sequencing • Lung cancer • Treatment

KEY POINTS

- Lung cancer genomes from smokers have a high burden of mutations. This high mutational burden poses a challenge for the discovery of low-frequency driver alterations.
- Sequencing a large number of tumor samples and combining genomic data from multiple cancer types for analysis can yield enough statistical power to identify low-frequency driver alterations in cancer genomes — some of which may be targetable.
- Although different subtypes of lung cancers share certain genomic alterations, the majority of these alterations tend to be histology specific. It is possible that the heterogeneity in mutational processes underlying malignant transformation and differences in the cell of origin account for this observation.
- The clonal architecture of cancers is complex. The role of clonal heterogeneity as a prognostic and predictive biomarker is currently being investigated.
- Whole-exome and whole-genome sequencing data have the potential to guide immunotherapy and cancer vaccine development.

INTRODUCTION

Lung cancer continues to remain a serious global problem and one of the leading causes of cancer-related death worldwide.[1] The past decade has witnessed significant advances in next-generation sequencing technologies, which have made it

Equal contribution (S. Devarakonda and A. Masood).
[a] Division of Oncology, Washington University School of Medicine, 660 South Euclid Avenue, St Louis, MO 63110, USA; [b] Division of Oncology, Alvin J Siteman Cancer Center, Washington University School of Medicine, 660 South Euclid Avenue, Box 8056, St. Louis, MO 63110, USA; [c] Section of Medical Oncology, Division of Oncology, Alvin J Siteman Cancer Center, Washington University School of Medicine, 660 South Euclid Avenue, Box 8056, St. Louis, MO 63110, USA
* Corresponding author.
E-mail address: rgovindan@wustl.edu

Hematol Oncol Clin N Am 31 (2017) 1–12
http://dx.doi.org/10.1016/j.hoc.2016.08.008
0889-8588/17/© 2016 Elsevier Inc. All rights reserved.

hemonc.theclinics.com

possible to study cancer genomes in unprecedented detail and gain a better understanding of the alterations that underlie cancer development and progression.[2–5] Comprehensive genomic analyses of lung cancer have been reported by several groups and consortia, such as The Cancer Genome Atlas (TCGA).[4–7] The aim of this review is to highlight some of the important findings reported in these studies and discuss their clinical significance.

SOMATIC MUTATIONS IN LUNG CANCER

Acquisition of somatic point mutations is one of the common mechanisms by which normal cells undergo malignant transformation. Cancer cells continually accrue a variety of mutations and are exposed to stresses, such as hypoxia, treatment, and attacks by the host immune system. As a result, cancer cells with mutations that confer upon them a survival advantage (often referred to as driver mutations) are selected over time.[8] Because driver mutations increase the survival fitness of cancer cells, these mutations are likely to be over-represented and recurrent in cancer samples that are obtained from different patients, compared with other bystander or passenger mutations that do not offer a growth advantage to the cancer cell.[8] Studies often use sophisticated statistical algorithms to identify significantly mutated genes.[3,9,10] These algorithms take into account several factors that influence mutation rate, such as gene size, background mutation rate, DNA repair mechanisms (genes that are more actively transcribed into RNA have lower mutation burdens due to transcription-coupled repair), and replication timing (genes that are replicated later during cell division are more prone to mutations).[9,10] Although these statistical predictions by themselves do not imply a biological role for genes in cancer, they can be extremely useful in identifying gene alterations for further functional studies.

Lung cancer genomes have a high burden of mutations, with approximately 8 mutations/megabase (Mb) or million base-pairs compared with other cancer types, such as pediatric tumors or acute leukemias.[9] This high mutation burden in lung cancers is attributed to cigarette smoke exposure and abnormal activity of cell intrinsic mutagenic processes, such as APOBEC cytidine deaminase enzymes, and poses a challenge for identifying low-frequency driver alterations from passenger alterations.[11] Exposure to cigarette smoke also results in a characteristic mutation pattern in tumors. Genomes of tumors from smokers are enriched for transversions, where a pyrimidine (cytosine or thymine) is replaced by a purine (adenine or guanine) or vice versa.[4] In contrast, genomes of lung adenocarcinomas (LUADs) from never-smokers have an approximately 10-fold lower mutation burden (0.6 mutations/Mb) and are enriched for transitions, where a purine is replaced by a purine or a pyrimidine by a pyrimidine.[12]

Using statistical algorithms, studies have reported recurrent mutations in tumor suppressors, such as *TP53, STK11, NF1, RB1, PTEN*, and *CDKN2A*, and oncogenes, such as *KRAS, EGFR, MET*, and *PIK3CA* in lung cancer.[4,5,13] While some of these alterations are shared by different subtypes of lung cancer, others are histology specific. For instance, LUADs are characterized by mutations in genes, such as *EGFR, KRAS, BRAF, ERBB2*, and *MET*, that activate the receptor tyrosine kinase (RTK)/RAS/RAF signaling pathway.[4] Unlike LUADs, small cell lung cancers (SCLCs) rarely show mutations in the RTK/RAS/RAF signaling pathway.[13,14] These tumors are typically characterized by comutation of the tumor suppressors, *TP53* and *RB1*, and alterations in genes that regulate neuroendocrine differentiation.[13] Similarly, although LUAD and squamous cell lung cancer (SQLC) share mutations in genes, such as *PIK3CA*,

CDKN2A, and TP53, SQLCs additionally demonstrate mutations that deregulate squamous differentiation.[5] In a recent analysis, only a 12% overlap was seen when genes mutated at a statistically significant level in 660 LUADs and 484 SQLCs were compared with each other.[3] More similarity was observed between significantly mutated genes in LUAD and other tumor types, such as glioblastoma and colorectal cancer, and between SQLC and head and neck squamous cell and bladder cancers, than between LUAD and SQLC in this study.[3] These findings suggest that genomic alterations tend to differ between different subtypes of lung cancer, possibly reflecting the differences in the cells from which these tumors arise and the distinct mutational processes that underlie the malignant transformation of these cells.[15]

Activating mutations in previously known RTK/RAS/RAF pathway genes, such as KRAS, EGFR, ERBB2, BRAF, and MET, were seen in approximately 62% of the 230 LUAD samples sequenced by TCGA.[4] Samples in which such known RTK/RAS/RAF pathway alterations were not detected were labeled "oncogene negative." When oncogene-positive and oncogene-negative samples were analyzed independently, other RTK/RAS/RAF pathway alterations, such as mutations in RIT1 and NF1, were found significantly enriched in the oncogene-negative sample subset, emphasizing the importance of such analyses in identifying new driver alterations. Similarly, analysis of combined genomic data from different tumor types (irrespective of the site of origin) can identify novel driver alterations by improving the statistical power to detect low-frequency alterations, because some cell survival pathways are commonly altered in all cancer types.[3,16] Such analyses could be particularly helpful in identifying low-frequency alterations in tumors with a high mutation burden, such as lung cancer.

Campbell and colleagues[3] analyzed SQLC and LUAD samples together and found 14 genes to be mutated at a statistically significant level, which were not identified when samples from either subtype were individually analyzed. Furthermore, on combining sequencing data from an additional 274 LUAD samples with samples from the TCGA data set, low-frequency alterations in RTK/RAS/RAF pathway genes, SOS1 and RASA1, and Rho kinase signaling genes, VAV1 and ARHGAP35, were identified in this study.[3] Because only a fraction of LUAD patients with RTK/RAS/RAF pathway alterations are targetable with currently approved therapies, such large-scale sequencing studies and analyses are likely to lead to the discovery of novel clinically useful targets.

COPY NUMBER ALTERATIONS

The human genome is diploid in nongerm cells, and, therefore, every cell has 2 copies of a gene (excluding genes on the sex chromosomes in men). Copy number alterations (CNAs) refer to deviations in this number.[8,17,18] CNAs can vary in size and, depending on the genomic region they involve, result in several-fold gain (amplification) of oncogenes and/or loss (deletion) of multiple tumor suppressors simultaneously, playing an important role in malignant transformation. CNAs are frequently observed in lung cancer genomes.[19]

Similar to somatic mutations, some CNAs are seen in all subtypes of lung cancers whereas others tend to be enriched in specific histologic subtypes. For instance, losses involving the short arm of chromosome 3 (3p) and tumor suppressors that are frequently mutated in lung cancer, such as CDKN2A and PTEN, are commonly observed in both SCLC and non-SCLCs (LUAD and SQLC).[20] The 3p region harbors multiple tumor suppressors, such as VHL, RASSF1A, FHIT, and FUS1.[20] On the other hand, amplification of a segment of the long arm of chromosome 3 is frequently observed in SQLCs.[5] This region contains genes, such as *SOX2, PIK3CA, HES1*, and *TP63*, which play a critical role in oncogenesis, development, and squamous differentiation. *SOX2* amplifications are also seen in SCLC.[14] *SOX2* is a transcription factor that plays a role in the development of lung epithelium and pluripotency and is considered to be a lineage-survival oncogene in SQLC.[21,22] Similarly, focal amplification of the region on chromosomal arm 14q that contains *NKX2-1 (TTF1)* is seen in approximately 14% of LUAD samples.[23–25] Similar to *SOX2* in SQLC, *NKX2-1* is considered a lineage-survival oncogene in LUAD.[25] Lung cancers also show amplifications in *TERT* (a ribonucleoprotein that is crucial for the synthesis of telomeric DNA); oncogenic transcription factors *MYC, MYCN,* and *MYCL1*; and RTKs, such as *PDGFRA, KIT, FGFR1,* and *MET*.[4,5,13,24]

Similar to mutations, combined analysis of LUADs and SQLCs can also allow the detection of recurrent low-frequency CNAs common to both subtypes. Recurrent amplifications around *MAPK1*, which participates in RAS/RTK/RAF signaling, and deletion of β2-microglobulin of (*B2M*), which is an integral part of the major histocompatibility complex, were observed in both LUADs and SQLCs when these samples were analyzed together.[3] Amplification peaks near RTK/RAS/RAF signaling genes, *FGFR1-WHSC1L1, PDGFRA-KIT-KDR,* and *MAPK1*, in oncogene-negative LUADs were observed at a statistically significant level in this analysis. Although some CNAs, such as *MET* amplification, can be targeted with tyrosine kinase inhibitors, the therapeutic significance of the vast majority of CNAs remains to be explored.[26]

CHROMOSOMAL REARRANGEMENTS

Translocations are structural rearrangements that bring 2 otherwise nonadjacent regions in the genome together.[8,27] When 2 otherwise separated genes are brought together, the translocation can result in the production of an aberrant fusion protein.[28,29] Fusion proteins contribute to oncogenesis by resulting in the inactivation of tumor suppressors (such as *TP73*) or abnormal activation of oncogenes.[13] For instance, translocations in oncogenes, such as *ALK, RET,* and *ROS1*, result in the activation of several signaling pathways that are crucial for cancer cell survival.[30] The discovery of RTK translocations in a subset of patients with lung cancer has allowed the targeting of these tumors with tyrosine kinase inhibitors, such as crizotinib, ceritinib, and alectinib, which has improved patient survival significantly.[31–33] These drugs are currently approved for use in patients with LUAD whose tumors contain *ALK* or *ROS1* fusions. Although there are no approved targeted therapies for tumors with *RET* fusions in lung cancer, there are reports to suggest responses with RET inhibitors, such as cabozantinib and vandetanib, that are approved for use in thyroid cancer (**Table 1**).[34,35]

Advances in RNA sequencing technologies have led to the discovery of several other low-frequency translocations in lung cancer genomes, a vast majority of which are nonrecurrent. Nevertheless, low-frequency recurrent fusions in *BRAF, NRG1, NTRK1,* and FGFR family of genes have been recently observed in certain subsets of patients with non-SCLC.[36–40] For example, fusions in *NTRK1* were observed in a small percentage of oncogene negative LUADs, and *NRG1* and *BRAF* fusions were observed in LUADs obtained from never-smokers. Similarly, fusions in oncogenes, such as the FGFR family of genes (*FGFR1, FGFR2,* and *FGFR3*) and *MYCL1*, have been reported in SQCCs and SCLCs, respectively.[14,41] Although there are no therapies that are currently approved for use in tumors with the vast majority of these rearrangements, there are some data to suggest that a few of these translocations maybe targetable with currently available tyrosine kinase inhibitors (see **Table 1**).

Table 1
Summary of currently Food and Drug Administration–approved therapies with proven or possible clinical activity (based on limited data/isolated case reports) in selected patients with lung cancer

Gene	Alteration	Food and Drug Administration–Approved Drugs with Proven Clinical Efficacy	Comments
EGFR	Mutation	Erlotinib, gefitinib, afatinib, and osimertinib	Osimertinib is currently approved for use in patients progressing on EGFR inhibitors who test positive for the T790M mutation.
BRAF	Mutation (V600E), gusion	Vemurafenib,[55,a] dabrafenib[56,a] +/– trametinib[57,a]	These drugs are currently approved for use in BRAF-mutated metastatic melanoma. The targetability of BRAF fusions in lung cancer is unknown. Responses to trametinib and combination therapy with sorafenib, bevacizumab, and temsirolimus have been reported in patients with other BRAF fusion–positive malignancies.[58]
ERBB2	Mutation (exon 20 insertion)	Trastuzumab,[59,60,a] afatinib[61,a]	Trastuzumab and lapatinib are approved for breast cancer and afatinib for EGFR-mutated lung cancer. Trastuzumab is also approved for use in gastric cancer.
MET	Amplification, mutation (exon 14 skipping)	Crizotinib,[43,62,a] cabozantinib[44,a]	Cabozantinib is approved for use in renal cell and medullary thyroid cancer. Crizotinib is approved for ALK and ROS1 rearranged lung cancer.
ALK	Fusion	Crizotinib, ceritinib, alectinib	Ceritinib and alectinib are approved in patients who are intolerant to or have progressed on crizotinib.
ROS1	Fusion	Crizotinib, ceritinib[63,a]	Crizotinib is currently the only drug approved for use in ROS1 rearranged lung cancer.
RET	Fusion	Vandetanib,[34,64,a] cabozantinib[35,a]	These drugs are currently approved for use in patients with medullary thyroid cancer.
NTRK1	Fusion	Crizotinib[36,a]	Stable disease was reported in one patient in this case report with crizotinib.
DDR2	Mutation	Dasatinib[65,a] +/– erlotinib[66,a]	This mutation was reported in SQLC. Dasatinib is approved for use in chronic myeloid leukemia.

[a] Off-label use.

SPLICING ALTERATIONS

Splicing is a mechanism by which introns between adjacent exons are removed from transcribed premessenger RNA, and the exons are joined together.[42] Cells possess the ability to vary the exons included in the final messenger RNA molecule in a process referred to as *alternate splicing*. This gives them the ability to synthesize different isoforms of the same protein from a single gene and achieve a remarkable degree of proteomic diversity. This process of alternate splicing is tightly regulated in the cell but often deregulated in cancer cells. Such deregulation allows cancer cells to manufacture aberrant versions of various proteins. Deregulation in splicing can be a consequence of mutations in genes that control splicing, such as *U2AF1*, or mutations in specific sequences within the gene, such as splice site mutations, that the splicing machinery uses to identify and process introns and exons.[4]

Aberrant splicing of oncogenes, such as *CTNNB1* (β-catenin) and *MET*, was observed in some of the LUAD samples sequenced by TCGA.[4] Although aberrant splicing in *CTNNB1* was associated with mutations in the splicing factor *U2AF1*, abnormal splicing of *MET* was predominantly due to splice site mutations within the gene. Splice site mutations in *MET* have been observed in approximately 3% of non-squamous lung cancers and result in the exclusion of exon 14 from *MET* messenger RNA.[43] Because this exon codes for a regulatory domain, the skipping of exon 14 can lead to persistent signaling through MET and thus favor oncogenesis. There are emerging clinical data to suggest clinical benefit with tyrosine kinase inhibitors, such as crizotinib and cabozantinib, in these tumors.[44]

CLONAL HETEROGENEITY AND IMPLICATIONS FOR THERAPY

In the 1970s, Peter Nowell proposed a hypothesis based on Darwinian natural selection that cancers evolve over time.[45] With the advent of next-generation sequencing technologies, it is now possible to study the clonal architecture of cancers and track their evolution, even at a single cell resolution.[46] Multiregion sequencing of tumor samples has clearly established that most tumors contain founder driver alterations that are ubiquitously detectable in all cells throughout the tumor, and subclonal private mutations that are confined to some regions of the tumor (**Fig. 1**).[47–50] The clonal architecture of a tumor can also be graphically represented in the form of a phylogenetic tree, in which founder clone aberrations map to the trunk and subclonal alterations map to the branches.

de Bruin and colleagues[48] sequenced 25 sites from 7 early-stage lung cancers, which allowed them to determine the clonal architecture of these tumors. This study observed various driver alterations in both clonal and subclonal distribution patterns within sequenced tumors. The probability of missing a high-confidence driver mutation on single-region sequencing was approximately 42% in this analysis, which has important implications for target discovery and treatment selection in the clinical setting.[48] The inability to distinguish founder from subclonal driver events could potentially lead to a suboptimal choice of therapy because, in theory, treatments targeting founder alterations are more likely to succeed than those targeting subclonal alterations that are confined to a single region of the tumor. This hypothesis is currently being evaluated in clinical studies, such as the DARWIN (Deciphering Antitumour Response and Resistance With INtratumour Heterogeneity) II trial (NCT02183883).

In a similar study, Zhang and colleagues[50] sequenced 48 regions from 11 early-stage resected LUADs and observed that only approximately 76% of the mutations were present in all regions of a given tumor. Driver mutations frequently mapped to the trunk in these tumors, suggesting that they were acquired early during the clonal

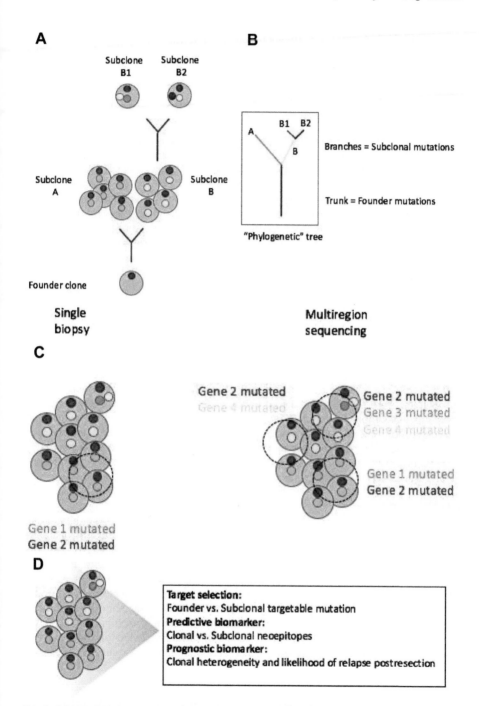

Fig. 1. Schematic representation of intratumor clonal heterogeneity and its potential clinical applications. (*A*) Shows the clonal relationship between different cells in a tumor, in which the founder alteration is depicted in red and subclonal alterations that are progressively accrued by cancer cells are shown in blue, yellow, green, and purple. (*B*) A representation of the clonal architecture of the tumor depicted in (*A*) in the form of a phylogenetic tree, where founder

evolution of these tumors. A correlation between the fraction of subclonal mutations and an increased likelihood of disease relapse was also observed in this study.[50] If validated in large prospective studies, intratumor heterogeneity may help serve as a prognostic biomarker to guide aggressive adjuvant therapies.

NEXT-GENERATION SEQUENCING AND IMMUNE-BASED THERAPIES

The ability to target the interactions between the tumor and host immune system has led to the development and approval of immune checkpoint inhibitors, such as nivolumab and pembrolizumab in lung cancer. Although the responses to these drugs can be durable and improve survival significantly in a subset of patients, not all patients who receive these drugs benefit from them.[51,52] The ability to sequence and comprehensively analyze the genomes of tumor samples from those achieving durable responses with these drugs is likely to offer a better understanding of the molecular factors that dictate response to immunotherapies. In this regard, a recent study demonstrated a correlation between high tumor mutation burden (such tumors are more likely to have mutated proteins that are perceived by the host immune system as foreign), DNA repair pathway mutations, and response to immunotherapy.[53]

Using computational algorithms that estimate the likelihood of a mutated protein in a cancer cell to be presented to the host immune system (neoepitope) and evoke an antitumor immune response, a recent analysis predicted that approximately 47% of LUADs and 53% of SQCCs contain 5 or more neoepitopes.[3] Apart from neoepitope burden, the clonality of neoepitopes in a tumor also plays a significant role in predicting for responses to immunotherapy. McGranahan and colleagues[49] demonstrated that tumors from patients achieving durable responses to checkpoint based immunotherapies were enriched for clonal neoepitopes, whereas tumors from poor responders were more likely to be enriched for subclonal neoepitopes. Multiregion sequencing of tumors is, therefore, likely to serve as a biomarker that may predict for responses to immunotherapy by offering an insight into the burden and clonality of neoepitopes in patient tumors (see **Fig. 1**). Such analyses also have the potential to facilitate the development of personalized antitumor vaccines.[54]

FUTURE DIRECTIONS

The development of targeted therapies and immunotherapies has significantly improved survival in a subset of patients with lung cancer. A majority of patients with lung cancer, however, continue to have dismal outcomes, and there is a critical need to develop novel therapeutic approaches to improve survival in these patients. The ability to sequence a large number of tumors and analyze the enormous amount of sequencing data generated from these experiments in a timely manner has dramatically improved the capacity to understand the molecular mechanisms that drive cancers and gain an insight into the vulnerabilities that can be exploited for treatment. It is likely that with the increasing number of sequenced tumors, several additional

---

alterations map to the trunk and subclonal alterations to the branches. (*C*) A representation of how a single biopsy obtained from a tumor site could potentially fail in identifying founder from subclonal alterations (gene 1 and gene 2), whereas such a distinction can easily be made through multiregion sequencing (because gene 2 is mutated in all tumor regions, it has a high probability of being a founder alteration). (*D*) Summarizes the potential clinical applications of multiregion sequencing of tumors.

low-frequency driver alterations, including some that might be targetable, will be discovered.

The ability to use next-generation sequencing technologies in the clinical setting is increasingly allowing personalizing therapies to individual patients and enrolling patients in biomarker-driven clinical trials. With the decreasing cost of sequencing, it is possible that the routine use of whole-exome/whole-genome sequencing as a diagnostic and prognostic test will soon become feasible. Apart from facilitating the identification of potential therapeutic targets, such testing is also likely to aid in the assessment of the clonal composition of a tumor, neoepitope burden and distribution, and how a tumor evolves during the course of treatment. Although it remains to be determined if these approaches will provide a meaningful survival benefit to patients with lung cancer, there is little doubt that next-generation sequencing technologies have dramatically furthered our understanding of this dreadful disease.

REFERENCES

1. Torre LA, Siegel RL, Jemal A. Lung cancer statistics. Adv Exp Med Biol 2016;893: 1–19.
2. Koboldt DC, Steinberg KM, Larson DE, et al. The next-generation sequencing revolution and its impact on genomics. Cell 2013;155:27–38.
3. Campbell JD, Alexandrov A, Kim J, et al. Distinct patterns of somatic genome alterations in lung adenocarcinomas and squamous cell carcinomas. Nat Genet 2016;48(6):607–16.
4. Collisson EA, Campbell JD, Brooks AN, et al, Cancer Genome Atlas Research Network. Comprehensive molecular profiling of lung adenocarcinoma. Nature 2014;511:543–50.
5. Hammerman PS, Lawrence MS, Voet D, et al. Cancer genome atlas research network. Comprehensive genomic characterization oaf squamous cell lung cancers. Nature 2012;489:519–25.
6. Tomczak K, Czerwińska P, Wiznerowicz M. The cancer genome atlas (TCGA): an immeasurable source of knowledge. Contemp Oncol (Pozn) 2015;19:A68–77.
7. Zhang J, Baran J, Cros A, et al. International cancer genome consortium data portal–a one-stop shop for cancer genomics data. Database (Oxford) 2011; 2011:bar026.
8. Vogelstein B, Papadopoulos N, Velculescu VE, et al. Cancer genome landscapes. Science 2013;339:1546–58.
9. Lawrence MS, Stojanov P, Polak P, et al. Mutational heterogeneity in cancer and the search for new cancer-associated genes. Nature 2013;499:214–8.
10. Dees ND, Zhang Q, Kandoth C, et al. MuSiC: identifying mutational significance in cancer genomes. Genome Res 2012;22:1589–98.
11. Alexandrov LB, Nik-Zainal S, Wedge DC, et al. Signatures of mutational processes in human cancer. Nature 2013;500:415–21.
12. Govindan R, Ding L, Griffith M, et al. Genomic landscape of non-small cell lung cancer in smokers and never-smokers. Cell 2012;150:1121–34.
13. George J, Lim JS, Jang SJ, et al. Comprehensive genomic profiles of small cell lung cancer. Nature 2015;524:47–53.
14. Rudin CM, Durinck S, Stawiski EW, et al. Comprehensive genomic analysis identifies SOX2 as a frequently amplified gene in small-cell lung cancer. Nat Genet 2012;44:1111–6.
15. Swanton C, Govindan R. Clinical implications of genomic discoveries in lung cancer. N Engl J Med 2016;374:1864–73.

16. Lawrence MS, Stojanov P, Mermel CH, et al. Discovery and saturation analysis of cancer genes across 21 tumour types. Nature 2014;505:495–501.
17. Ozer HG, Usubalieva A, Dorrance A, et al. Identification of medium-sized copy number alterations in whole-genome sequencing. Cancer Inform 2014;13: 105–11.
18. Stratton MR, Campbell PJ, Futreal PA. The cancer genome. Nature 2009;458: 719–24.
19. Zack TI, Schumacher SE, Carter SL, et al. Pan-cancer patterns of somatic copy number alteration. Nat Genet 2013;45:1134–40.
20. Zabarovsky ER, Lerman MI, Minna JD. Tumor suppressor genes on chromosome 3p involved in the pathogenesis of lung and other cancers. Oncogene 2002;21: 6915–35.
21. Karachaliou N, Rosell R, Viteri S. The role of SOX2 in small cell lung cancer, lung adenocarcinoma and squamous cell carcinoma of the lung. Transl Lung Cancer Res 2013;2:172–9.
22. Bass AJ, Watanabe H, Mermel CH, et al. SOX2 is an amplified lineage-survival oncogene in lung and esophageal squamous cell carcinomas. Nat Genet 2009;41:1238–42.
23. Gao J, Aksoy BA, Dogrusoz U, et al. Integrative analysis of complex cancer genomics and clinical profiles using the cBioPortal. Sci Signal 2013;6:pl1.
24. Weir BA, Woo MS, Getz G, et al. Characterizing the cancer genome in lung adenocarcinoma. Nature 2007;450:893–8.
25. Yamaguchi T, Hosono Y, Yanagisawa K, et al. NKX2-1/TTF-1: an enigmatic oncogene that functions as a double-edged sword for cancer cell survival and progression. Cancer Cell 2013;23:718–23.
26. Camidge D, Ou SHI, Shapiro G, et al. Efficacy and safety of crizotinib in patients with advanced c-MET-amplified non-small cell lung cancer (NSCLC). J Clin Oncol 2014;32(5s) [suppl; abstract: 8001].
27. Nambiar M, Raghavan SC. How does DNA break during chrom osomal translocations? Nucleic Acids Res 2011;39:5813–25.
28. Parker BC, Zhang W. Fusion genes in solid tumors: an emerging target for cancer diagnosis and treatment. Chin J Cancer 2013;32:594–603.
29. Kumar-Sinha C, Kalyana-Sundaram S, Chinnaiyan AM. Landscape of gene fusions in epithelial cancers: seq and ye shall find. Genome Med 2015;7:129.
30. Takeuchi K, Soda M, Togashi Y, et al. RET, ROS1 and ALK fusions in lung cancer. Nat Med 2012;18:378–81.
31. Shaw AT, Kim DW, Nakagawa K, et al. Crizotinib versus chemotherapy in advanced ALK-positive lung cancer. N Engl J Med 2013;368:2385–94.
32. Shaw AT, Engelman JA. Ceritinib in ALK-rearranged non-small-cell lung cancer. N Engl J Med 2014;370:2537–9.
33. Shaw AT, Gandhi L, Gadgeel S, et al. Alectinib in ALK-positive, crizotinib-resistant, non-small-cell lung cancer: a single-group, multicentre, phase 2 trial. Lancet Oncol 2016;17:234–42.
34. Falchook GS, Ordóñez NG, Bastida CC, et al. Effect of the RET Inhibitor vandetanib in a patient with ret fusion-positive metastatic non-small-cell lung cancer. J Clin Oncol 2016;34:e141–4.
35. Drilon A, Wang L, Hasanovic A, et al. Response to Cabozantinib in patients with RET fusion-positive lung adenocarcinomas. Cancer Discov 2013;3: 630–5.
36. Vaishnavi A, Capelletti M, Le AT, et al. Oncogenic and drug-sensitive NTRK1 rearrangements in lung cancer. Nat Med 2013;19:1469–72.

37. Seo JS, Ju YS, Lee WC, et al. The transcriptional landscape and mutational profile of lung adenocarcinoma. Genome Res 2012;22:2109–19.
38. Shim HS, Kenudson M, Zheng Z, et al. Unique genetic and survival characteristics of invasive mucinous adenocarcinoma of the lung. J Thorac Oncol 2015;10: 1156–62.
39. Nakaoku T, Tsuta K, Ichikawa H, et al. Druggable oncogene fusions in invasive mucinous lung adenocarcinoma. Clin Cancer Res 2014;20:3087–93.
40. Jang JS, Lee A, Li J, et al. Common oncogene mutations and novel SND1-BRAF transcript fusion in lung adenocarcinoma from never smokers. Sci Rep 2015;5: 9755.
41. Wu YM, Su F, Kalyana-Sundaram S, et al. Identification of targetable FGFR gene fusions in diverse cancers. Cancer Discov 2013;3(6):636–47.
42. Zhang J, Manley JL. Misregulation of Pre-mRNA alternative splicing in cancer. Cancer Discov 2013;3:1228–37.
43. Awad MM, Oxnard GR, Jackman DM, et al. MET Exon 14 mutations in non-small-cell lung cancer are associated with advanced age and stage-dependent met genomic amplification and c-met overexpression. J Clin Oncol 2016;34: 721–30.
44. Paik PK, Drilon A, Fan PD, et al. Response to MET inhibitors in patients with stage IV lung adenocarcinomas harboring MET mutations causing exon 14 skipping. Cancer Discov 2015;5:842–9.
45. Nowell PC. The clonal evolution of tumor cell populations. Science 1976;194: 23–8.
46. Navin NE. The first five years of single-cell cancer genomics and beyond. Genome Res 2015;25:1499–507.
47. Gerlinger M, Rowan AJ, Horswell S, et al. Intratumor heterogeneity and branched evolution revealed by multiregion sequencing. N Engl J Med 2012;366:883–92.
48. de Bruin EC, McGranahan N, Mitter R, et al. Spatial and temporal diversity in genomic instability processes defines lung cancer evolution. Science 2014; 346:251–6.
49. McGranahan N, Furness AJ, Rosenthal R, et al. Clonal neoantigens elicit T cell immunoreactivity and sensitivity to immune checkpoint blockade. Science 2016;351:1463–9.
50. Zhang J, Fujimoto J, Zhang J, et al. Intratumor heterogeneity in localized lung adenocarcinomas delineated by multiregion sequencing. Science 2014;346: 256–9.
51. Borghaei H, Paz-Ares L, Horn L, et al. Nivolumab versus docetaxel in advanced nonsquamous non-small-cell lung cancer. N Engl J Med 2015;373:1627–39.
52. Garon EB, Rizvi NA, Hui R, et al. Pembrolizumab for the treatment of non-small-cell lung cancer. N Engl J Med 2015;372:2018–28.
53. Rizvi NA, Hellmann MD, Snyder A, et al. Cancer immunology. Mutational landscape determines sensitivity to PD-1 blockade in non-small cell lung cancer. Science 2015;348:124–8.
54. Carreno BM, Magrini V, Becker-Hapak M, et al. Cancer immunotherapy. A dendritic cell vaccine increases the breadth and diversity of melanoma neoantigen-specific T cells. Science 2015;348:803–8.
55. Gautschi O, Pauli C, Strobel K, et al. A patient with BRAF V600E lung adenocarcinoma responding to vemurafenib. J Thorac Oncol 2012;7:e23–4.
56. Planchard D, Kim TM, Mazieres J, et al. Dabrafenib in patients with BRAF(V600E)-positive advanced non-small-cell lung cancer: a single-arm, multicentre, open-label, phase 2 trial. Lancet Oncol 2016;17(5):642–50.

57. Planchard D, Groen H, Kim T, et al. Interim results of a phase II study of the BRAF inhibitor (BRAFi) dabrafenib (D) in combination with the MEK inhibitor trametinib (T) in patients (pts) with BRAF V600E mutated (mut) metastatic non-small cell lung cancer (NSCLC). J Clin Oncol 2015;33 [suppl; abstract: 8006].

58. Ross JS, Wang K, Chmielecki J, et al. The distribution of BRAF gene fusions in solid tumors and response to targeted therapy. Int J Cancer 2016;138:881–90.

59. Cappuzzo F, Bemis L, Varella-Garcia M. HER2 mutation and response to trastuzumab therapy in non-small-cell lung cancer. N Engl J Med 2006;354:2619–21.

60. Mazières J, Peters S, Lepage B, et al. Lung cancer that harbors an HER2 mutation: epidemiologic characteristics and therapeutic perspectives. J Clin Oncol 2013;31:1997–2003.

61. De Grève J, Teugels E, Geers C, et al. Clinical activity of afatinib (BIBW 2992) in patients with lung adenocarcinoma with mutations in the kinase domain of HER2/neu. Lung Cancer 2012;76:123–7.

62. Waqar SN, Morgensztern D, Sehn J. MET mutation associated with responsiveness to crizotinib. J Thorac Oncol 2015;10:e29–31.

63. Subbiah V, Hong DS, Meric-Bernstam F. Clinical activity of ceritinib in ROS1-rearranged non-small cell lung cancer: Bench to bedside report. Proc Natl Acad Sci U S A 2016;113(11):E1419–20.

64. Gautschi O, Zander T, Keller FA, et al. A patient with lung adenocarcinoma and RET fusion treated with vandetanib. J Thorac Oncol 2013;8:e43–4.

65. Pitini V, Arrigo C, Di Mirto C, et al. Response to dasatinib in a patient with SQCC of the lung harboring a discoid-receptor-2 and synchronous chronic myelogenous leukemia. Lung Cancer 2013;82:171–2.

66. Hammerman PS, Sos ML, Ramos AH, et al. Mutations in the DDR2 kinase gene identify a novel therapeutic target in squamous cell lung cancer. Cancer Discov 2011;1:78–89.

Lung Cancer Biomarkers

Pamela Villalobos, MD, Ignacio I. Wistuba, MD*

KEYWORDS

- Lung cancer • Genotyping • Biomarkers • Molecular targets

KEY POINTS

- The molecular characterization of lung cancer has changed the classification and treatment of these tumors, becoming an essential component of pathologic diagnosis and therapy decisions.
- The success of targeted therapies and new immunotherapy approaches has created a new paradigm of personalized therapy in lung cancer.
- Pathologists should be able to precisely handle tissue adequacy in terms of quantity and quality and maintaining tumor cells for detection of molecular alterations.
- This article focuses on clinically relevant cancer biomarkers as targets for therapy, and potential new targets for drug development.

INTRODUCTION

Lung cancer has shown a decrease in incidence and mortality in recent decades; however, it remains one of the cancers with the highest incidence and ranks first in cancer-related deaths in the United States.[1] An estimated 221,200 new cases and 158,040 deaths are expected to occur in 2015, representing approximately 13% of all cancers diagnosed and 27% of all cancer deaths.[2] Despite advances in early detection and standard treatment, most patients are diagnosed at an advanced stage and have a poor prognosis, with an overall 5-year survival rate of 10% to 15%.[3] Lung cancer is a heterogeneous disease comprising several subtypes with pathologic and clinical relevance.[4] The recognition of histologic subtypes of non–small cell lung carcinoma (NSCLC), namely adenocarcinoma, squamous cell carcinoma, and large cell lung carcinoma as the most frequent subtypes, has become important as a determinant of therapy in this disease.[5] In addition, in recent years, the identification of molecular abnormalities in a large proportion of patients with lung cancer has allowed the emergence of personalized targeted therapies and has opened new horizons and created new expectations for these patients.[6] The use of predictive biomarkers to

Disclosure Statement: The authors have nothing to disclose.
Department of Translational Molecular Pathology, The University of Texas MD Anderson Cancer Center, 2130 Holcombe Boulevard, Unit 2951, Houston, TX 77030, USA
* Corresponding author.
E-mail address: iiwistuba@mdanderson.org

identify tumors that could respond to targeted therapies has meant a change in the paradigm of lung cancer diagnosis.[5]

This paradigm change affects all stakeholders in the fight against lung cancer including pathologists. Currently, several multiplex genotyping platforms for the detection of oncogene mutations, gene amplifications, and rearrangement are moving to the clinical setting. Genome-wide molecular investigations using next-generation sequencing (NGS) technologies have been evaluated in the research setting, with promising results. Further investigations in NSCLC are required for a better understanding of the implications of intratumor heterogeneity and the roles of tumor suppressor genes and epigenetic events with no known driver mutations. NGS in the clinical setting will provide comprehensive information cheaper and faster by using small amounts of tissue. Pathologists should be able to precisely handle tissue adequacy in terms of quantity and quality and maintaining tumor cells for detection of molecular alterations. The recent clinical successes of immunotherapy approaches to lung cancer have posed additional challenges to the scientific community and pathologists to develop predictive biomarkers of response to these therapies and have highlighted the need for proper procurement and processing of tissue specimens from patients with lung cancer.

This article focuses on the major predictive biomarkers in NSCLC, with special emphasis on their clinical and molecular importance, and the current status of molecular testing for these biomarkers.

HISTOLOGIC SUBTYPING OF NON–SMALL CELL LUNG CARCINOMA

The advent of molecular profiling and targeted therapy has renewed interest in the classification of NSCLC into major subtypes, such as adenocarcinoma, squamous cell carcinoma, and large cell lung carcinoma.[7] Other subtypes, including sarcomatoid carcinoma and neuroendocrine large cell carcinoma, represent a very minor proportion of the total NSCLC cases.[7] The most recent histologic classification of lung cancer published by the World Health Organization in 2015 incorporates relevant genetics and immunohistochemistry (IHC) aspects of different tumor subtypes (**Fig. 1**).[7] Lung cancers are increasingly diagnosed and staged by transthoracic core needle biopsy and fine-needle aspiration, transbronchial needle aspiration, endobronchial ultrasound-guided transbronchial needle aspiration, and endoscopic ultrasound-guided fine-needle aspiration. It is well established that poorly differentiated adenocarcinoma and squamous cell carcinoma of the lung can appear indistinguishable by routine microscopy, particularly in small biopsy and cytology specimens. In these small specimens, particularly in poorly differentiated tumors, there is a need to integrate morphology with IHC analysis to make a precise diagnosis. This includes the examination of IHC expression of thyroid transcription factor and the novel aspartic proteinase of the pepsin family A (napsin A) for adenocarcinoma and p40 and cytokeratin 5/6 for squamous cell carcinoma.[8] In addition, histochemical staining of mucin is useful for the diagnosis of adenocarcinoma histology. The correct histologic diagnosis of these specimens is important, but it is also imperative to exercise judicial use of the tissue to maximize the yield for molecular testing (**Table 1**).

GENOMIC BIOMARKERS IN NON–SMALL CELL LUNG CARCINOMA

Advances in elucidating the molecular biology of lung cancer have led to the identification of several potential biomarkers that could be relevant in the clinical management of patients with NSCLC.

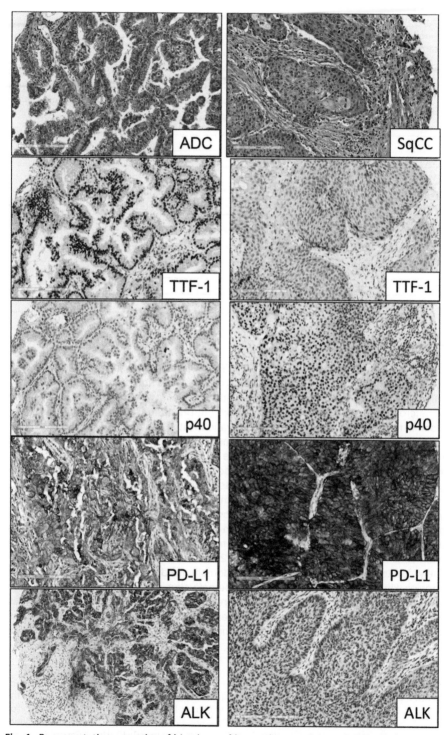

Fig. 1. Representative examples of histology of lung adenocarcinoma (ADC) and squamous cell carcinoma (SqCC) histology and biomarker analysis using IHC. ADC tumor tissue shows

Table 1
Frequency of the main molecular alterations in lung adenocarcinoma and squamous cell carcinoma

Gene	Alteration	Adenocarcinoma Frequency, %	Squamous Cell Carcinoma Frequency, %
EGFR	Mutation	10	3
ALK	Rearrangement	4–7	None
ROS	Rearrangement	1–2	None
KRAS	Mutation	25–35	5
MET	Mutation	8	3
MET	Amplification	4	1
NTRK1	Rearrangement	3	None
FGFR	Amplification	3	20
HER2	Mutation	1.6–4	None
BRAF	Mutation	1–3	0.3
PIK3CA	Mutation	2	7
RET	Rearrangement	1–2	None
DDR2	Mutation	0.5	3–4
PTEN	Deletion	—	16

Epidermal Growth Factor Receptor

The epidermal growth factor receptor (EGFR) is a tyrosine kinase receptor member of the ERBB family. The *EGFR* gene is located on the short arm of chromosome 7 at position 12.[9] When the extracellular ligand binds to EGFR, it generates homodimerization or heterodimerization of the receptor, leading to phosphorylation of sites in the cytoplasmic tyrosine kinase and activation of various intracellular pathways, including the phosphatidylinositol 3-kinase (PI3K)/AKT/mammalian target of rapamycin (mTOR) and RAS/RAF/mitogen-activated protein kinase (MAPK) pathways, which lead to cell proliferation, metastasis, and prevention of apoptosis.[10] EGFR is overexpressed in 62% of NSCLCs, and its expression has been associated with poor prognosis.[11] Approximately 10% of patients with adenocarcinoma of the lung in the United States and 30% to 50% in East Asia have lung tumors associated with *EGFR* mutations.[11] These mutations occur within exons 18 to 21, which encode for a portion of the EGFR kinase domain.[10] Approximately 90% of *EGFR* mutations occur as in-frame deletions in exon 19 or as missense mutations in exon 21 (44% and 41% of all mutations, respectively).[4] Activating mutations in the kinase domain of EGFR trigger ligand-independent tyrosine kinase activation, leading to hyperactivation of downstream antiapoptotic signaling pathways.[10] *EGFR* mutations are found more often in adenocarcinomas with lepidic features from female never-smokers.[10] The high response rates (55%–78%) to treatment with tyrosine kinase inhibitors (TKIs), such as gefitinib,

---

positive expression for thyroid transcription factor (TTF)-1 (nuclear), programmed death-ligand 1 (PD-L1; membrane and cytoplasm), and anaplastic lymphoma kinase (ALK; cytoplasm); p40 shows negative expression. SqCC shows positive expression for p40 (nuclear) and PD-L1 (membrane and cytoplasm); p40 and ALK expression are negative (original magnification ×20).

erlotinib, and afatinib, in patients with *EGFR*-mutant tumors, and the significantly greater progression-free survival (PFS) of these patients, have made EGFR TKIs the standard treatment of patients with these mutations.[6] However, most of these patients develop resistance and relapse in a short time, because of the occurrence of a new mutation (T790 M) in exon 20 of the EGFR kinase domain (50%), amplification of the *MET* oncogene (21%), or mutations of *PI3KCA*.[4]

EGFR mutations are identified mostly with the use of gene sequencing methodologies and real-time polymerase chain reaction (PCR)-based assays. Both methods have been reported to have high performance and sensitivity in the detection of these mutations in formalin-fixed and paraffin-embedded tissues.[4] Detection of *EGFR* mutations by an IHC-based approach with specific antibodies against mutant proteins has been attempted but showed variable sensitivity and significant variability between studies.[12]

Anaplastic Lymphoma Kinase

Anaplastic lymphoma kinase (ALK) is a tyrosine kinase receptor member of the insulin receptor superfamily. The *ALK* gene is located on the short arm of chromosome 2 at position 23.[13] *ALK* gene rearrangement was originally identified in anaplastic large cell lymphoma[14] and was subsequently described in a subset of NSCLC tumors harboring a fusion of *ALK* and echinoderm microtubule-associated protein-like 4 (*EML4*) genes.[4] This rearrangement encodes for a chimeric protein with constitutive kinase activity, which promotes malignant growth and proliferation.[14] The *EML4-ALK* fusion has been detected in 3.7% to 7% of NSCLCs,[10,14] usually in adenocarcinomas with signet-ring cells or cribriform histology features, and is more common in young patients who have never smoked.[14] There are several *EML4-ALK* rearrangement variants and also *ALK* fusion with other less frequent partners, such as kinesin family member 5B (*KIF5B*), TRK-fused gene (*TFG*), kinesin light chain 1 (*KLC1*), and huntingtin-interacting protein 1 (*HIP1*) genes, resulting in oncogenic transformation.[13,15] It has been shown that *EGFR*, Kirsten rat sarcoma viral oncogene homolog gene (*KRAS*), and *ALK* molecular alterations are mutually exclusive events[4]; nevertheless, they have been described in up to 2.7% of lung adenocarcinoma cases with concurrent molecular alterations.[16] The *ALK* fusion defines a distinct subpopulation of patients with lung adenocarcinoma who are highly responsive (57%–74%) to ALK inhibitors, such as crizotinib. Patients treated with crizotinib demonstrated significantly better median PFS and response rate compared with patients who received chemotherapy.[17] As a result, testing for *ALK* rearrangements in patients with advanced lung adenocarcinoma is recommended in current clinical practice guidelines.[5,10] However, despite initial responses, a fraction of the patients develop acquired resistance to crizotinib, because of secondary mutations within the kinase domain of EML4-ALK; these include L1196 M, C1156Y, and F1174 L, among others.[18,19] Several second-generation ALK inhibitors that target ALK-positive NSCLC, such as alectinib, ceritinib, and AP26133, have been developed and are currently under evaluation in clinical trials.[20]

Current diagnostic approaches to detect *ALK* fusion genes and their results include break-apart fluorescence in situ hybridization (FISH), IHC, and reverse-transcription PCR (RT-PCR).[21] Break-apart FISH has been established in clinical trials as the standard method for confirmation of *ALK* status.[22] FISH and IHC have shown high concordance in several reports, especially with the development of IHC antibodies (clones 5A4 and D5F3) with better sensitivities and specificities (83%–100%) for the detection of ALK rearrangement.[23,24] As a result, IHC detection of the ALK protein is being considered as an adequate screening tool to test NSCLC samples for ALK rearrangements or as a tool to evaluate cases that are not interpretable by FISH.[25,26] Nevertheless, other studies reveal major discordances, suggesting the need to combine both tests to optimize detection.[22] Other methods, such as RT-PCR and NGS, are in use but have not been examined systematically compared with FISH as a predictor of response to ALK inhibitors.[27,28]

Kirsten Rat Sarcoma Viral Oncogene Homolog

KRAS is an oncogene located on the long arm of chromosome 12 at position 12.1.[29] It is a member of the RAS family of membrane-associated G proteins and encodes for a protein with intrinsic GTPase activity, which is involved in a variety of cellular responses including proliferation, cytoskeletal reorganization, and survival.[30] KRAS acts downstream of several tyrosine kinases receptors, including EGFR, and is associated with activation of the RAS/RAF/MAP kinase (MEK)/extracellular signal-regulated kinase (ERK) and RAS/MAPK signaling pathways.[10] *KRAS* mutations occur in 25% to 35% of patients with NSCLC, principally adenocarcinomas with a solid pattern,[31] and are found more often in white patients compared with Asians, in former or current smokers, but without sex predilection.[32] Mutations in the form of single-nucleotide missense variants are found in codons 12 and 13 in approximately 95% of cases.[4,32] In never-smokers, the most common *KRAS* mutations are G12D and G12 V, whereas G12 C is the most common mutation associated with smoking.[31,32] The presence of *KRAS* mutation may be associated with unfavorable outcome[33] and could be a negative predictor of responsiveness to chemotherapy.[34] In addition, it is associated with an increased likelihood of having a second primary tumor[35] and is a predictor of resistance to targeted therapy with EGFR-TKIs, such as gefitinib or erlotinib, in patients with NSCLC.[36]

Because *KRAS*, *EGFR*, and *ALK* molecular alterations are mutually exclusive, it has been suggested that *KRAS* testing could be a surrogate assay to exclude *EGFR*- and *ALK*-positive cases[10]; however, this approach is not currently recommended. Although there are no targeted therapies approved for patients with lung cancer and *KRAS* mutation, several clinical trials aimed at downstream signaling targets are under way. Different phase 2 trials have reported improvements in PFS and response rate with the combination of selumetinib (MEK1/MEK2 inhibitor) and docetaxel compared with docetaxel alone[37] and promising results with sorafenib (RAS/RAF pathway inhibitor), with a disease control rate of approximately 50%.[38] Conversely, trametinib (MEK1/MEK2 inhibitor) did not show advantages over docetaxel in patients with NSCLC.[39]

ROS Proto-oncogene 1, Receptor Tyrosine Kinase

ROS proto-oncogene 1, receptor tyrosine kinase (ROS1) is a tyrosine kinase receptor member of the insulin receptor family and is located on the long arm of chromosome 6 at position 22. ROS1 plays a role in epithelial cell differentiation during the development of a variety of organs, but no ligand for this receptor has been identified.[40] *ROS1* rearrangements were originally described in glioblastoma and have also been reported in cholangiocarcinoma and ovarian cancer.[41] Approximately 1% to 2% of NSCLCs harbor *ROS1* rearrangements,[41] and several fusion partners including *CD74*, solute carrier family 34, member 2 (*SLC34A2*), leucine-rich repeats and immunoglobulin-like domains 3 (*LRIG3*), ezrin (*EZR*), syndecan 4 (*SDC4*), tropomyosin 3 (*TPM3*), and *FIG* have been reported in these tumors. All of these fusions result in a chimeric protein that has been reported to be oncogenic.[40,41] *ROS1*-rearranged NSCLC typically occurs in young, female, never-smokers with a histologic diagnosis of adenocarcinoma[40,41] and is usually mutually exclusive with other oncogenic drivers

(*EGFR, KRAS, ALK*).[41] Clinical trials have reported that patients with advanced NSCLC harboring *ROS1* rearrangement have benefited from crizotinib treatment, showing response rates up to 80%.[40,42] Ongoing phase 1 and 2 studies are investigating the activity of crizotinib and ceritinib (ALK inhibitor) in *ROS1*-rearranged NSCLC.[43,44] ROS1 testing is indispensable for identifying patients who could benefit from crizotinib treatment. The National Comprehensive Cancer Network 2014 guidelines recommend that all patients with advanced triple-negative (*EGFR, ALK*, and *KRAS*) lung adenocarcinoma be tested for other molecular markers including *ROS1*.[5]

There is not a gold standard method, but currently available diagnostic methods include FISH, RT-PCR, and IHC.[45] FISH is the only method approved by the US Food and Drug Administration to detect *ALK*-rearranged NSCLC and has been used in clinical trials as the standard method for confirmation of *ROS1* rearrangement; nevertheless, it is an expensive and laborious technique. Because *ROS1*-rearranged lung cancer is rare, assessment of ROS1 protein expression by IHC may be used as a screening tool for the identification of candidates suitable for ROS1-targeted therapy. In fact, studies have found that ROS1 IHC (D4D6 clone) has a high sensitivity (100%) and specificity (92%–97%) for ROS1 rearrangements compared with FISH.[45]

Human Epidermal Growth Factor Receptor 2

The human EGFR 2 gene *HER2* (*ERBB2*) is a proto-oncogene located on chromosome 17 at position 12.[46] It encodes for a tyrosine kinase receptor member of the ERBB receptor family.[47] HER2 lacks a specific ligand. Nevertheless, it can be combined with other ERBB receptors to form a heterodimer.[48] This allows for the activation of important signal transduction pathways, including the MAPK and PI3K pathways, involved in cell proliferation, differentiation, and migration.[47] HER2 expression and/or amplification are found in many cancers including breast and gastric cancer.[48] Overexpression of HER2 has been reported in 7% to 34.9% of NSCLCs and has been associated with poor prognosis in patients with these tumors.[47] Activating mutations of *HER2* have been found in 1.6% to 4% of lung cancers.[47,49] These mutations occur in the four exons of the tyrosine kinase domain (exons 18–21) and are found more often in adenocarcinomas in female, Asian, never-smokers, or light smokers. *HER2* mutations are almost always mutually exclusive with other driver oncogene alterations in lung cancer described previously.[49] Different studies reinforce the importance of screening lung adenocarcinomas for *HER2* mutation as a method to select patients who could benefit from *HER2*-targeted therapies (afatinib and trastuzumab), which have shown response rates of approximately 50%.[50] Several clinical trials of targeted agents, such as trastuzumab, neratinib, and pyrotinib, among others, are being conducted in patients with *HER2* mutation.[47] HER2 mutations are usually assessed via sequencing approaches.

RET Proto-oncogene

The *RET* proto-oncogene is located on the long arm of chromosome 10 at position 11.2. It encodes for a tyrosine kinase receptor for the glial cell line–derived neurotrophic factor family of ligands and is involved in cell proliferation, migration, and differentiation, and neuronal navigation.[51] *RET* chromosomal rearrangements were originally described in papillary thyroid carcinoma.[51] Approximately 1% to 2% of NSCLCs harbor *RET* fusions, and several fusion partners, including kinesin family member 5B (*KIF5B*; 90%), coiled-coil domain containing 6 (*CCDC6*), nuclear receptor coactivator 4 (*NCOA4*), and tripartite motif-containing 33 (*TRIM33*), have been described.[52,53] *RET*-rearranged NSCLC typically occurs in adenocarcinomas with more poorly differentiated solid features in young never-smokers, and it is mutually exclusive with known driver oncogenes.[52,54] In vitro studies showed that *RET* fusions lead to oncogenic transformation, which can be inhibited by multitargeted kinase inhibitors, such as vandetanib, sorafenib, and sunitinib.[54] Preliminary studies with cabozantinib (MET and vascular endothelial growth factor receptor 2 inhibitor) in *RET*-rearranged lung adenocarcinoma are promising.[53]

FISH is currently the standard diagnostic assay for detection of *RET* chromosomal rearrangements. RT-PCR is usually insufficient for the detection of new partners or isoforms, and *RET* IHC has shown low sensitivity and specificity for *RET* rearrangements.[52,54] Sequencing approaches, including NGS methodologies, are also frequently used to detect *RET* translocations.

MET Proto-oncogene

The *MET* gene is located on the long arm of chromosome 7 at position 31.[55] This oncogene encodes for a tyrosine kinase receptor (hepatocyte growth factor receptor), which activates multiple signaling pathways that play fundamental roles in cell proliferation, survival, motility, and invasion.[4] Pathologic activation of *MET* includes mutation, gene amplification, and protein overexpression.[56] MET alterations were first reported in patients with renal papillary carcinoma and mutations in the MET kinase domain leading to constitutive activation of the receptor.[57] In lung cancer, *MET* mutations are found in the extracellular semaphorin and juxtamembrane domains, occurring in 3% of squamous cell lung cancers and 8% of lung adenocarcinomas.[56] *MET* amplifications are found in 4% of lung adenocarcinomas and 1% of squamous cell lung cancers and are associated with sensitivity to MET inhibitors.[56] In NSCLC, MET and hepatocyte growth factor protein expression, along with high *MET* gene copy number, have been described as poor prognosis factors.[58,59] Activating point mutations affecting splice sites of exon 14 of the *MET* gene (*MET*ex14), which occur in 4% of lung adenocarcinomas, represent a possible oncogenic driver and identify a subset of patients who may benefit from MET inhibitors, such as capmatinib and crizotinib.[56] This novel alteration is usually assayed by NGS methodology.

B-RAF Proto-oncogene, Serine/Threonine Kinase

The B-RAF proto-oncogene, serine/threonine kinase (*BRAF*) oncogene is located on the long arm of chromosome 7 at position 34. It encodes for a serine/threonine kinase, which is involved in the RAS/RAF/MEK/ERK signaling pathway.[60] When activated by oncogenic mutations, BRAF phosphorylates MEK and promotes cell growth, proliferation, and survival.[60] The highest incidence of *BRAF* mutation is in malignant melanoma (27%–70%), followed by papillary thyroid cancer, colorectal cancer, and serous ovarian cancer.[61] *BRAF* mutations have also been reported in 1% to 3% of NSCLCs.[60] In contrast to melanoma, only half of *BRAF* mutations in NSCLC are V600 E mutations. Other non-V600 E mutations reported in NSCLC include G469 A (~35%) and D594 G (~10%). All BRAF mutations are mutually exclusive with other driver alterations, such as those of *EGFR, KRAS*, and *ALK*.[60,62] *BRAF*-mutated NSCLC has been reported to be mostly adenocarcinoma, and in contrast to patients with *EGFR* mutations or *ALK* rearrangements who are mostly never-smokers, patients with *BRAF* mutations are mostly current or former smokers.[62] Nevertheless, patients with NSCLC and *BRAF* V600 E mutations have a worse prognosis and lower response to platinum-based chemotherapy than patients with wild-type *BRAF*. These patients have benefited from treatment with BRAF and MEK inhibitors.[63] BRAF inhibitors, such as vemurafenib and dabrafenib, have high and selective activity against the V600E-mutant BRAF kinase, with overall responses rates from 33% to 42%.[63,64] BRAF and MEK inhibitors targeting *BRAF* mutation–positive NSCLC, such as trametinib, selumetinib, and dasatinib, among others, are currently under evaluation in clinical trials.

Phosphatidylinositol-4,5-Bisphosphate 3-Kinase Catalytic Subunit Alpha

PI3Ks are heterodimeric lipid kinases composed of catalytic and regulatory subunits and are part of several downstream pathways involved in cell growth, transformation, adhesion, apoptosis, survival, and motility.[65] The *PIK3CA* gene is located on the long arm of chromosome 3 at position 26.3. It encodes for the catalytic subunit p110 alpha of P13Ks.[66] *PKI3CA* amplifications, deletions, and somatic missense mutations have been reported in many tumors including lung cancers. In fact, *PIK3CA* is one of the most commonly mutated oncogenes, along with *KRAS*, in human cancers.[67] Mutations are found in 1% to 4% of patients with NSCLC, usually affecting exons 9 and 20 (80%).[4,65,67–69] These mutations are not mutually exclusive with other driver alterations and have been reported more frequently in lung squamous cell carcinoma compared with adenocarcinoma (6.5% vs 1.5%).[69] However, *PIK3CA* mutations have not shown association with any clinicopathologic features.[65,68,69] Squamous cell carcinomas with *PIK3CA* gains are not accompanied by other genetic alterations, suggesting that this gene may play an important role in the pathogenesis of squamous cell cancers.[65] Studies have shown that *PIK3CA* mutations in *EGFR*-mutated lung cancer confer resistance to EGFR-TKIs and are a negative prognostic predictor in patients with NSCLC treated with EGFR-TKIs.[70] *PI3KCA* alterations and their downstream effectors, such as phosphatase and tensin homolog, mTOR, and AKT, are potential therapeutic targets for NSCLC therapy and are being evaluated in clinical trials for lung cancer.[71] Alterations in *PI3KCA* are detected using sequencing approaches, mostly NGS assays.

Neurotrophic Receptor Tyrosine Kinase 1

The neurotrophic receptor tyrosine kinase 1 (*NTRK1*) proto-oncogene is located on chromosome 1q21 to 22 and encodes for a receptor tyrosine kinase, also known as tropomyosin-related kinase (TRK) A, belonging to the TRK superfamily of receptor tyrosine kinases (117). *NTRK1* is involved in the regulation of cell growth and differentiation via activation of several signal transduction pathways including MAPK, PI3K, and phospholipase C-gamma.[72] *NTRK1* rearrangements have been found in colon cancer, thyroid cancer, and glioblastoma multiforme.[72] In lung cancer, approximately 3% of adenocarcinomas harbor *NTRK1* fusions, and some fusion partners, including myosin phosphatase RHO-interacting protein (*MPRIP*)-*NTRK1* and *CD74-NTRK1*, have been reported.[73] All of these fusions result in constitutive TRKA kinase activity, which has been reported to be oncogenic.[73] In early phase 1 studies, NTRK inhibitors, such as entrectinib and LOXO-101, have shown promising results in patients with solid tumors harboring NTRK fusions.[74]

Fibroblast Growth Factor Receptor

The fibroblast growth factor receptor (*FGFR*) gene is located on chromosome 8 at position 12 and encodes for a tyrosine kinase receptor belonging to the FGFR family. The FGFR family includes four receptor tyrosine kinases (FGFRs 1–4). When ligand-receptor binding occurs, FGFR dimerizes and phosphorylates FGFR substrate 2-alpha (FRS2α), leading to activation of different pathways, including the RAS/MAPK and PI3K/AKT/mTOR pathways, promoting cell survival, motility, invasiveness, and proliferation.[75,76] In cancer, *FGFR* gene amplifications, somatic missense mutations, and chromosomal translocations are the most frequent mechanisms of activation.[76] *FGFR* has been identified as an oncogenic driver in breast, gastric, endometrial, urothelial, and brain tumors, among others.[76] In lung cancer, the incidence of *FGFR1* amplification is significantly higher in squamous cell carcinoma (20%) compared with adenocarcinoma (3%) and is more frequent in current smokers compared with former and never-smokers. Other specific clinic-demographic features also correlate with *FGFR1* amplification.[75,77] Some studies have recognized *FGFR* amplification as an independent negative prognostic factor in patients with NSCLC,[78] whereas other studies have shown the opposite.[75] In addition, *FGFR* amplifications may be found in concurrence with other tumor genetic alterations including *TP53* and *PIK3CA* mutation and platelet-derived growth factor receptor A (*PDGFRA*) amplification.[77] Somatic *FGFR* mutations in lung tumors usually occur in *FGFR2* and *FGFR3* and have been detected in 6% of lung squamous cell carcinomas.[79] Multiple FGFR inhibitors, such as ponatinib, a multitargeted kinase inhibitor that displays potent pan–anti-FGFR activity, are in development, with promising results in cell lines and xenograft models.[80] Phase 1 and 2 clinical trials of FGFR inhibitors (eg, dovitinib, nintedanib, ponatinib, and AZD4547) are ongoing in patients with NSCLC.[81] *FGFR* gene copy number is usually assayed by FISH; however, members of this family are frequently part of NGS testing panels.

Discoidin Domain Receptor Tyrosine Kinase 2

The discoidin domain receptor tyrosine kinase 2 gene (*DDR2*) is located on the long arm of chromosome 1 at position 23.3 and encodes for a tyrosine kinase receptor that is expressed in mesenchymal tissues and that binds fibrillar collagen as ligand. DDR2 activates important signaling pathways including SRC, SRC homology domain-containing, Janus kinase, ERK1/2, and PI3K and promotes cell migration, proliferation, and survival.[82] In cancer, *DDR2* mutations have been reported in melanoma and uterine, gastric, bladder, and colorectal cancers.[83] In lung cancer, *DDR2* mutations occur in 3% to 4% of lung squamous cell carcinomas[84] compared with 0.5% of adenocarcinomas[85] and are only present in smokers.[86] No other significant association with clinicopathologic status has been found.[84] At least 11 different *DDR2* mutations have been identified[84] distributed throughout the gene and include the extracellular-binding discoidin domain and the cytoplasmic kinase domain.[82,84] *DDR2* mutations have been associated with response to dasatinib (a multitargeted kinase inhibitor) in preclinical models and early phase clinical trials. Phase 2 clinical trials of dasatinib in patients with lung squamous cell carcinoma are under way.[82,84]

IMMUNOTHERAPY MARKERS IN LUNG CANCER

Historically, lung cancer has not been considered immunogenic because of several failed attempts with cytokines and vaccines. Nevertheless, over the past few years, immunotherapy has re-emerged strongly with the development of checkpoint inhibitors as treatments for NSCLC. Immune checkpoints are inhibitory pathways with the functions of maintaining self-tolerance and modulating immune responses.[87] Immune checkpoint proteins that have been studied more comprehensively in many types of cancer, including lung cancer, are cytotoxic T-lymphocyte-associated antigen 4 (CTLA-4) and the programmed death-ligand 1 receptor (PD-1), which are expressed mainly on T cells, and programmed death-ligand 1 (PD-L1), which is expressed on tumor cells and tumor inflammatory infiltrate including macrophages, dendritic cells, and T cells.[88] Many other checkpoint molecules, such as T-cell immunoglobulin and mucin domain-containing protein 3, B- and T-lymphocyte-associated protein, V-domain Ig suppressor of T-cell activation, and lymphocyte-activation gene 3, have been identified and are currently being evaluated as potential targets for cancer immunotherapy.[89]

Cytotoxic T-Lymphocyte-Associated Antigen 4

Monoclonal antibodies that inhibit CTLA-4, such as ipilimumab, are available to prevent the binding of CTLA-4 with its ligands (CD80/CD86), leading to reactivation of the antitumor immune response mediated by specific T cells.[88] A phase 2 study of ipilimumab in combination with chemotherapy in patients with advanced NSCLC showed promising results, with a significant improvement in PFS versus a control group treated with chemotherapy alone.[90] A phase 3 trial of ipilimumab in combination with chemotherapy in patients with squamous histology NSCLC is ongoing.[91] Currently, there is no biomarker to predict response to CTLA-4 therapy.

Programmed Death-Ligand 1 Receptor

Several monoclonal antibodies targeting the interaction between PD-1 and its ligands PD-L1 and PD-L2 are available. There are different ways to block the PD-1 pathway; one is to use antibodies directed against PD-1 or by blocking its ligand PD-L1.[92] Clinical trials in NSCLC have shown sustained responses in approximately 20% of unselected patients to treatment with monoclonal antibodies against PD-1, such as nivolumab and pembrolizumab, and with antibodies against PD-L1, such as MPDL3280 A. The Food and Drug Administration has approved the use of nivolumab in advanced NSCLC on or after platinum-based chemotherapy and pembrolizumab as second-line treatment of NSCLC after chemotherapy.[93,94] A recent study has reported that greater nonsynonymous mutation burden is associated with improved objective response, durable clinical benefit, and PFS in patients with NSCLC treated with pembrolizumab.[95] Furthermore, IHC PD-L1 positivity in NSCLC has been identified as a potential predictor of response to anti-PD-1 and anti-PD-L1 monoclonal antibody therapy[96] and also as a prognostic biomarker.[97] Other studies reported that PD-L1 overexpression cannot be currently considered a robust predictive biomarker for response to immunotherapy or a prognostic biomarker.[98] These discrepancies may be caused by assay variability and interpretive subjectivity differences for the evaluation of PD-L1 expression, including differences in detection methods, IHC antibody clones, and cutoff values for determining PD-L1 positivity, and heterogeneity in PD-L1 expression and site of PD-L1 expression (tumor cells and tumor immune cells).[99,100] Further studies are needed to compare different assays and to clarify and standardize testing protocols to confirm the suitability of PD-L1 expression as a biomarker.

REFERENCES

1. Siegel R, Naishadham D, Jemal A. Cancer statistics, 2013. CA Cancer J Clin 2013;63(1):11–30.
2. American Cancer Society. Cancer facts & figures 2015. Available at: http://www.cancer.org/research/cancerfactsstatistics/cancerfactsfigures2015/index. Accessed May 25, 2016.
3. Cagle PT, Allen TC, Olsen RJ. Lung cancer biomarkers: present status and future developments. Arch Pathol Lab Med 2013;137(9):1191–8.
4. Fujimoto J, Wistuba II. Current concepts on the molecular pathology of non-small cell lung carcinoma. Semin Diagn Pathol 2014;31(4):306–13.
5. Kerr KM, Bubendorf L, Edelman MJ, et al, Panel Members. Second ESMO consensus conference on lung cancer: pathology and molecular biomarkers for non-small-cell lung cancer. Ann Oncol 2014;25(9):1681–90.
6. Mok TS. Personalized medicine in lung cancer: what we need to know. Nat Rev Clin Oncol 2011;8(11):661–8.

7. Travis WD, Bambrilla E, Burke AP, et al, editors. WHO classification of tumours of the lung, pleura, thymus and heart (IARC WHO classification of tumours). 4th edition. Geneva (Switzerland): World Health Organization; 2015.

8. Travis WD, Brambilla E, Riely GJ. New pathologic classification of lung cancer: relevance for clinical practice and clinical trials. J Clin Oncol 2013;31(8): 992–1001.

9. Khalil FK, Altiok S. Advances in EGFR as a predictive marker in lung adenocarcinoma. Cancer Control 2015;22(2):193–9.

10. Sholl LM. Biomarkers in lung adenocarcinoma: a decade of progress. Arch Pathol Lab Med 2015;139(4):469–80.

11. Sharma SV, Bell DW, Settleman J, et al. Epidermal growth factor receptor mutations in lung cancer. Nat Rev Cancer 2007;7(3):169–81.

12. Fan X, Liu B, Xu H, et al. Immunostaining with EGFR mutation-specific antibodies: a reliable screening method for lung adenocarcinomas harboring EGFR mutation in biopsy and resection samples. Hum Pathol 2013;44(8): 1499–507.

13. Zhao Z, Verma V, Zhang M. Anaplastic lymphoma kinase: role in cancer and therapy perspective. Cancer Biol Ther 2015;16(12):1691–701.

14. Chatziandreou I, Tsioli P, Sakellariou S, et al. Comprehensive molecular analysis of NSCLC; clinicopathological associations. PLoS One 2015;10(7):e0133859.

15. Fang DD, Zhang B, Gu Q, et al. HIP1-ALK, a novel ALK fusion variant that responds to crizotinib. J Thorac Oncol 2014;9(3):285–94.

16. Sholl LM, Aisner DL, Varella-Garcia M, et al, LCMC Investigators. Multi-institutional oncogenic driver mutation analysis in lung adenocarcinoma: the Lung Cancer Mutation Consortium experience. J Thorac Oncol 2015;10(5):768–77.

17. Solomon BJ, Mok T, Kim DW, et al, PROFILE 1014 Investigators. First-line crizotinib versus chemotherapy in ALK-positive lung cancer. N Engl J Med 2014; 371(23):2167–77.

18. Choi YL, Soda M, Yamashita a, et al, ALK Lung Cancer Study Group. EML4-ALK mutations in lung cancer that confer resistance to ALK inhibitors. N Engl J Med 2010;363(18):1734–9.

19. Sasaki T, Okuda K, Zheng W, et al. The neuroblastoma-associated F1174L ALK mutation causes resistance to an ALK kinase inhibitor in ALK-translocated cancers. Cancer Res 2010;70(24):10038–43.

20. Sullivan I, Planchard D. ALK inhibitors in non-small cell lung cancer: the latest evidence and developments. Ther Adv Med Oncol 2016;8(1):32–47.

21. Toyokawa G, Seto T. Anaplastic lymphoma kinase rearrangement in lung cancer: its biological and clinical significance. Respir Investig 2014;52(6):330–8.

22. Cabillic F, Gros A, Dugay F, et al. Parallel FISH and immunohistochemical studies of ALK status in 3244 non-small-cell lung cancers reveal major discordances. J Thorac Oncol 2014;9(3):295–306.

23. Martinez P, Hernández-Losa J, Montero MÁ, et al. Fluorescence in situ hybridization and immunohistochemistry as diagnostic methods for ALK positive non-small cell lung cancer patients. PLoS One 2013;8(1):e52261.

24. Sholl LM, Weremowicz S, Gray SW, et al. Combined use of ALK immunohistochemistry and FISH for optimal detection of ALK-rearranged lung adenocarcinomas. J Thorac Oncol 2013;8(3):322–8.

25. Yi ES, Boland JM, Maleszewski JJ, et al. Correlation of IHC and FISH for ALK gene rearrangement in non-small cell lung carcinoma: IHC score algorithm for FISH. J Thorac Oncol 2011;6(3):459–65.

26. Paik JH, Choe G, Kim H, et al. Screening of anaplastic lymphoma kinase rearrangement by immunohistochemistry in non-small cell lung cancer: correlation with fluorescence in situ hybridization. J Thorac Oncol 2011;6(3):466–72.
27. Wallander ML, Geiersbach KB, Tripp SR, et al. Comparison of reverse transcription-polymerase chain reaction, immunohistochemistry, and fluorescence in situ hybridization methodologies for detection of echinoderm microtubule-associated proteinlike 4-anaplastic lymphoma kinase fusion-positive non-small cell lung carcinoma: implications for optimal clinical testing. Arch Pathol Lab Med 2012;136(7):796–803.
28. Pekar-Zlotin M, Hirsch FR, Soussan-Gutman L, et al. Fluorescence in situ hybridization, immunohistochemistry, and next-generation sequencing for detection of EML4-ALK rearrangement in lung cancer. Oncologist 2015;20(3):316–22.
29. McBride OW, Swan DC, Tronick SR, et al. Regional chromosomal localization of N-ras, K-ras-1, K-ras-2 and myb oncogenes in human cells. Nucleic Acids Res 1983;11(23):8221–36.
30. Edkins S, O'Meara S, Parker A, et al. Recurrent KRAS codon 146 mutations in human colorectal cancer. Cancer Biol Ther 2006;5(8):928–32.
31. Kempf E, Rousseau B, Besse B, et al. KRAS oncogene in lung cancer: focus on molecularly driven clinical trials. Eur Respir Rev 2016;25(139):71–6.
32. Dogan S, Shen R, Ang DC, et al. Molecular epidemiology of EGFR and KRAS mutations in 3,026 lung adenocarcinomas: higher susceptibility of women to smoking-related KRAS-mutant cancers. Clin Cancer Res 2012;18(22): 6169–77.
33. Ying M, Zhu XX, Zhao Y, et al. KRAS mutation as a biomarker for survival in patients with non-small cell lung cancer, a meta-analysis of 12 randomized trials. Asian Pac J Cancer Prev 2015;16(10):4439–45.
34. Macerelli M, Caramella C, Faivre L, et al. Does KRAS mutational status predict chemoresistance in advanced non-small cell lung cancer (NSCLC)? Lung Cancer 2014;83(3):383–8.
35. Shepherd FA, Domerg C, Hainaut P, et al. Pooled analysis of the prognostic and predictive effects of KRAS mutation status and KRAS mutation subtype in early-stage resected non-small-cell lung cancer in four trials of adjuvant chemotherapy. J Clin Oncol 2013;31(17):2173–81.
36. Pao W, Wang TY, Riely GJ, et al. KRAS mutations and primary resistance of lung adenocarcinomas to gefitinib or erlotinib. PLoS Med 2005;2(1):e17.
37. Jänne PA, Shaw AT, Pereira JR, et al. Selumetinib plus docetaxel for KRAS-mutant advanced non-small-cell lung cancer: a randomised, multicentre, placebo-controlled, phase 2 study. Lancet Oncol 2013;14(1):38–47.
38. Dingemans AM, Mellema WW, Groen HJ, et al. A phase II study of sorafenib in patients with platinum-pretreated, advanced (Stage IIIb or IV) non-small cell lung cancer with a KRAS mutation. Clin Cancer Res 2013;19(3):743–51.
39. Blumenschein GR Jr, Smit EF, Planchard D, et al. A randomized phase II study of the MEK1/MEK2 inhibitor trametinib (GSK1120212) compared with docetaxel in KRAS-mutant advanced non-small-cell lung cancer (NSCLC)[†]. Ann Oncol 2015; 26(5):894–901.
40. Bergethon K, Shaw AT, Ou SH, et al. ROS1 rearrangements define a unique molecular class of lung cancers. J Clin Oncol 2012;30(8):863–70.
41. Yoshida A, Kohno T, Tsuta K, et al. ROS1-rearranged lung cancer: a clinicopathologic and molecular study of 15 surgical cases. Am J Surg Pathol 2013;37(4): 554–62.

42. Mazières J, Zalcman G, Crinò L, et al. Crizotinib therapy for advanced lung adenocarcinoma and a ROS1 rearrangement: results from the EUROS1 cohort. J Clin Oncol 2015;33(9):992–9.

43. ClinicalTrials.gov #NCT01964157. An open-label, multicenter, phase II study of LDK378 in patients with non-small cell lung cancer harboring ROS1 rearrangement. Available at: https://clinicaltrials.gov/ct2/show/NCT01964157?term=An+Open-label%2C+Multicenter%2C+Phase+II+Study+of+LDK378+in+Patients+With+Non-small+Cell+Lung+Cancer+Harboring+ROS1+Rearrangement&rank=1. Accessed May 25, 2016.

44. ClinicalTrials.gov #NCT02183870. EUCROSS: European trial on crizotinib in ROS1 translocated lung cancer (EUCROSS). Available at: https://clinicaltrials.gov/ct2/show/NCT02183870?term=EUCROSS%3A+European+Trial+on+Crizotinib+in+ROS1+Translocated+Lung+Cancer&rank=1. Accessed May 25, 2016.

45. Cao B, Wei P, Liu Z, et al. Detection of lung adenocarcinoma with ROS1 rearrangement by IHC, FISH, and RT-PCR and analysis of its clinicopathologic features. Onco Targets Ther 2015;9:131–8.

46. Popescu NC, King CR, Kraus MH. Localization of the human erbB-2 gene on normal and rearranged chromosomes 17 to bands q12-21.32. Genomics 1989;4(3):362–6.

47. Ricciardi GR, Russo A, Franchina T, et al. NSCLC and HER2: between lights and shadows. J Thorac Oncol 2014;9(12):1750–62.

48. Bu S, Wang R, Pan Y, et al. Clinicopathologic characteristics of patients with HER2 insertions in non-small cell lung cancer. Ann Surg Oncol 2016. [Epub ahead of print].

49. Shigematsu H, Takahashi T, Nomura M, et al. Somatic mutations of the HER2 kinase domain in lung adenocarcinomas. Cancer Res 2005;65(5):1642–6.

50. Mazières J, Peters S, Lepage B, et al. Lung cancer that harbors an HER2 mutation: epidemiologic characteristics and therapeutic perspectives. J Clin Oncol 2013;31(16):1997–2003.

51. Knowles PP, Murray-Rust J, Kjaer S, et al. Structure and chemical inhibition of the RET tyrosine kinase domain. J Biol Chem 2006;281(44):33577–87.

52. Wang R, Hu H, Pan Y, et al. RET fusions define a unique molecular and clinicopathologic subtype of non-small-cell lung cancer. J Clin Oncol 2012;30(35):4352–9.

53. Drilon A, Wang L, Hasanovic A, et al. Response to cabozantinib in patients with RET fusion-positive lung adenocarcinomas. Cancer Discov 2013;3(6):630–5.

54. Lipson D, Capelletti M, Yelensky R, et al. Identification of new ALK and RET gene fusions from colorectal and lung cancer biopsies. Nat Med 2012;18(3):382–4.

55. Zhen Z, Giordano S, Longati P, et al. Structural and functional domains critical for constitutive activation of the HGF-receptor (Met). Oncogene 1994;9(6):1691–7.

56. Paik PK, Drilon A, Fan PD, et al. Response to MET inhibitors in patients with stage IV lung adenocarcinomas harboring MET mutations causing exon 14 skipping. Cancer Discov 2015;5(8):842–9.

57. Schmidt L, Duh FM, Chen F, et al. Germline and somatic mutations in the tyrosine kinase domain of the MET proto-oncogene in papillary renal carcinomas. Nat Genet 1997;16(1):68–73.

58. Masuya D, Huang C, Liu D, et al. The tumour-stromal interaction between intratumoral c-Met and stromal hepatocyte growth factor associated with tumour growth and prognosis in non-small-cell lung cancer patients. Br J Cancer 2004;90(8):1555–62.

59. Beau-Faller M, Ruppert AM, Voegell AC, et al. MET gene copy number in non-small cell lung cancer: molecular analysis in a targeted tyrosine kinase inhibitor naïve cohort. J Thorac Oncol 2008;3(4):331–9.
60. Cardarella S, Ogino A, Nishino M, et al. Clinical, pathologic, and biologic features associated with BRAF mutations in non-small cell lung cancer. Clin Cancer Res 2013;19(16):4532–40.
61. Garnett MJ, Marais R. Guilty as charged: B-RAF is a human oncogene. Cancer Cell 2004;6(4):313–9.
62. Paik PK, Arcila ME, Fara M, et al. Clinical characteristics of patients with lung adenocarcinomas harboring BRAF mutations. J Clin Oncol 2011;29(15):2046–51.
63. Planchard D, Kim TM, Mazieres J, et al. Dabrafenib in patients with BRAFV600E-positive advanced non-small-cell lung cancer: a single-arm, multicentre, open-label, phase 2 trial. Lancet Oncol 2016;17(5):642–50.
64. Hyman DM, Puzanov I, Subbiah V, et al. Vemurafenib in multiple nonmelanoma cancers with BRAF V600 mutations. N Engl J Med 2015;373(8):726–36.
65. Yamamoto H, Shigematsu H, Nomura M, et al. PIK3CA mutations and copy number gains in human lung cancers. Cancer Res 2008;68(17):6913–21.
66. Karakas B, Bachman KE, Park BH. Mutation of the PIK3CA oncogene in human cancers. Br J Cancer 2006;94(4):455–9.
67. Samuels Y, Velculescu VE. Oncogenic mutations of PIK3CA in human cancers. Cell Cycle 2004;3(10):1221–4.
68. Endoh H, Yatabe Y, Kosaka T, et al. PTEN and PIK3CA expression is associated with prolonged survival after gefitinib treatment in EGFR-mutated lung cancer patients. J Thorac Oncol 2006;1(7):629–34.
69. Kawano O, Sasaki H, Endo K, et al. PIK3CA mutation status in Japanese lung cancer patients. Lung Cancer 2006;54(2):209–15.
70. Chen JY, Cheng YN, Han L, et al. Predictive value of K-ras and PIK3CA in non-small cell lung cancer patients treated with EGFR-TKIs: a systemic review and meta-analysis. Cancer Biol Med 2015;12(2):126–39.
71. Thomas A, Rajan A, Lopez-Chavez A, et al. From targets to targeted therapies and molecular profiling in non-small cell lung carcinoma. Ann Oncol 2013;24(3):577–85.
72. Alberti L, Carniti C, Miranda C, et al. RET and NTRK1 proto-oncogenes in human diseases. J Cell Physiol 2003;195(2):168–86.
73. Vaishnavi A, Capelletti M, Le AT, et al. Oncogenic and drug-sensitive NTRK1 re-arrangements in lung cancer. Nat Med 2013;19(11):1469–72.
74. Passiglia F, Caparica R, Giovannetti E, et al. The potential of neurotrophic tyrosine kinase (NTRK) inhibitors for treating lung cancer. Expert Opin Investig Drugs 2016;25(4):385–92.
75. Jiang T, Gao G, Fan G, et al. FGFR1 amplification in lung squamous cell carcinoma: a systematic review with meta-analysis. Lung Cancer 2015;87(1):1–7.
76. Dienstmann R, Rodon J, Prat A, et al. Genomic aberrations in the FGFR pathway: opportunities for targeted therapies in solid tumors. Ann Oncol 2014;25(3):552–63.
77. Weiss J, Sos ML, Seidel D, et al. Frequent and focal FGFR1 amplification associates with therapeutically tractable FGFR1 dependency in squamous cell lung cancer. Sci Transl Med 2010;2(62):62ra93.
78. Seo AN, Jin Y, Lee HJ, et al. FGFR1 amplification is associated with poor prognosis and smoking in non-small-cell lung cancer. Virchows Arch 2014;465(5):547–58.

79. Liao RG, Jung J, Tchaicha J, et al. Inhibitor-sensitive FGFR2 and FGFR3 mutations in lung squamous cell carcinoma. Cancer Res 2013;73(16):5195–205.
80. Gozgit JM, Wong MJ, Moran L, et al. Ponatinib (AP24534), a multitargeted pan-FGFR inhibitor with activity in multiple FGFR-amplified or mutated cancer models. Mol Cancer Ther 2012;11(3):690–9.
81. Tiseo M, Gelsomino F, Alfieri R, et al. FGFR as potential target in the treatment of squamous non small cell lung cancer. Cancer Treat Rev 2015;41(6):527–39.
82. Payne LS, Huang PH. Discoidin domain receptor 2 signaling networks and therapy in lung cancer. J Thorac Oncol 2014;9(6):900–4.
83. Beauchamp EM, Woods BA, Dulak AM, et al. Acquired resistance to dasatinib in lung cancer cell lines conferred by DDR2 gatekeeper mutation and NF1 loss. Mol Cancer Ther 2014;13(2):475–82.
84. Hammerman PS, Sos ML, Ramos AH, et al. Mutations in the DDR2 kinase gene identify a novel therapeutic target in squamous cell lung cancer. Cancer Discov 2011;1(1):78–89.
85. Ding L, Getz G, Wheeler DA, et al. Somatic mutations affect key pathways in lung adenocarcinoma. Nature 2008;455(7216):1069–75.
86. An SJ, Chen ZH, Su J, et al. Identification of enriched driver gene alterations in subgroups of non-small cell lung cancer patients based on histology and smoking status. PLoS One 2012;7(6):e40109.
87. Pardoll DM. The blockade of immune checkpoints in cancer immunotherapy. Nat Rev Cancer 2012;12(4):252–64.
88. Seetharamu N, Budman DR, Sullivan KM. Immune checkpoint inhibitors in lung cancer: past, present and future. Future Oncol 2016;12(9):1151–63.
89. Swatler J, Kozlowska E. Immune checkpoint-targeted cancer immunotherapies. Postepy Hig Med Dosw 2016;70:25–42 [Abstract in English; Article in Polish].
90. Lynch TJ, Bondarenko I, Luft A, et al. Ipilimumab in combination with paclitaxel and carboplatin as first-line treatment in stage IIIB/IV non-small-cell lung cancer: results from a randomized, double-blind, multicenter phase II study. J Clin Oncol 2012;30(17):2046–54.
91. Carrizosa DR, Gold KA. New strategies in immunotherapy for non-small cell lung cancer. Transl Lung Cancer Res 2015;4(5):553–9.
92. Brahmer JR. Immune checkpoint blockade: the hope for immunotherapy as a treatment of lung cancer? Semin Oncol 2014;41(1):126–32.
93. Garon EB, Rizvi NA, Hui R, et al, KEYNOTE-001 Investigators. Pembrolizumab for the treatment of non-small-cell lung cancer. N Engl J Med 2015;372(21):2018–28.
94. Gettinger SN, Horn L, Gandhi L, et al. Overall survival and long-term safety of nivolumab (anti-programmed death 1 antibody, BMS-936558, ONO-4538) in patients with previously treated advanced non-small-cell lung cancer. J Clin Oncol 2015;33(18):2004–12.
95. Rizvi NA, Hellmann MD, Snyder A, et al. Cancer immunology. Mutational landscape determines sensitivity to PD-1 blockade in non-small cell lung cancer. Science 2015;348(6230):124–8.
96. Borghaei H, Paz-Ares L, Horn L, et al. Nivolumab versus docetaxel in advanced nonsquamous non-small-cell lung cancer. N Engl J Med 2015;373(17):1627–39.
97. Sun JM, Zhou W, Choi YL, et al. Prognostic significance of programmed cell death ligand 1 in patients with non-small-cell lung cancer: a large cohort study of surgically resected cases. J Thorac Oncol 2016;11(7):1003–11.

98. Sorensen SF, Zhou W, Dolled-Filhart M, et al. PD-L1 expression and survival among patients with advanced non-small cell lung cancer treated with chemotherapy. Transl Oncol 2016;9(1):64–9.
99. Velcheti V, Schalper KA, Carvajal DE, et al. Programmed death ligand-1 expression in non-small cell lung cancer. Lab Invest 2014;94(1):107–16.
100. Taube JM, Anders RA, Young GD, et al. Colocalization of inflammatory response with B7-h1 expression in human melanocytic lesions supports an adaptive resistance mechanism of immune escape. Sci Transl Med 2012;4(127):127ra37.

Neoadjuvant and Adjuvant Therapy for Non–Small Cell Lung Cancer

Jody C. Chuang, MD, PhD[a], Ying Liang, MD, PhD[b], Heather A. Wakelee, MD[c],*

KEYWORDS

- Adjuvant chemotherapy • Neoadjuvant chemotherapy
- Postoperative radiation therapy

KEY POINTS

- The use of 4 cycles of cisplatin-based adjuvant chemotherapy is the standard of care for patients with resected stage II and IIIA non–small cell lung cancer.
- Neoadjuvant chemotherapy can also be considered but lacks the same level of data as adjuvant treatment.
- Good methods for selection of patients who are most likely to benefit from chemotherapy have yet to be determined.
- Ongoing adjuvant trials are exploring biomarkers of chemotherapy benefit, molecularly targeted agents, postoperative radiation therapy, and immunotherapy agents.

BACKGROUND

Lung cancer cure rates have increased slowly over the last decades, despite tremendous advances in our understanding of the molecular biology of the disease, screening, and improvements in local therapy options. Median 5-year survival rate,

Disclosure Statement: Dr H.A. Wakelee has consulting relationships with Peregrine, ACEA, Pfizer, Helsinn, Genentech (uncompensated) and performs research (with funds paid to her institution) with Clovis, Exelixis, AstraZeneca/MedImmune, Genentech/Roche, BMS, Gilead, Novartis, Xcovery, Pfizer, Celgene, Gilead, Pharmacyclics, and Eli Lilly and Company. Drs J.C. Chuang and Y Liang have nothing to disclose.

[a] Divisions of Hematology and Oncology, Department of Medicine, Stanford Hospital and Clinics, 875 Blake Wilbur Drive, Stanford, CA 94305, USA; [b] First Division, Department of Medical Oncology, Sun Yat-sen University Cancer Center, State Key Laboratory of Oncology in South China, Collaborative Innovation Center for Cancer Medicine, No 651, Dongfeng East Road, 16th Floor, Building No 2, Guangzhou, Guangdong 510060, China; [c] Division of Oncology, Department of Medicine, Stanford Cancer Institute, Stanford University, 875 Blake Wilbur Drive, Room 2233, Stanford, CA 94305-5826, USA
* Corresponding author.
E-mail address: Hwakelee@stanford.edu

Hematol Oncol Clin N Am 31 (2017) 31–44
http://dx.doi.org/10.1016/j.hoc.2016.08.011
0889-8588/17/© 2016 Elsevier Inc. All rights reserved.

as an indicator of cure rates, ranges from just more than 50% for stage IA disease to less than 30% for stage IIIA disease.[1]

For the early stages of disease, complete surgical resection remains the most effective initial therapy for patients. Recent data also support the use of stereotactic radiation therapy in patients who are not good operative candidates, although trials to compare it with surgery in operative candidates suffer from poor accrual, leaving that question unanswered. Multiple attempts to improve outcomes from surgery with the addition of chemotherapy either before (neoadjuvant) or after (adjuvant) use of targeted therapies and postoperative radiation have been investigated.

ADJUVANT CHEMOTHERAPY

Although the benefit of adjuvant chemotherapy in other malignancies has been known for decades, this approach in non–small cell lung cancer (NSCLC) has only been a standard since positive trial results in 2003. Earlier outcome data and case series from single academic centers were viewed with some skepticism given concerns of selection bias. In 1995, an individual patient meta-analysis published by the Non–Small Cell Lung Cancer Collaborative Group (NSCLCCG) reported a survival detriment with the earliest adjuvant trials, which used long-term alkylating agent-based regimens. But the cisplatin-based regimens adopted in the early 1980s showed more promise.[2] Analysis of data from more than 1300 patients enrolled in 8 trials of adjuvant cisplatin-based therapy showed a trend toward survival benefit at 5 years with a 5% improvement over observation (overall survival hazard ratio [OS HR], 0.87; 95% confidence interval [CI], 0.74–1.02, $P = .08$). Multiple randomized phase III trials followed to confirm these results, although results of the first trials were negative. The Eastern Cooperative Oncology Group 3590 (Intergroup 0115) study, the European Big Lung Trial, and the Adjuvant Lung Project Italy (ALPI) all failed to show a survival benefit, although they were well-conducted, randomized, phase III trials of adjuvant cisplatin-based regimens.[3–5] In these trials, patients with completed resected NSCLC were randomly assigned to approximately 3 months of cisplatin-based chemotherapy, initiated within 2 months of surgical resection. ALPI was large enough (1209 patients) to detect a benefit such as what was seen in the NSCLCCG meta-analysis, but the study was negative with an OS HR of 0.96 (95% CI, 0.81–1.13; $P = .589$).[5]

Starting in 2003, other studies started to detect the level of benefit predicted in the meta-analysis. The International Adjuvant Lung Cancer Trial (IALT) (n = 1867)[6] reported in 2004 a 4% 5-year survival benefit (44.5% vs 40.4%) and an OS HR of 0.86 (95% CI, 0.76–0.98; $P<.03$). Patients enrolled on this trial were randomly assigned to observation or adjuvant chemotherapy with cisplatin and either etoposide, vindesine, or vinblastine. In 2009, the long-term follow-up results were presented with an OS HR of 0.91 (95% CI, 0.81–1.02; $P = .10$), although the disease-free survival (DFS) benefit persisted (HR, 0.88; 95% CI, 0.78–0.98; $P = .02$).[7] These results, however, did not alter the use of adjuvant cisplatin-based chemotherapy, especially in light of other positive studies.

Two other adjuvant chemotherapy trials maintained the significantly improved survival benefits even with long-term follow-up. These trials used only the cisplatin/vinorelbine doublet. The National Cancer Institute of Canada Clinical Trials Group JBR.10 trial[8] enrolled 482 completed resected stage IB-II patients in North America and has continued to show a significant survival advantage for adjuvant chemotherapy group compared with observation with a median of 9.3 years of follow-up (HR, 0.78; 95% CI, 0.61–0.99; $P = .04$).[9] The absolute survival benefit at 5 years was 11% in the final analysis of JBR.10. The Adjuvant Navelbine International Trialist Association (ANITA) study[10] randomly assigned 840 patients (39% stage IIIA) with an OS HR of 0.80 (95% CI, 0.66–0.96; P = .017) and an absolute OS benefit favoring the chemotherapy group at 5 years of 8.6%.

Two large meta-analyses were conducted on the studies discussed above. The Lung Adjuvant Cisplatin Evaluation (LACE) analysis[11] included 4584 patients from ALPI, IALT, ANITA, JBR.10, and the European Big Lung Trial. The authors reported a 5.4% absolute survival benefit at 5 years, with a median of 5.1 years of follow-up, corresponding to an OS HR of 0.89 (95% CI, 0.82–0.96; P = .005) in favor of the chemotherapy arm. When broken down by stage, no benefit was found for stage IA (OS HR, 1.41; 95% CI, 0.96–2.09) or stage IB (OS HR, 0.93; 95% CI, 0.78–1.10). In patients with lymph node involvement, however, the benefit was significant with both stage II and III groups having an OS HR of 0.83 (95% CI, 0.73–0.95). The updated NSCLCCG[12] postoperative chemotherapy meta-analysis included individual data on 8447 patients and also confirmed the 4% absolute survival increase (95% CI, 3%–6%) at 5 years from 60% to 64% (HR, 0.86; 95% CI, 0.81–0.92; P<.0001). Guidelines continue to endorse the use of adjuvant cisplatin-based chemotherapy for stage II and IIIA NSCLC after complete resection, supported by the results of the 2 meta-analyses.[13,14]

The use of adjuvant cisplatin-based chemotherapy doublets for patients with stage I NSCLC remains controversial. Many studies and clinical practice use a 4-cm cut-point for adjuvant chemotherapy, based on subset analyses of 2 trials. When the stage IB patients in JBR.10 were divided into those with tumors at least 4 cm in size and those with smaller tumors, the OS HR was 1.73(P = .06) for the smaller tumors (<4 cm) but OS HR was 0.66 (P = .13) for the larger tumors, implying potential chemotherapy benefit.[9] The OS HR for the patients with tumors at least 4 cm in size was also 0.66 (P = .04) in a similar analysis done from CALGB9633 (further described in detail below).[15] A more recent retrospective analysis of nearly 30,000 patients from the National Cancer Database also showed improved median and 5-year survival in patients with resected T2N0M0 NSCLC who received adjuvant chemotherapy compared with those who did not. In the National Cancer Database analysis, the benefit of adjuvant chemotherapy was even seen in patients with tumor 3.1 to 3.9 cm in size.[16]

CHEMOTHERAPY CHOICE

Other controversy surrounds the use of the chemotherapeutic agent to pair with cisplatin. In the LACE meta-analysis, cisplatin/vinorelbine was associated with a substantially superior survival benefit compared with the other regimens used.[17] In a small phase II adjuvant trial, cisplatin/pemetrexed was better tolerated than cisplatin/vinorelbine, but efficacy data were inconclusive.[18] Recent data from the large adjuvant trial E1505 confirm that, given a choice, many practitioners in the United States prefer other platinum doublets. The E1505 trial found that investigators were choosing from among all 4 chemotherapy options (cisplatin/vinorelbine 25%, cisplatin/gemcitabine 19%, cisplatin/docetaxel 23%, and cisplatin/pemetrexed 33%).[19] A subset analysis found no significant differences in outcome among the 4 regimens, although cisplatin/pemetrexed resulted in less grade 3/4/5 toxicity overall compared with the others. Nevertheless, the study was not randomized for chemotherapy choice and was not powered for this subset analysis.[19] The ongoing JIPANG trial in Japan is randomly assigning patients to cisplatin/pemetrexed or cisplatin/vinorelbine and will provide prospective data to better resolve the question of whether there is a meaningful difference based on which chemotherapy doublet is used.

Limited data exist to support the substitution of carboplatin for cisplatin, yet this is done regularly in the United States, especially in the elderly. The largest clinical trial experience and only randomized data with this approach are from the CALGB-9633 trial,[15] which included 344 stage IB patients. The final analysis of the trial was negative with an OS HR of 0.83 (90% CI, 0.64–1.08; $P = .125$), although it was more of a benefit in patients with larger tumors as mentioned above. In practice, carboplatin use in the adjuvant setting should be reserved for patients who are unable to tolerate cisplatin.

Besides adjuvant cisplatin-based doublet chemotherapy, substantial evidence supports other strategies such as with oral chemotherapeutics. In Asia, particularly Japan, the combination of uracil and tegafur (a prodrug of 5-fluorouricil) has been studied extensively and is used for stage I tumors based on an OS benefit in stage I patients with tumors greater than 2 cm in size.[20,21] The ongoing JCOG-0707 trial is comparing uracil/tegafur with S-1, an oral agent composed of tegafur and gimeracil.

ELDERLY PATIENTS

Certain subsets of patients deserve mention, particularly the elderly. About a third of patients enrolled on JBR.10 were 65 years or older, and this subgroup had a significant OS benefit from adjuvant chemotherapy (HR, 0.61; 95% CI, 0.38–0.98; $P = .04$).[22] In a broader evaluation of all trials included in the LACE meta-analysis, the 414 patients (9%) who were at least 70 years old had no increase in severe toxicity rates but only a trend toward a survival benefit with adjuvant chemotherapy (HR, 0.90; 95% CI, 0.70–1.16; $P = .29$).[23] A Canadian analysis of population-based data from the Ontario cancer registry identified a significant increase in use of adjuvant chemotherapy in the elderly after 2004 to 2006, with a resultant increase in 4-year survival.[24] Of note, 70% of the elderly who received adjuvant chemotherapy in that analysis received cisplatin.

NEOADJUVANT CHEMOTHERAPY

The data in support of neoadjuvant chemotherapy are more limited, partially because larger trials examining neoadjuvant therapy were halted early when the positive adjuvant trial results were known and surgery alone control arms were no longer thought to be appropriate. One of the largest studies, Chemotherapy for Early Stages Trial, randomly assigned 270 patients with stages IB, II, and IIIA NSCLC to 3 cycles of induction chemotherapy with cisplatin and gemcitabine followed by surgery versus surgery alone.[25] Both DFS (HR, 0.70; $P = .003$) and OS (HR, 0.63; $P = .02$) were significantly in favor of the chemotherapy arm, although this benefit was limited to those patients with stage IIB/IIIA disease. The largest trial (N = 624) to directly compare neoadjuvant with adjuvant with no chemotherapy for resected early-stage lung cancer was restricted to stage IA (at least 2 cm in size), IB, II, and T3N1 disease. The Neo-adjuvant versus Adjuvant Taxol/Carbo Hope (NATCH) trial used carboplatin/paclitaxel chemotherapy and included a high percentage of stage I patients, which may explain why no significant differences were found between the 3 arms, although 5-year DFS rates favored the chemotherapy arms.[26] Therefore, a look at the meta-analyses may provide a better understanding of neoadjuvant chemotherapy. An analysis of 590 patients from 6 randomized trials published from 1990 to 2003 concluded that neoadjuvant chemotherapy led to a nonsignificant improvement in OS (HR 0.65, 95% CI, 0.41–1.04).[27] In 2010 a meta-analysis of 13 randomized trials reported an OS HR of 0.84 (95% CI, 0.77–0.92; $P = .0001$) in favor of the neoadjuvant chemotherapy.[28] The largest meta-analyses based on individual patient data are from 15 randomized studies of neoadjuvant chemotherapy (N = 2385) and reported an OS HR of

0.87 (95% CI, 0.78–0.96; $P = .007$), corresponding to a 5% absolute survival benefit at 5 years In keeping with what is seen in the adjuvant trial meta-analyses.[29]

CHEMOTHERAPY BIOMARKERS

The discovery of appropriate biomarkers for selection of patients for adjuvant chemotherapy has been challenging. Numerous prognostic gene signatures have been reported, with 1 predictive marker developed in the JBR.10 trial but not used in practice.[30] The DNA repair enzyme ERCC1 was thought to be a biomarker of cisplatin benefit on IALT,[31] but subsequent work refuted those findings and led to closure of the French intergroup TASTE trial designed on ERCC1 testing.[32] The Spanish Lung Cancer Group also attempted to better select chemotherapy based on analysis of enzymes involved in DNA repair but also failed to show a benefit with this approach.[33] The Italian ITACA trial results are awaited as the last trial investigating this approach to chemotherapy selection.[34]

MOLECULARLY TARGETED THERAPY

With the rapid increase in our knowledge about molecular drivers of NSCLC and the benefits of targeted treatment in advanced disease, the logical extension was to study the targeted agents in earlier stages of lung cancer to attempt an increase in cure rates. The most extensive experience is the epidermal growth factor receptor (EGFR) tyrosine kinase inhibitors (TKIs). Compared with first-line chemotherapy treatment, patients with advanced-stage NSCLC harboring EGFR mutations have higher response and longer progression-free survival (PFS) when treated with EGFR-targeted TKIs with randomized phase III data in that setting with gefitinib, erlotinib, and afatinib. In multiple trials for metastatic NSCLC with activating mutations in EGFR, the EGFR TKIs produce superior response and PFS compared with platinum doublet chemotherapy in treatment naïve patients.[35–43] Other than in subset analysis, however, an OS benefit has not been demonstrated, likely because of crossover. The lack of a survival benefit is an issue in the adjuvant setting, where cure is the goal.[44,45] Similar outcomes with significant response and PFS improvements with the anaplastic lymphoma kinase (ALK) inhibitor crizotinib compared with chemotherapy have been reported in patients with tumors harboring translocations of ALK.[46,47]

The idea of using targeted TKI therapy in the adjuvant therapy is not unique to lung cancer. For patients with resected early-stage HER2-positive breast cancer, the use of the HER2 antibody trastuzumab for 1 year improves OS,[48] and the use of adjuvant imatinib for patients with resected gastrointestinal stromal tumor is an established standard after trials proved this approach improves OS.[49] Results with targeted adjuvant therapy in early-stage lung cancer, however, have been more complicated.

The earliest data for adjuvant TKI therapy in resected lung cancer were retrospective analyses and nonrandomized studies. A retrospective Chinese study identified 138 patients with completely resected early-stage adenocarcinoma with EGFR-mutated disease and showed no differences in recurrence risk or survival compared with a matched cohort that differed in EGFR mutation status. The investigators also looked at the 31 patients with EGFR-mutant lung cancer who received EGFR TKI therapy compared with the 107 who did not. Those who received adjuvant EGFR TKIs had longer DFS than those who did not ($P = .033$) but no median OS difference ($P = .258$). Nevertheless, there was a longer 3-year OS in those receiving EGFR TKI (92.5% vs 81%).[50] Another large retrospective cohort of patients from Memorial Sloan Kettering Cancer Center with completely resected early stage (I–III) EGFR-mutant lung adenocarcinoma were evaluated for outcomes based on whether they received adjuvant

EGFR TKI therapy.[51] This was a nonrandomized approach in which approximately one-third of evaluated patients (n = 56) received perioperative EGFR TKI therapy. In a multivariate analysis controlling for known prognostic factors (sex, stage, type of surgery, and adjuvant platinum chemotherapy), the authors reported a 2-year DFS of 89% for patients treated with adjuvant TKI compared with 72% in those not treated with an adjuvant TKI (HR, 0.53; 95% CI, 0.28–1.03; P = .06). The OS HR was 0.62 (95% CI, 0.26–1.51; P = .296).

The largest nonrandomized prospective study, the SELECT study, investigated adjuvant erlotinib in resected early-stage (IA–IIIA) EGFR mutation–positive NSCLC patients.[52] The 100 enrolled patients received erlotinib 150 mg daily for 2 years after completion of optional adjuvant chemotherapy, and with a median follow-up of 3 years, the 2-year DFS was 90% (97% stage I, 73% stage II, and 92% stage III).

These encouraging data led to randomized trials, although many were initiated before the importance of EGFR mutations in selection of therapy was well established. NCIC CTG BR19 was a randomized, double-blind, placebo-controlled trial of 2 years of adjuvant gefitinib or placebo for completely resected NSCLC.[53] Because the patients were not selected for EGFR mutations, the subset with EGFR mutations was very small (n = 15), with no clear benefit of gefitinib shown.[53] The larger phase III, randomized RADIANT trial looked at adjuvant erlotinib for resected early-stage NSCLC patients (who could have received prior adjuvant chemotherapy) selected for EGFR expression by immunohistochemistry and fluorescence in situ hybridization but not by EGFR mutation status.[54] The study was powered for a primary endpoint of DFS in the full data set, with secondary analyses including DFS and OS in patients with del19 or L858R EGFR activating mutations. Nearly 1000 patients were enrolled, and no statistically significant differences were found in DFS or OS in the overall group. For the subset of 161 patients with activating EGFR mutations, however, the DFS did favor erlotinib (HR, 0.61; 95% CI, 0.384–0.981; P = .0391). The study was designed such that no endpoint would be considered statistically significant if the primary endpoint was negative; thus, the EGFR mutation subset results are not statistically significant. Of further concern, at the time of publication, the OS results, although not mature, did not favor the erlotinib arm in the EGFR mutation–positive subset. Thus, the use of adjuvant EGFR TKI therapy should still be restricted to clinical trial use. Multiple trials are ongoing in North America and Asia further exploring this option and looking at the use of adjuvant ALK inhibitors in patients with resected early-stage ALK-positive NSCLC (**Table 1**).

Other attempts at targeted therapy have been less promising. The Easter Cooperative Oncology Group–ACRIN E1505 trial studied the addition of adjuvant bevacizumab to chemotherapy and did not show a benefit in DFS or OS.[55] The MAGRIT trial failed to show a benefit to the addition of the MAGE-A3 vaccine.[56]

ONGOING MOLECULARLY TARGETED TRIALS

Some of the questions to be addressed in ongoing trials are:

1. Whether targeted TKI therapy leads to an OS benefit, which arguably remains the most appropriate endpoint in an adjuvant setting where cure is the goal
2. Duration of therapy
3. Whether TKIs should be used in addition to or instead of adjuvant platinum-based chemotherapy

The ALCHEMIST trial is enrolling patients with resected early-stage (IB–IIIA) NSCLC across the United States NCI National Clinical Trials Network (**Fig. 1**). Eligible patients

Table 1
Ongoing phase III adjuvant EGFR TKI trials

Trial	Stage	Selected Patients	N	Adjuvant Treatment	Treatment Duration	Primary Endpoint(a)
C-TONG 1104 NCT01405079	II–IIIA (N1-N2)	EGFR del 19 exon or L858R	220	Gefitinib vs cisplatin/vinorelbine	2 y vs 4 cycles	3-y DFS
GASTO1002 NCT01996098	IIA–IIIA	EGFR del 19 or L858R	477	Chemotherapy followed by icotinib vs observation	6 mo vs 12 mo vs none	5-y DFS
BD-IC-IV-59 NCT02125240	II–IIIA	Adenocarcinoma, del19 or L858R	300	Chemotherapy followed by icotinib vs placebo	—	2-y DFS
WJOG6401L IMPACT	II–IIIA	EGFR-mutant del19 or L858R	230	Gefitinib vs cisplatin/vinorelbine	2 y vs 4 cycles	5-y DFS
ALCHEMIST A081105	I–III	EGFR-mutant del19 or L858R	450	Erlotinib vs placebo	2 y	OS

Abbreviation: N, number of estimated enrollment.

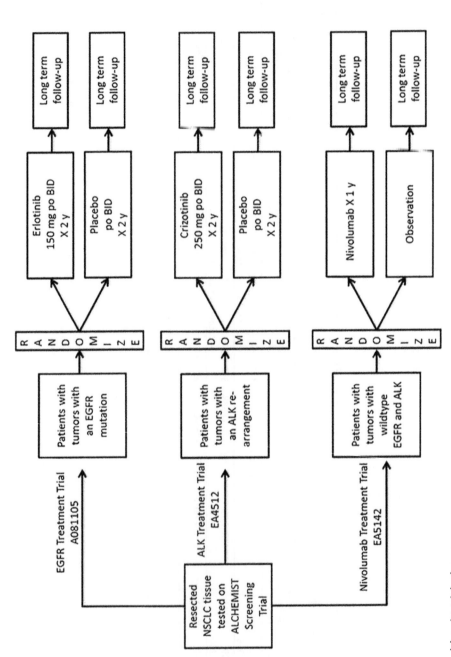

Fig. 1. US alchemist trial schema.

are screened for EGFR-activating mutations and ALK translocations, and if those are identified, patients are then entered into the appropriate substudy and randomly assigned after completion of all planned adjuvant chemotherapy or radiation therapy. Those without actionable mutations are eligible for the ANVIL substudy discussed in the immunotherapy section. The phase III EGFR trial (NCT02193282) aims to enroll 410 patients and is powered to find an OS HR of 0.67 favoring 2 years of erlotinib over placebo. The phase III ALK trial (NCT02201992) aims to 378 patients and is powered to find an OS HR of 0.67 favoring 2 years of crizotinib therapy over placebo.

In Asia, multiple trials are exploring adjuvant EGFR TKIs for patients with resected stage II to IIIA tumors with activating EGFR mutations. Both the ADJUVANT (C-TONG 1104) trial in China and IMPACT WJOG6410L in Japan are phase III trials in this setting comparing gefitinib with cisplatin/vinorelbine using DFS as the primary endpoint (see **Table 1**). Other trials are exploring variations on this theme using gefitinib or icotinib and either after or instead of adjuvant chemotherapy. In the United States, a randomized phase II study is asking the question of duration of adjuvant TKI-treated disease looking at afatinib for 3 months versus 2 years in patients with resected stage I to III EGFR-mutated NSCLC.

A study focused on duration of therapy with adjuvant EGFR TKI but without addressing the question of utility compared with no adjuvant EGFR TKI is currently ongoing in the United States at a limited number of academic sites (NCT01746251). Patients with resected stage I–III NSCLC with EGFR mutations are randomly assigned to receive afatinib for 3 months versus 2 years.

RADIATION THERAPY

Preoperative radiation therapy has no standard role for early-stage NSCLC. Postoperative radiation therapy (PORT), however, remains highly controversial but is often used in stage III NSCLC. The PORT meta-analysis, updated more than a decade ago to include a total of 10 studies,[57] showed harm with PORT for stage I or II resected NSCLC but neither benefit nor harm in the setting of N2 disease. Controversy over this modality has continued. A subset analysis from the ANITA adjuvant trial suggested that PORT was beneficial for patients with resected N2 disease and additive when given after adjuvant chemotherapy in that setting but had no benefit for earlier-stage patients.[10] Radiation use was not randomized in the trial. Further studies have included a retrospective analysis from the Surveillance, Epidemiology, and End Results (SEER) database of nearly 7500 patients and also concluded that this approach was harmful in the setting of resected stage I to II NSCLC but may be beneficial for patients with involved N2 nodes.[58] It is hoped that the controversy will be resolved with results of the ongoing Lung Adjuvant Radiotherapy Trial, a phase III trial that is randomly assigning patients with resected N2 disease to receive PORT or not (NCT00410683).

SUMMARY AND FUTURE DIRECTIONS

The use of 4 cycles of cisplatin-based adjuvant chemotherapy is now the standard of care for patients with resected stage II and IIIA NSCLC. The use in stage IB remains controversial but is often considered for larger tumors (at least 4 cm in size). Cisplatin/vinorelbine has the most extensive data in support of its use, but recent data suggest that other regimens used for metastatic NSCLC may be considered. Neoadjuvant chemotherapy lacks the same level of data as adjuvant treatment, but meta-analyses of this approach support its use. Selection of patients who are most likely to benefit from chemotherapy remains elusive. PORT is considered for many

Table 2
Ongoing PD-1/PD-L1 adjuvant trials

Drug/Trial	Description	Stages Entered		Primary Endpoint
Nivolumab ALCHEMIST/ANVIL	US NCI, observation as control	IB (4 cm) – IIIA After adjuvant chemotherapy and/or radiation	Phase 3 Allows PD-L1+ and PD-L1 -	OS/DFS
Atezolizumab Impower010	Global, placebo controlled	IB (4 cm) – IIIA After adjuvant chemotherapy	Phase 3 Restricted to PD-L1+	DFS
MEDI4736	Global, placebo controlled	IB (4 cm) – IIIA After adjuvant chemotherapy	Phase 3 Allows PD-L1+ and PD-L1 -	DFS
Pembrolizumab Keynote-091	ETOP/EORTC, placebo controlled	IB (4 cm) – IIIA After adjuvant chemotherapy	Phase 3 Allows PD-L1+ and PD-L1 -	DFS

Abbreviations: ETOP/EORTC, European Thoracic Oncology Platform/European Organisation for the Research and Treatment of Cancer; US NCI, United States National Cancer Institute.

patients with resected N2 NSCLC, but this remains controversial with the ongoing LungART trial designed to give prospective randomized data on this topic.

Areas of ongoing research include targeted tyrosine kinase inhibitor use in patients with resected NSCLC harboring an activating mutation in EGFR or translocation in ALK. Trials to date support an improvement in DFS but no OS benefit, and multiple ongoing studies seek to find the truth regarding the utility of this approach. Another area of investigation for adjuvant therapy is with the immunotherapy checkpoint agents. The PD-1 inhibitors nivolumab and pembrolizumab are approved for the second-line treatment of advanced-stage NSCLC; thus, these agents are under investigation for earlier stages of disease **(Table 2)**.[59–61] Chemotherapy has helped improve outcomes, but continued investigations with novel approaches are necessary to continue to improve cure rates for patients with resected early stage NSCLC.

REFERENCES

1. Groome PA, Bolejack V, Crowley JJ, et al. The IASLC lung cancer staging project: validation of the proposals for revision of the T, N, and M descriptors and consequent stage groupings in the forthcoming (seventh) edition of the TNM classification of malignant tumours. J Thorac Oncol 2007;2:694–705.

2. Chemotherapy in non-small cell lung cancer: a meta-analysis using updated data on individual patients from 52 randomised clinical trials. Non-small Cell Lung Cancer Collaborative Group. BMJ 1995;311:899–909.

3. Keller SM, Adak S, Wagner H, et al. A randomized trial of postoperative adjuvant therapy in patients with completely resected stage II or IIIA non-small-cell lung cancer. Eastern Cooperative Oncology Group. N Engl J Med 2000;343:1217–22.

4. Waller D, Peake MD, Stephens RJ, et al. Chemotherapy for patients with non-small cell lung cancer: the surgical setting of the big lung Trial. Eur J Cardiothorac Surg 2004;26:173–82.

5. Scagliotti GV, Fossati R, Torri V, et al. Randomized study of adjuvant chemotherapy for completely resected stage I, II, or IIIA non-small-cell Lung cancer. J Natl Cancer Inst 2003;95:1453–61.

6. Arriagada R, Bergman B, Dunant A, et al. Cisplatin-based adjuvant chemotherapy in patients with completely resected non-small-cell lung cancer. N Engl J Med 2004;350:351–60.
7. Arriagada R, Dunant A, Pignon JP, et al. Long-term results of the international adjuvant lung cancer trial evaluating adjuvant Cisplatin-based chemotherapy in resected lung cancer. J Clin Oncol 2010;28:35–42.
8. Winton T, Livingston R, Johnson D, et al. Vinorelbine plus cisplatin vs. Observation in resected non-small-cell lung cancer. N Engl J Med 2005;352:2589–97.
9. Butts CA, Ding K, Seymour L, et al. Randomized phase III trial of vinorelbine plus cisplatin compared with observation in completely resected stage IB and II non-small-cell lung cancer: updated survival analysis of JBR-10. J Clin Oncol 2010; 28:29–34.
10. Douillard JY, Rosell R, De Lena M, et al. Adjuvant vinorelbine plus cisplatin versus observation in patients with completely resected stage IB-IIIA non-small-cell lung cancer (adjuvant navelbine international trialist association [ANITA]): a randomised controlled trial. Lancet Oncol 2006;7:719–27.
11. Pignon JP, Tribodet H, Scagliotti GV, et al. Lung adjuvant cisplatin evaluation: A pooled analysis by the LACE collaborative group. J Clin Oncol 2008;26(21): 3552–9.
12. NM-aC Group, Arriagada R, Auperin A, et al. Adjuvant chemotherapy, with or without postoperative radiotherapy, in operable non-small-cell lung cancer: two meta-analyses of individual patient data. Lancet 2010;375:1267–77.
13. Ettinger DS, Bepler G, Bueno R, et al. Non-small cell lung cancer clinical practice guidelines in oncology. J Natl Compr Canc Netw 2006;4:548–82.
14. Pisters KM, Evans WK, Azzoli CG, et al. Cancer care ontario and American society of clinical oncology adjuvant chemotherapy and adjuvant radiation therapy for stages I-IIIA resectable non small-cell lung cancer guideline. J Clin Oncol 2007; 25:5506–18.
15. Strauss GM, Herndon JE 2nd, Maddaus MA, et al. Adjuvant paclitaxel plus carboplatin compared with observation in stage IB non-small-cell lung cancer: CALGB 9633 with the cancer and leukemia group B, radiation therapy oncology group, and north central cancer treatment group study groups. J Clin Oncol 2008;26:5043–51.
16. Morgensztern D, Du L, Waqar SN, et al. Adjuvant Chemotherapy for Patients with T2N0M0 Non-small-cell Lung Cancer (NSCLC). J Thorac Oncol 2016. http://dx. doi.org/10.1016/j.jtho.2016.05.022.
17. Douillard JY, Tribodet H, Aubert D, et al. Adjuvant cisplatin and vinorelbine for completely resected non-small cell lung cancer: subgroup analysis of the Lung Adjuvant Cisplatin Evaluation. J Thorac Oncol 2010;5:220–8.
18. Kreuter M, Vansteenkiste J, Fischer JR, et al. Randomized phase 2 trial on refinement of early-stage NSCLC adjuvant chemotherapy with cisplatin and pemetrexed versus cisplatin and vinorelbine: the TREAT study. Ann Oncol 2013;24:986–92.
19. Wakelee HA, Dahlberg SE, Keller SM, et al. E1505: Adjuvant chemotherapy+/-bevacizumab for early stage NSCLC: Outcomes ased on chemotherapy subsets. J Clinical Oncology Proceedings ASCO 2016 2016 [abstract: 8507].
20. Kato H, Ichinose Y, Ohta M, et al. A randomized trial of adjuvant chemotherapy with uracil-tegafur for adenocarcinoma of the lung. N Engl J Med 2004;350: 1713–21.
21. Hamada C, Tanaka F, Ohta M, et al. Meta-analysis of postoperative adjuvant chemotherapy with tegafur-uracil in non-small-cell lung cancer. J Clin Oncol 2005;23:4999–5006.

22. Pepe C, Hasan B, Winton TL, et al. Adjuvant vinorelbine and cisplatin in elderly patients: National Cancer Institute of Canada and Intergroup Study JBR.10. J Clin Oncol 2007;25:1553–61.

23. Fruh M, Rolland E, Pignon JP, et al. Pooled analysis of the effect of age on adjuvant cisplatin-based chemotherapy for completely resected non-small-cell lung cancer. J Clin Oncol 2008;26:3573–81.

24. Cuffe S, Booth CM, Peng Y, et al. Adjuvant chemotherapy for non-small-cell lung cancer in the elderly: a population-based study in Ontario, Canada. J Clin Oncol 2012;30:1813–21.

25. Scagliotti GV, Pastorino U, Vansteenkiste JF, et al. Randomized phase III study of surgery alone or surgery plus preoperative cisplatin and gemcitabine in stages IB to IIIA non-small-cell lung cancer. J Clin Oncol 2012;30:172–8.

26. Felip E, Rosell R, Maestre JA, et al. Preoperative chemotherapy plus surgery versus surgery plus adjuvant chemotherapy versus surgery alone in early-stage non-small-cell lung cancer. J Clin Oncol 2010;28:3138–45.

27. Berghmans T, Paesmans M, Meert AP, et al. Survival improvement in resectable non-small cell lung cancer with (neo)adjuvant chemotherapy: results of a meta-analysis of the literature. Lung Cancer 2005;49:13–23.

28. Song WA, Zhou NK, Wang W, et al. Survival benefit of neoadjuvant chemotherapy in non-small cell lung cancer: an updated meta-analysis of 13 randomized control trials. J Thorac Oncol 2010;5:510–6.

29. NSCLC Meta-analysis Collaborative Group. Preoperative chemotherapy for non-small-cell lung cancer: a systematic review and meta-analysis of individual participant data. Lancet 2014;383:1561–71.

30. Zhu CQ, Ding K, Strumpf D, et al. Prognostic and predictive gene signature for adjuvant chemotherapy in resected non-small-cell lung cancer. J Clin Oncol 2010;28:4417–24.

31. Olaussen KA, Dunant A, Fouret P, et al. DNA repair by ERCC1 in non-small-cell lung cancer and cisplatin-based adjuvant chemotherapy. N Engl J Med 2006; 355:983–91.

32. Friboulet L, Olaussen KA, Pignon JP, et al. ERCC1 isoform expression and DNA repair in non-small-cell lung cancer. N Engl J Med 2013;368:1101–10.

33. Massuti B, Rodriguez-Paniagua JM, Cobo Dols M, et al. Results Ph III trial customized adjuvant CT after resection of NSCLC with lymph node metastases SCAT: a Spanish lung cancer group trial. Journal of Thoracic Oncology Proceedings WCLC 2015 2015 [abstract: oral 04.05].

34. Novello S, Grohe C, Geissler M, et al. Preliminary results of the international tailored chemotherapy adjuvant trial: The ITACA trial. Journal of Thoracic Oncology Proceedings WCLC 2015 2015 [abstract: oral04.05].

35. Mok TS, Wu YL, Thongprasert S, et al. Gefitinib or carboplatin-paclitaxel in pulmonary adenocarcinoma. N Engl J Med 2009;361:947–57.

36. Fukuoka M, Wu YL, Thongprasert S, et al. Biomarker analyses and final overall survival results from a phase III, randomized, open-label, first-line study of gefitinib versus carboplatin/paclitaxel in clinically selected patients with advanced non-small-cell lung cancer in Asia (IPASS). J Clin Oncol 2011;29:2866–74.

37. Mitsudomi T, Morita S, Yatabe Y, et al. Gefitinib versus cisplatin plus docetaxel in patients with non-small-cell lung cancer harbouring mutations of the epidermal growth factor receptor (WJTOG3405): an open label, randomised phase 3 trial. Lancet Oncol 2010;11:121–8.

38. Inoue A, Kobayashi K, Maemondo M, et al. Updated overall survival results from a randomized phase III trial comparing gefitinib with carboplatin-paclitaxel for

chemo-naive non-small cell lung cancer with sensitive EGFR gene mutations (NEJ002). Ann Oncol 2013;24:54–9.

39. Zhou C, Wu YL, Chen G, et al. Erlotinib versus chemotherapy as first-line treatment for patients with advanced EGFR mutation-positive non-small-cell lung cancer (OPTIMAL, CTONG-0802): a multicentre, open-label, randomised, phase 3 study. Lancet Oncol 2011;12:735–42.

40. Rosell R, Carcereny E, Gervais R, et al. Erlotinib versus standard chemotherapy as first-line treatment for European patients with advanced EGFR mutation-positive non-small-cell lung cancer (EURTAC): a multicentre, open-label, randomised phase 3 trial. Lancet Oncol 2012;13:239–46.

41. Sequist LV, Yang JC, Yamamoto N, et al. Phase III study of afatinib or cisplatin plus pemetrexed in patients with metastatic lung adenocarcinoma with EGFR mutations. J Clin Oncol 2013;31:3327–34.

42. Yang JC, Hirsh V, Schuler M, et al. Symptom control and quality of life in LUX-Lung 3: a phase III study of afatinib or cisplatin/pemetrexed in patients with advanced lung adenocarcinoma with EGFR mutations. J Clin Oncol 2013;31: 3342–50.

43. Wu YL, Zhou C, Hu CP, et al. Afatinib versus cisplatin plus gemcitabine for first-line treatment of Asian patients with advanced non-small-cell lung cancer harbouring EGFR mutations (LUX-Lung 6): an open-label, randomised phase 3 trial. Lancet Oncol 2014;15(2):213–22.

44. Yang JC-H, Sequist LV, schuler M, et al. Overall survival (OS) in patients (pts) with advanced non-small cell lung cancer (NSCLC) harboring common (Del19/L858R) epidermal growth factor receptor mutations (EGFR mut): Pooled analysis of two large open-label phase III studies (LUX-Lung 3 [LL3] and LUX-Lung 6 [LL6]) comparing afatinib with chemotherapy (CT). J Clin Oncol 32 2014 [abstract: 8004].

45. Yang JC, Wu YL, Schuler M, et al. Afatinib versus cisplatin-based chemotherapy for EGFR mutation-positive lung adenocarcinoma (LUX-Lung 3 and LUX-Lung 6): analysis of overall survival data from two randomised, phase 3 trials. Lancet Oncol 2015;16:141–51.

46. Shaw AT, Kim DW, Nakagawa K, et al. Crizotinib versus chemotherapy in advanced ALK-positive lung cancer. N Engl J Med 2013;368:2385–94.

47. Solomon BJ, Mok T, Kim DW, et al. First-line crizotinib versus chemotherapy in ALK-positive lung cancer. N Engl J Med 2014;371:2167–77.

48. Smith I, Procter M, Gelber RD, et al. 2-year follow-up of trastuzumab after adjuvant chemotherapy in HER2-positive breast cancer: a randomised controlled trial. Lancet 2007;369:29–36.

49. Joensuu H, Eriksson M, Sundby Hall K, et al. One vs three years of adjuvant imatinib for operable gastrointestinal stromal tumor: a randomized trial. JAMA 2012; 307:1265–72.

50. Lv C, An C, Feng Q, et al. A retrospective study of stage I to IIIa lung adenocarcinoma after resection: what is the optimal adjuvant modality for patients with an EGFR mutation? Clin Lung Cancer 2015;16(6):e173–81.

51. Janjigian YY, Park BJ, Zakowski MF, et al. Impact on disease-free survival of adjuvant erlotinib or gefitinib in patients with resected lung adenocarcinomas that harbor EGFR mutations. J Thorac Oncol 2011;6:569–75.

52. Neal JW, Pennell NA, Govindan R, et al. The SELECT study: a multicenter phase II trial of adjuvant erlotinib in resected epidermal growth factor receptor (EGFR) mutation-positive non-small cell lung cancer (NSCLC). J Clin Oncol 2012;30.

53. Goss GD, O'Callaghan C, Lorimer I, et al. Gefitinib versus placebo in completely resected non-small-cell lung cancer: results of the NCIC CTG BR19 study. J Clin Oncol 2013;31:3320–6.
54. Kelly K, Altorki NK, Eberhardt WEE, et al. A randomized, double-blind phase 3 trial of adjuvant erlotinib (E) versus placebo (P) following complete tumor resection with or without adjuvant chemotherapy in patients (pts) with stage IB-IIIA EGFR positive (IHC/FISH) non-small cell lung cancer (NSCLC): RADIANT results. 2014; ASCO Annual Meeting Abstract # 7501, 2014.
55. Wakelee HA, Dahlberg SE, Keller SM, et al. Randomized phase III trial of adjuvant chemotherapy with or without bevacizumab in resected non-small cell lung cancer (NSCLC): Results of E1505. Journal of Thoracic Oncology Proceedings WCLC 2015 2015 [abstract: plen04.03].
56. Vansteenkiste JF, Cho BC, Vanakesa T, et al. Efficacy of the MAGE-A3 cancer immunotherapeutic as adjuvant therapy in patients with resected MAGE-A3-positive non-small-cell lung cancer (MAGRIT): a randomised, double-blind, placebo-controlled, phase 3 trial. Lancet Oncol 2016;17:822–35.
57. Burdett S, Stewart L. Group PM-a: Postoperative radiotherapy in non-small-cell lung cancer: update of an individual patient data meta-analysis. Lung Cancer 2005;47:81–3.
58. Lally BE, Zelterman D, Colasanto JM, et al. Postoperative radiotherapy for stage II or III non-small-cell lung cancer using the surveillance, epidemiology, and end results database. J Clin Oncol 2006;24:2998–3006.
59. Brahmer J, Reckamp KL, Baas P, et al. Nivolumab versus docetaxel in advanced squamous-cell non-small-cell lung cancer. N Engl J Med 2015;373:123–35.
60. Borghaei H, Paz-Ares L, Horn L, et al. Nivolumab versus docetaxel in advanced nonsquamous non-small-cell lung cancer. N Engl J Med 2015;373:1627–39.
61. Herbst RS, Baas P, Kim DW, et al. Pembrolizumab versus docetaxel for previously treated, PD-L1-positive, advanced non-small-cell lung cancer (KEYNOTE-010): a randomised controlled trial. Lancet 2016;387:1540–50.

Treatment of Locally Advanced Non–Small Cell Lung Cancer

 CrossMark

Kit Tam, MD[a], Megan Daly, MD[b], Karen Kelly, MD[a],*

KEYWORDS

- Non–small cell lung cancer • Chemoradiation • Locally advanced disease

KEY POINTS

- Stage III non–small cell lung cancer (NSCLC) is a heterogeneous disease.
- Concurrent chemoradiation with platinum/etoposide and carboplatin/paclitaxel is the standard of care for unresectable disease.
- 60 Gy standard fractionation remains the standard of care for radiation dose.
- Integration of novel immunotherapeutic and molecular targeted therapies is a promising area of investigation.

INTRODUCTION

Stage III NSCLC comprises the most heterogeneous group of patients and accounts for one-third of all patients diagnosed with lung cancer. Despite this heterogeneity, chemoradiation is the treatment of choice for the majority of patients. The 2-year and 5-year overall survival (OS) rates are estimated at 55% and 36%, respectively, for patients with stage IIIA disease and 34% and 19%, respectively, for patients with stage IIIB disease.[1]

PATIENT EVALUATION

To accurately classify a patient within this diverse stage, a comprehensive work-up is imperative. After a thorough history and physical examination, staging focuses on the pathologic and radiographic assessment of primary and/or nodal disease and assessment of a patient's physiologic reserve and expected tolerance to planned therapies.

Disclosures: None (K. Tam, M. Daly). Royalties: UpToDate Author; Advisor: AstraZeneca, Ariad, Boehringer Ingelheim, Clovis, Genentech, Lilly, Synta; Research: AbbVie, Celgene, EMD Serono, Genentech, Gilead, Lilly, Millennium, Novartis (K. Kelly).
[a] University of California Davis Medical Center, 4501 X Street, Suite 3016, Sacramento, CA 95817, USA; [b] University of California Davis Medical Center, 4501 X Street, Suite G-140, Sacramento, CA 95817, USA
* Corresponding author.
E-mail address: karkelly@ucdavis.edu

Hematol Oncol Clin N Am 31 (2017) 45–57
http://dx.doi.org/10.1016/j.hoc.2016.08.009

Initial imaging includes a computerized tomography (CT) of the chest to delineate local and regional disease and anatomic relationship to normal thoracic structures, whole-body positron emission tomography (PET)/CT for regional and distant staging, and a brain magnetic resonance imaging (MRI) to evaluate for intracranial metastases. Pathologic disease confirmation should be obtained from the most accessible tumor site, whether primary or nodal. Primary tumors may be accessed by CT-guided fine-needle aspiration or core biopsy, surgically via video-assisted thoracoscopic surgery, or by endobronchial ultrasound–guided fine-needle aspiration for centrally located tumors adjacent to bronchus. Nodal deposits may be accessed via endobronchial ultrasound (levels 2R/2L, 4R/4L, 7, and 10R/10L), esophageal ultrasound (levels 5, 7, 8, and 9), mediastinoscopy, mediastinotomy, or video-assisted thoracoscopic surgery.

If surgical management is being considered, comprehensive pathologic mediastinal staging is recommended (**Fig. 1**) especially because the rates of both false-positive and false-negative PET/CT interpretations for mediastinal nodes remain high. A meta-analysis of 28 studies, including 3255 patients, identified sensitivity and specificity of 0.67 and 0.87, respectively, for PET/CT in the nodal staging of NSCLC.[2] Patients with bulky, multistation mediastinal adenopathy less commonly undergo comprehensive pathologic nodal staging and are managed nonsurgically. Biopsy of

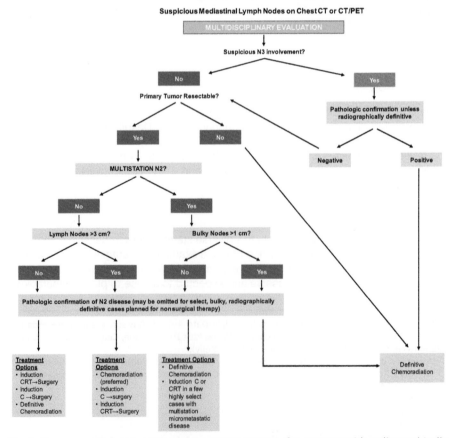

Fig. 1. Recommended evaluation and treatment strategy for patients with radiographically suspicious mediastinal nodes. C, chemotherapy; CRT, chemoradiotherapy.

radiographically borderline nodes in nonoperative patients, however, may also have an impact on radiation therapy target delineation for definitive chemoradiation.

For patients under consideration for surgical resection, assessment of performance status, pulmonary reserve, and comorbidities is crucial. Pulmonary function tests with spirometry and diffusion capacity are a standard component of a presurgical work-up and are a helpful baseline prior to nonsurgical therapy. Threshold values for resectability vary among surgeons, but an estimated postoperative forced expiratory volume in the first second of expiration or diffusing capacity of the lungs for carbon monoxide of less than 30% indicates an increased risk for complications after resection. Low-technology exercise tests, including stair climbing and shuttle walk, as well as cardio-pulmonary exercise tests, are also used to determine expected operative risk.[3]

RESECTABLE STAGE III NON–SMALL CELL LUNG CANCER

The role of surgery in the treatment of stage III NSCLC remains controversial. A small body of evidence suggests that a subset of patients with pathologic N2 disease may benefit from surgery after induction chemoradiotherapy or chemotherapy. The most persuasive data come from a subset analysis of the North America Intergroup trial (INT0139; Radiation Therapy Oncology Group [RTOG] 9039)[4]; 429 patients were randomized to receive 2 cycles of cisplatin/etoposide (PE) concurrently with 45 Gy radiation followed by surgery or continued radiation to 61 Gy. There was no survival difference between the 2 arms but a subset analysis by the extent of surgery showed a significant survival advantage for patients undergoing lobectomy, with a median survival (MS) of 34 months after lobectomy versus 22 months for the nonsurgical arm ($P = .002$) and a 5-year OS of 36% versus 18%, respectively. Patients undergoing pneumonectomy had a nonsignificant but numerically worse outcome, with an MS of 19 months with surgery compared with 29 months without surgery and 5-year OS rates of 22% versus 24%, respectively. A higher than expected perioperative mortality in the pneumonectomy arm of 26% contributed to these results. In addition to the extent of surgical resection, retrospective analyses show that the number and size of involved nodes and nodal response to induction are important factors. Lymph node(s) greater than or equal to 1 cm on CT (clinical N2 disease), multistation involvement, or nodes greater than 3 cm portend survival decrements,[5] and mediastinal tumor clearance with induction therapy is associated with prolonged survival.[4,6,7] In INT0139, patients who cleared their mediastinal disease (N0) had an MS of 34.4 months compared with 26.4 months for patients with N1–N3 or unknown N status.[4] Based on these data, it is recommended that patients undergo repeat pathologic evaluation of the mediastinum prior to definitive surgery; if disease is found, the resection should be aborted and the patient should receive or complete definitive chemoradiation.

The optimal induction regimen is unknown. A randomized phase III trial conducted by the Swiss Group for Clinical Cancer Research evaluated induction docetaxel and cisplatin versus docetaxel plus cisplatin followed by radiotherapy in resectable pathologically proved stage III N2 disease.[8] There was no difference in event-free survival between the arms, suggesting chemotherapy alone was sufficient prior to resection. The trial had several limitations, however, including its small sample size, 11 years of accrual, sequential radiotherapy design, and lack of an OS endpoint. Several attempts to conduct randomized trials comparing the 2 approaches have failed due to poor accrual. Current guidelines allow for chemotherapy alone or chemoradiation as the induction regimen. For patients treated without neoadjuvant radiotherapy, adjuvant postoperative radiotherapy (PORT) may be considered after surgical management of N2 disease. A large meta-analysis, including 2128 patients from

9 randomized trials, identified a survival decrement to the use of PORT for N0–N1 patients with no apparent survival impact for N2 disease, although many of the analyzed trials used outdated radiation techniques, including cobalt.[9] Subsequent population-based studies using modern radiation techniques have suggested a small OS benefit to the use of PORT for N2 disease.[10,11] It is anticipated that the currently accruing Lung Adjuvant Radiotherapy Trial trial in Europe, in which resected N2 patients are randomized between PORT and no PORT, should provide a definitive answer to this question. All patients should be discussed at a multidisciplinary tumor board and a tailored treatment plan devised.

UNRESECTABLE STAGE III NON–SMALL CELL LUNG CANCER

A majority of patients with stage III disease are unresectable. Radiation as monotherapy cures fewer than 10% of patients.[12] Multiple studies show that patients with unresectable disease may achieve long-term survival when radiation therapy is combined with chemotherapy (**Table 1**). The landmark study performed by Dillman and colleagues[13] demonstrated a 4-month improvement in MS and a doubling of long-term survivors after induction chemotherapy with cisplatin and vinblastine followed by thoracic radiation compared with radiation therapy alone. RTOG and the Eastern Cooperative Oncology Group conducted a confirmatory trial that favored the combination arm. The results were also corroborated by a French multicenter randomized study.[14] Based on the positive results from these 3 trials, the addition of chemotherapy to radiotherapy became the standard of care for the management of locally advanced NSCLC.

Timing of Chemotherapy and Radiotherapy

The next set of studies investigated timing of chemotherapy and radiation (**Table 2**). The West Japan Thoracic Oncology Group was the first to demonstrate that concurrent compared with sequential chemoradiation significantly improved response rate and survival.[15] Confirmatory trials performed by cooperative groups in France,[16] the Czech Republic,[18] and the United States (RTOG 9410),[19] also showed a survival

Table 1						
Phase III trials comparing induction chemotherapy followed by radiation therapy versus radiation therapy alone						
Author, Reference	N	Treatment	Median Survival (mo)	2 y Overall Survival (%)	5 y Overall Survival (%)	P Value
Dillman et al,[13] 1990	78	Cisplatin-vinblastine + radiation therapy	13.8	26	19	P = .0066
	77	RT alone	9.7	13	7	
Sause et al,[14] 2000	149	Cisplatin-vinblastine + radiation therapy	13.2	32	8	P = .04
	152	RT alone	11.4	21	5	
Le Chevalier et al,[17] 1994	176	Cisplatin-vindesine-cyclophosphamide-lomustine + radiation therapy	12	21	11[a]	P = .08
	177	Radiation therapy alone	10	14	5[a]	

[a] 3-Year data.

Table 2
Phase III trials comparing concurrent versus sequential chemoradiation

Author, Reference	N	Treatment	OR (%)	Median Survival (mo)	2 y Overall Survival (%)	5 y Overall Survival (%)	P Value
Furuse et al,[15] 1999	156	Concurrent	84	16.5	34.6	15.8	P = .03998
	158	Sequential	66.4	13.3	27.4	8.9	
Fournel et al,[16] 2005	100	Concurrent	49	16.3	39	21[b]	P = .24
	101	Sequential	54	14.5	26	14[b]	
Zatloukal et al,[18] 2004	52	Concurrent	80	16.6	34.2	18.6[a]	P = .023
	50	Sequential	47	12.9	14.3	9.5[a]	
Curran et al,[19] 2011	193	Concurrent	70	17	—	16	P = .46
	195	Sequential	61	14.6	—	10	

Abbreviation: OR, overal response.
[a] 3-Year data.
[b] 4-Year data.

benefit for the concurrent approach. A meta-analysis of concurrent versus sequential chemoradiation data from 6 randomized trials involving 1205 patients with median follow-up of 6 years demonstrated a significant survival benefit for concurrent chemoradiation (hazard ratio 0.84; 95% CI, 0.74–0.95; $P = .004$), with an absolute benefit of 5.7% at 3 years and 4.5% at 5 years.[20] Based on these results, concurrent therapy is considered standard for good-performance status patients. Sequential chemoradiation remains an option for patients with a marginal performance status, and poor-performance patients are typically treated with radiation alone.

Selection of Chemotherapy Regimen

All cytotoxic chemotherapy agents used to treat metastatic lung cancer exhibit radiosensitizing properties. Based on a small study evaluating PE with concurrent radiation that demonstrated a doubling of survival compared with historical data and the encouraging results with this combination in a Southwest Oncology Group (SWOG) trial in limited-stage small cell lung cancer,[21,22] PE was chosen for subsequent phase III studies. Trials evaluating second-generation agents (taxanes, vinorelbine, gemcitabine, and irinotecan) in combination with cisplatin or carboplatin concurrently with radiation[23–25] were also conducted. Weekly paclitaxel and carboplatin emerged as a well-tolerated and efficacious regimen. The most recent phase III randomized trial evaluating the modern regimen pemetrexed and cisplatin followed by pemetrexed consolidation versus standard chemoradiotherapy with PE in patients with nonsquamous histology was stopped early for futility (**Table 3**)[26] after randomization and treatment of 555 patients. OS for the pemetrexed and cisplatin arm was found not superior to the PE arm. As a result of these studies, concurrent weekly paclitaxel and carboplatin or cyclic PE remain the most commonly administered regimens.

Role of Induction, Consolidation, and Maintenance Systemic Therapy

Despite improvements in both MS and OS using concurrent chemoradiation, efforts to improve the still high rates of distant failure using induction or consolidation chemotherapy were undertaken (**Table 4**). The Cancer and Leukemia Group B 39801 randomized patients to chemoradiation alone with weekly carboplatin and paclitaxel or 2 cycles of induction carboplatin and paclitaxel followed by the identical chemoradiotherapy.[27] The results failed to show a benefit for induction chemotherapy. An induction approach is, however, a plausible strategy to evaluate in patients whose tumors

Table 3
Phase III trials of integration of newer cytotoxic and targeted agents into chemoradiotherapy

Trial, Reference	N	Treatment	Median Survival (mo)	95% CI	2 y Overall Survival (%)	3 y Overall Survival (%)	P Value
RTOG 0617[34]	217	Standard-dose radiation therapy (60 Gy)	28.7	24.1–36.9	57.6	—	P = .04
	207	High-dose radiation therapy (74 Gy)	20.3	17.7–25	44.6	—	
	237	With cetuximab	25	20.2–30.5	52.3	—	P = .29
	228	No cetuximab	24	19.8–28.6	50.1	—	
PROCLAIM[25]	301	Concurrent chemoradiation with pemetrexed-cisplatin followed by consolidation pemetrexed	26.8	0.79–1.2	52	40	P = .831
	297	Concurrent chemoradiation with PE followed by consolidation chemotherapy	25	—	52	37	

have an epidermal growth factor receptor (EGFR) sensitizing mutation or an anaplastic lymphoma kinase (ALK) fusion given the exceptional efficacy of tyrosine kinase inhibitors in stage IV disease. The RTOG 1306 is an ongoing randomized phase II trial of induction erlotinib or crizotinib for 12 weeks followed by standard treatment using weekly paclitaxel/carboplatin or cyclic PE with radiation versus standard treatment alone.

Table 4
Phase III trials comparing induction, consolidation, and maintenance therapies to concurrent chemoradiation alone

Author/Trial	N	Treatment	Median Survival (mo)	95% CI	2 y Overall Survival (%)	3 y Overall Survival (%)	P Value
CALGB 39801 (induction)	184	Induction followed by concurrent chemoradiation	14	11–16	31	23	P = .3
	182	Concurrent chemoradiation	12	10–16	29	19	
Hanna (consolidation)	73	Concurrent chemoradiation followed by 3 cycles of docetaxel	21.2	—	—	27.1	P = .883
	74	Observation	23.2	—	—	26.1	
S0023 (maintenance)	118	Gefitinib	23	17–29	46	—	P = .013
	125	Placebo	35	25–40	59	—	
START (maintenance)	829	Tecemotide	25.6	22.5–29.2	51	40	P = .123
	410	Placebo	22.3	19.6–25.5	46	37	

The role of consolidation therapy was initially studied by SWOG. They reported an impressive 26-month MS and 3-year OS of 37% in 83 patients with stage IIIB disease after standard PE with radiation therapy followed by 3 cycles of docetaxel.[28] A randomized phase III trial, however, by the Hoosier Oncology Group and US Oncology Network using the identical SWOG regimen did not demonstrate a survival advantage for consolidation docetaxel.[29] Although there is no evidence to support consolidation chemotherapy, most physicians consider consolidation therapy if weekly radiosensitizing paclitaxel/carboplatin is used to address potential micrometastatic disease.

Building on the docetaxel consolidation backbone, SWOG undertook an evaluation of maintenance gefitinib. The S0023 trial randomized patients to gefitinib or placebo after concurrent chemoradiation with PE followed by docetaxel. Patients treated with gefitinib had inferior survival that remains unexplained but was not due to toxicity.[30] Another randomized study, the START (Stimulating Targeted Antigenic Response to NSCLC trial, evaluated tecemotide, a MUC1 antigen-specific immunotherapy that induces a T-cell response to MUC1, a commonly overexpressed antigen on lung cancer cells. Patients were randomized to maintenance tecemotide after concurrent or sequential chemoradiation. OS was similar in the 2 arms.[31]

Radiation Dose and Fractionation

Multiple early phase I and II nonrandomized trials suggested safety and efficacy of radiation dose escalation with thoracic radiation as monotherapy for NSCLC.[32] RTOG 0117 was designed to determine the maximum tolerated radiation dose in the setting of concurrent chemotherapy.[33] A maximum tolerated dose of 74 Gy in 37 fractions was identified using 3-D conformal radiation therapy (3DCRT) with concurrent paclitaxel and carboplatin. This dose was found well tolerated with a low rate of acute and late toxicities.

This dose fractionation schedule was then tested in a phase III randomized comparison with 60 Gy in 30 fractions with concurrent carboplatin and paclitaxel, RTOG 0617 (see **Table 3**). After the phase II study RTOG 0324 identified an impressive median OS of 22.7 months with the addition of cetuximab,[34] RTOG 0617 was modified to 2 × 2 factorial design to also evaluate the addition of cetuximab to chemoradiation. An interim analysis did not reveal benefit to high-dose radiation therapy (74 Gy) and the high-dose arms were closed. The randomization to cetuximab arms continued to completion and found similar OS with or without cetuximab. Further analysis of the radiation dose comparison suggested potential harm from 74 Gy.[35] In light of these results, 60 Gy in standard fractionation remains the standard-of-care dose for the treatment of locally advanced NSCLC with concurrent chemotherapy.

Radiation Techniques

Radiotherapy techniques for locally advanced lung cancer have markedly evolved over the past 2 decades. Historically, 2-D radiation therapy was used to treat locally advanced NSCLC, using simple field arrangements based on bony anatomic landmarks on plain films. CT-based simulation has gradually replaced 2-D radiation therapy planning, allowing accurate target delineation on axial CT slices and use of 3DCRT planning with multiple conformal beams shaped to the target volume. 4-D CT, a technique in which images are acquired at each table position for a full respiratory cycle, has been widely implemented to allow accurate assessment of respiratory tumor motion. Target delineation is also enhanced by the routine use of PET/CT staging. With improved imaging, there has been a reduction in the use of elective nodal irradiation in recent years, and retrospective and population-based studies do not suggest an excess of isolated regional failures with this approach.[36,37]

Planning techniques have transitioned from 2-D to 3-D, with more recent implementation of intensity-modulated radiotherapy (IMRT). IMRT uses inverse planning with modulated beams to conformally sculpt dose around irregular target volumes (**Fig. 2**). Planning studies suggest the potential for IMRT to reduce dose to critical structures, including heart, lung, and spinal cord.[38] Clinical data supporting its routine use for locally advanced NSCLC, however, are limited. Several retrospective studies suggest reduced rates of pneumonitis after treatment with IMRT.[39,40] A nonrandomized, exploratory analysis from RTOG 0617 identified significantly less decline in patient-reported quality of life after treatment with IMRT compared with 3DCRT up to 1 year after completion of treatment.[41] Several population-based studies have failed, however, to demonstrate a clear survival or toxicity benefit to IMRT for the treatment of NSCLC.[42–44] There are no completed, prospective randomized trials comparing IMRT to 3DCRT for any thoracic malignancy.

TREATMENT COMPLICATIONS

Although it is difficult to isolate the side effects from each component, chemotherapy is typically associated with cytopenias and nausea and vomiting. Radiation is associated with esophagitis, cough, pneumonitis, fatigue, dermatitis, and myelosuppression. Late toxicities from radiation include chronic lung fibrosis, esophageal strictures, cardiac toxicity, brachial plexopathy, and rarely radiation-induced myelopathy

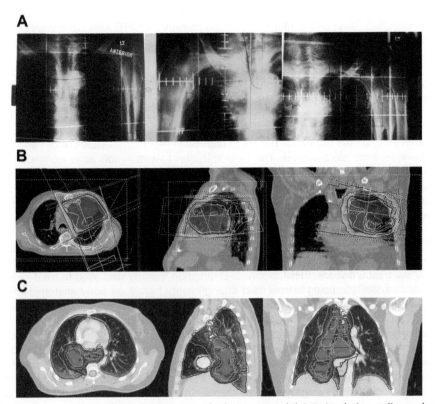

Fig. 2. The evolution of radiation planning for lung cancer. (*A*) 2-D simulation radiographs. (*B*) 3DCRT conformal plan using CT with 3 fields. (*C*) IMRT plan.

of the spinal cord. Overall both regimens are safe and tolerable. Chemotherapy side effects can be managed with dose reductions, dose delays, and supportive care measures. Granulocyte stimulating factors are a contraindication with concurrent therapy.

Esophagitis is typically the most prominent acute side effect observed with thoracic radiotherapy. Management is symptom directed, including antacids; topical anesthetics, such as viscous lidocaine; and narcotic and non-narcotic pain medications. Radiation pneumonitis is a common and potentially fatal subacute complication that manifests with shortness of breath, cough, and low-grade fevers. Risk factors include volume of lung receiving greater than or equal to 20 Gy (V20), the volume of lung receiving 5 Gy (V5), mean lung dose,[45,46] the use of carboplatin/paclitaxel chemotherapy, and increasing age.[47] Symptomatic radiation pneumonitis is managed with oral prednisone over a slow taper of 4 to 8 weeks, with supplemental oxygen as necessary. Historically, limited attention was given to cardiac dosimetry during treatment because cardiac complications were believed to predominantly manifest years to decades after treatment. A secondary analysis of RTOG 0617 identified the volume of the heart receiving 5 Gy (V5) and 30 Gy (V30) as major predictors of mortality.[35] These results suggest cardiac dosimetry should be a significant consideration in the treatment planning process.

SURVEILLANCE

Unfortunately, a majority of patients develop distant metastases, local recurrence, or both. The current National Comprehensive Cancer Network guidelines recommend a history and physical examination and chest CT every 6 to 12 months for 2 years followed by a low-dose CT annually thereafter, noting that patients with residual imaging abnormalities after treatment may require more frequent imaging. National Comprehensive Cancer Network guidelines suggest PET/CT or brain MRI is not warranted, although PET/CT may be useful to differentiate radiation fibrosis or consolidation from malignancy identified on CT. Localized recurrences are occasionally amenable to definitive intent reirradiation, but long-term disease control is rare.[48] Whether earlier detection of local failure would increase cure rates remains speculative. Distant metastases are treated with the appropriate systemic regimen.

SUMMARY

Stage III NSCLC is the most challenging stage of lung cancer to treat due to its heterogeneous makeup. Additional factors, such as comorbidities, cardiopulmonary reserve, and performance status, add to this complexity. It is essential that stage III patients undergo multidisciplinary evaluation and treatment planning to ensure optimal therapy is selected for each patient.

Although there have not been therapeutic advances in the treatment of stage III NSCLC in recent years, there is a renewed optimism for near-term advances based on exciting new therapies to treat metastatic disease and in radiation planning and delivery. Thus, the continued evaluation of integrating novel systemic agents and defining optimal radiation doses and schedules remain the backbone of research efforts. The proved benefit of immunotherapy in stage IV lung cancer warrants evaluation in earlier stages of lung cancer. The PACIFIC study is a randomized phase III, double-blinded, international trial to evaluate the efficacy and safety of durvalumab, an antiprogrammed death ligand 1 antibody in patients with unresectable stage III NSCLC who have not progressed after definitive, platinum-based, concurrent chemoradiation. It is likely that immune checkpoint inhibitors are the first of many novel immune agents that will be evaluated in the coming years. Another interesting class of agents being examined is DNA repair inhibitors. SWOG is conducting a phase I/II trial evaluating the addition of the poly-ADP-ribose polymerase inhibitor veliparib to concurrent chemoradiation as a potential chemosensitizer and radiosensitizer. In addition, the discovery of predictive biomarkers and imaging tools that would allow tailoring therapy is being pursued.

Despite the disappointing results from RTOG 0617, there remains substantial interest in dose escalation for locally advanced NSCLC, given the high rates of locoregional failure and associated symptom burden. Hypofractionation, the delivery of larger than the conventional 2 Gy daily fractions to achieve a higher biologic effective dose, is one area of particular interest. The currently accruing RTOG 1106 uses modest hypofractionation with 2.2 Gy fractions over the first 21 fractions, coupled with midtreatment target volume reduction and adaptive replanning, followed by a hypofractionated boost dose individualized based on normal tissue dose-volume metrics. In aggregate, current prospective trials seek to bring systemic advances realized for metastatic disease to patients with locally advanced NSCLC and to personalize local therapy based on patient and tumor-specific metrics.

REFERENCES

1. Goldstraw P, Chansky K, Crowley J, et al. The IASLC Lung Cancer Staging Project: proposals for revision of the TNM stage groupings in the forthcoming (Eighth) edition of the TNM classification for lung cancer. J Thorac Oncol 2016;11(1): 39–51.
2. Pak K, Park S, Cheon GJ, et al. Update on nodal staging in non-small cell lung cancer with integrated positron emission tomography/computed tomography: a meta-analysis. Ann Nucl Med 2015;29(5):409–19.
3. Brunelli A, Kim AW, Berger KI, et al. Physiologic evaluation of the patient with lung cancer being considered for resectional surgery: diagnosis and management of lung cancer, 3rd ed: American College of Chest Physicians evidence-based clinical practice guidelines. Chest 2013;143(5 Suppl):e166S–90S.
4. Albain KS, Swann RS, Rusch VW, et al. Radiotherapy plus chemotherapy with or without surgical resection for stage III non-small-cell lung cancer: a phase III randomised controlled trial. Lancet 2009;374(9687):379–86.
5. Andre F, Grunenwald D, Pignon JP, et al. Survival of patients with resected N2 non-small-cell lung cancer: evidence for a subclassification and implications. J Clin Oncol 2000;18(16):2981–9.
6. Decaluwe H, De Leyn P, Vansteenkiste J, et al. Surgical multimodality treatment for baseline resectable stage IIIA-N2 non-small cell lung cancer. Degree of mediastinal lymph node involvement and impact on survival. Eur J Cardiothorac Surg 2009;36(3):433–9.
7. Suntharalingam M, Paulus R, Edelman MJ, et al. Radiation therapy oncology group protocol 02-29: a phase II trial of neoadjuvant therapy with concurrent chemotherapy and full-dose radiation therapy followed by surgical resection and consolidative therapy for locally advanced non-small cell carcinoma of the lung. Int J Radiat Oncol Biol Phys 2012;84(2):456–63.
8. Pless M, Stupp R, Ris HB, et al. Induction chemoradiation in stage IIIA/N2 non-small-cell lung cancer: a phase 3 randomised trial. Lancet 2015;386(9998): 1049–56.
9. Postoperative radiotherapy in non-small-cell lung cancer: systematic review and meta-analysis of individual patient data from nine randomised controlled trials. PORT Meta-analysis Trialists Group. Lancet 1998;352(9124):257–63.

10. Lally BE, Detterbeck FC, Geiger AM, et al. The risk of death from heart disease in patients with nonsmall cell lung cancer who receive postoperative radiotherapy: analysis of the surveillance, epidemiology, and end results database. Cancer 2007;110(4):911–7.

11. Corso CD, Rutter CE, Wilson LD, et al. Re-evaluation of the role of postoperative radiotherapy and the impact of radiation dose for non-small-cell lung cancer using the National Cancer Database. J Thorac Oncol 2015;10(1):148–55.

12. Perez CA, Pajak TF, Rubin P, et al. Long-term observations of the patterns of failure in patients with unresectable non-oat cell carcinoma of the lung treated with definitive radiotherapy. Report by the Radiation Therapy Oncology Group. Cancer 1987;59(11):1874–81.

13. Dillman RO, Seagren SL, Propert KJ, et al. A randomized trial of induction chemotherapy plus high-dose radiation versus radiation alone in stage III non-small-cell lung cancer. N Engl J Med 1990;323(14):940–5.

14. Sause W, Kolesar P, Taylor S IV, et al. Final results of phase III trial in regionally advanced unresectable non-small cell lung cancer: Radiation Therapy Oncology Group, Eastern Cooperative Oncology Group, and Southwest Oncology Group. Chest 2000;117(2):358–64.

15. Furuse K, Fukuoka M, Kawahara M, et al. Phase III study of concurrent versus sequential thoracic radiotherapy in combination with mitomycin, vindesine, and cisplatin in unresectable stage III non-small-cell lung cancer. J Clin Oncol 1999;17(9):2692–9.

16. Fournel P, Robinet G, Thomas P, et al. Randomized phase III trial of sequential chemoradiotherapy compared with concurrent chemoradiotherapy in locally advanced non-small-cell lung cancer: Groupe Lyon-Saint-Etienne d'Oncologie Thoracique-Groupe Francais de Pneumo-Cancerologie NPC 95-01 Study. J Clin Oncol 2005;23(25):5910–7.

17. Le Chevalier T, Arriagada R, Quoix E. Radiotherapy alone versus combined chemotherapy and radiotherapy in unresectable non-small cell lung carcinoma. Lung Cancer 1994;10(Suppl 1):S239–44.

18. Zatloukal P, Petruzelka L, Zemanova M, et al. Concurrent versus sequential chemoradiotherapy with cisplatin and vinorelbine in locally advanced non-small cell lung cancer: a randomized study. Lung Cancer 2004;46(1):87–98.

19. Curran WJ Jr, Paulus R, Langer CJ, et al. Sequential vs. concurrent chemoradiation for stage III non-small cell lung cancer: randomized phase III trial RTOG 9410. J Natl Cancer Inst 2011;103(19):1452–60.

20. Auperin A, Le Péchoux C, Rolland E, et al. Meta-analysis of concomitant versus sequential radiochemotherapy in locally advanced non-small-cell lung cancer. J Clin Oncol 2010;28(13):2181–90.

21. Friess GG, Baikadi M, Harvey WH. Concurrent cisplatin and etoposide with radiotherapy in locally advanced non-small cell lung cancer. Cancer Treat Rep 1987; 71(7–8):681–4.

22. McCracken JD, Janaki LM, Crowley JJ, et al. Concurrent chemotherapy/radiotherapy for limited small-cell lung carcinoma: a Southwest Oncology Group Study. J Clin Oncol 1990;8(5):892–8.

23. Yamamoto N, Nakagawa K, Nishimura Y, et al. Phase III study comparing second- and third-generation regimens with concurrent thoracic radiotherapy in patients with unresectable stage III non-small-cell lung cancer: West Japan Thoracic Oncology Group WJTOG0105. J Clin Oncol 2010;28(23):3739–45.

24. Belani CP, Choy H, Bonomi P, et al. Combined chemoradiotherapy regimens of paclitaxel and carboplatin for locally advanced non-small-cell lung cancer: a

randomized phase II locally advanced multi-modality protocol. J Clin Oncol 2005; 23(25):5883–91.

25. Vokes EE, Perry MC, Kindler HL, et al. The cancer and leukemia group B respiratory committee. Clin Cancer Res 2006;12(11 Pt 2):3581s–8s.

26. Senan S, Brade A, Wang LH, et al. PROCLAIM: randomized phase III trial of pemetrexed-cisplatin or etoposide-cisplatin plus thoracic radiation therapy followed by consolidation chemotherapy in locally advanced nonsquamous non-small-cell lung cancer. J Clin Oncol 2016;34(9):953–62.

27. Vokes EE, Herndon JE 2nd, Kelley MJ, et al. Induction chemotherapy followed by chemoradiotherapy compared with chemoradiotherapy alone for regionally advanced unresectable stage III non-small-cell lung cancer: Cancer and Leukemia Group B. J Clin Oncol 2007;25(13):1698–704.

28. Gandara DR, Chansky K, Albain KS, et al. Consolidation docetaxel after concurrent chemoradiotherapy in stage IIIB non-small-cell lung cancer: phase II Southwest Oncology Group Study S9504. J Clin Oncol 2003;21(10):2004–10.

29. Hanna N, Neubauer M, Yiannoutsos C, et al. Phase III study of cisplatin, etoposide, and concurrent chest radiation with or without consolidation docetaxel in patients with inoperable stage III non-small-cell lung cancer: the Hoosier Oncology Group and U.S. Oncology. J Clin Oncol 2008;26(35):5755–60.

30. Kelly K, Chansky K, Gaspar LE, et al. Phase III trial of maintenance gefitinib or placebo after concurrent chemoradiotherapy and docetaxel consolidation in inoperable stage III non-small-cell lung cancer: SWOG S0023. J Clin Oncol 2008;26(15):2450–6.

31. Butts C, Socinski MA, Mitchell PL, et al. Tecemotide (L-BLP25) versus placebo after chemoradiotherapy for stage III non-small-cell lung cancer (START): a randomised, double-blind, phase 3 trial. Lancet Oncol 2014;15(1):59–68.

32. Cox JD, Azarnia N, Byhardt RW, et al. A randomized phase I/II trial of hyperfractionated radiation therapy with total doses of 60.0 Gy to 79.2 Gy: possible survival benefit with greater than or equal to 69.6 Gy in favorable patients with Radiation Therapy Oncology Group stage III non-small-cell lung carcinoma: report of Radiation Therapy Oncology Group 83-11. J Clin Oncol 1990;8(9):1543–55.

33. Bradley JD, Moughan J, Graham MV, et al. A phase I/II radiation dose escalation study with concurrent chemotherapy for patients with inoperable stages I to III non-small-cell lung cancer: phase I results of RTOG 0117. Int J Radiat Oncol Biol Phys 2010;77(2):367–72.

34. Blumenschein GR Jr, Paulus R, Curran WJ, et al. Phase II study of cetuximab in combination with chemoradiation in patients with stage IIIA/B non-small-cell lung cancer: RTOG 0324. J Clin Oncol 2011;29(17):2312–8.

35. Bradley JD, Paulus R, Komaki R, et al. Standard-dose versus high-dose conformal radiotherapy with concurrent and consolidation carboplatin plus paclitaxel with or without cetuximab for patients with stage IIIA or IIIB non-small-cell lung cancer (RTOG 0617): a randomised, two-by-two factorial phase 3 study. Lancet Oncol 2015;16(2):187–99.

36. Fernandes AT, Shen J, Finlay J, et al. Elective nodal irradiation (ENI) vs. involved field radiotherapy (IFRT) for locally advanced non-small cell lung cancer (NSCLC): a comparative analysis of toxicities and clinical outcomes. Radiother Oncol 2010;95(2):178–84.

37. Sulman EP, Komaki R, Klopp AH, et al. Exclusion of elective nodal irradiation is associated with minimal elective nodal failure in non-small cell lung cancer. Radiat Oncol 2009;4:5.

38. Grills IS, Yan D, Martinez AA, et al. Potential for reduced toxicity and dose esca-lation in the treatment of inoperable non-small-cell lung cancer: a comparison of intensity-modulated radiation therapy (IMRT), 3D conformal radiation, and elec-tive nodal irradiation. Int J Radiat Oncol Biol Phys 2003;57(3):875–90.
39. Ling DC, Hess CB, Chen AM, et al. Comparison of toxicity between intensity-modulated radiotherapy and 3-dimensional conformal radiotherapy for locally advanced non-small-cell lung cancer. Clin Lung Cancer 2016;17(1):18–23.
40. Yom SS, Liao Z, Liu HH, et al. Initial evaluation of treatment-related pneumonitis in advanced-stage non-small-cell lung cancer patients treated with concurrent chemotherapy and intensity-modulated radiotherapy. Int J Radiat Oncol Biol Phys 2007;68(1):94–102.
41. Movsas B, Hu C, Sloan J, et al. Quality of life analysis of a radiation dose-escalation study of patients with non-small-cell lung cancer: a secondary analysis of the radiation therapy oncology group 0617 randomized clinical trial. JAMA On-col 2016;2(3):359–67.
42. Chen AB, Li L, Cronin A, et al. Comparative effectiveness of intensity-modulated versus 3D conformal radiation therapy among medicare patients with stage III lung cancer. J Thorac Oncol 2014;9(12):1788–95.
43. Harris JP, Murphy JD, Hanlon AL, et al. A population-based comparative effec-tiveness study of radiation therapy techniques in stage III non-small cell lung can-cer. Int J Radiat Oncol Biol Phys 2014;88(4):872–84.
44. Shirvani SM, Jiang J, Gomez DR, et al. Intensity modulated radiotherapy for stage III non-small cell lung cancer in the United States: predictors of use and associ-ation with toxicities. Lung Cancer 2013;82(2):252–9.
45. Dang J, Li G, Ma L, et al. Predictors of grade $>/=$ 2 and grade $>/=$ 3 radiation pneumonitis in patients with locally advanced non-small cell lung cancer treated with three-dimensional conformal radiotherapy. Acta Oncol 2013;52(6):1175–80.
46. Khalil AA, Hoffmann L, Moeller DS, et al. New dose constraint reduces radiation-induced fatal pneumonitis in locally advanced non-small cell lung cancer patients treated with intensity-modulated radiotherapy. Acta Oncol 2015;54(9):1343–9.
47. Palma DA, Senan S, Tsujino K, et al. Predicting radiation pneumonitis after che-moradiation therapy for lung cancer: an international individual patient data meta-analysis. Int J Radiat Oncol Biol Phys 2013;85(2):444–50.
48. Drodge CS, Ghosh S, Fairchild A. Thoracic reirradiation for lung cancer: a litera-ture review and practical guide. Ann Palliat Med 2014;3(2):75–91.

First-Line Systemic Therapy for Non–Small Cell Lung Cancer

Rebecca S. Heist, MD, MPH

KEYWORDS

- Non–small cell lung cancer • Systemic therapy • First-line

KEY POINTS

- Platinum-based combination is the cornerstone of first-line systemic therapy.
- Emerging data suggest that immunotherapy with PD-1 inhibition has a role in first line treatment in selected patients.
- Addition of agents, such as bevacizumab or necitumumab, has benefit in selected populations.
- Switch maintenance and continuation maintenance therapies have shown benefit after completion of platinum combination therapy.

INTRODUCTION

Lung cancer remains the leading cause of cancer-related death in the United States.[1] Although recent advances in screening for lung cancer facilitate early detection and improve survival, currently most lung cancers are detected in advanced stages. For patients with metastatic disease, systemic therapy is the cornerstone of treatment. Many advances have been made in the first-line systemic treatment of non–small cell lung cancer (NSCLC), and current treatment approaches are markedly different from what they were several years ago.

PATIENT EVALUATION OVERVIEW

Evaluation of a patient with metastatic NSCLC includes patient-centered and cancer-centered factors. Optimal management requires knowledge of a patient's medical history, comorbidities, and performance status (PS), and the histologic and molecular subtype of the cancer itself. In terms of patient-centered factors, the patient's PS is a critical component to deciding on how well they will tolerate systemic therapy. Medical issues including cardiovascular history, diabetes, and other significant medical

Department of Thoracic Oncology, Massachusetts General Hospital, 32 Fruit Street, Yawkey 7B, Boston, MA 02114, USA
E-mail address: rheist@partners.org

Hematol Oncol Clin N Am 31 (2017) 59–70
http://dx.doi.org/10.1016/j.hoc.2016.08.001
0889-8588/17/© 2016 Elsevier Inc. All rights reserved.

hemonc.theclinics.com

problems must be factored into decision making. Symptoms, such as hemoptysis, are important to elicit because some therapies are contraindicated in that setting. In terms of cancer-centered factors, histologic and molecular subtype of the cancer are important for choosing first-line systemic treatment options. At the very least, nonsquamous or squamous histologic subtype of the NSCLC must be established. Broad genomic testing is becoming widely available, and patients with sensitizing *EGFR* mutations or *ALK and ROS1* rearrangements are best managed with targeted therapy as first-line treatment. The optimal management of these select molecularly defined patients is discussed elsewhere. This article focuses on the management of patients without these specific molecular alterations.

TREATMENT
First-Line Treatment with Platinum Combinations

Platinum-based combination chemotherapy is the standard of care for the first-line treatment of metastatic NSCLC. Results from Keynote-024 have not yet been formally presented, but the press release suggests that among patients with high levels of PD-L1 expression, first-line PD-1 therapy with pembrolizumab is more effective than platinum-based chemotherapy. The data from this study are still pending at the time of this article but will likely change the first-line therapy paradigm for patients without actionable gene alterations. A meta-analysis published in 1995 showed that cisplatin-based regimens had benefit over best supportive care in the treatment of metastatic NSCLC, whereas regimens with alkylators showed no benefit.[2] For many years, the treatment of patients with metastasis was informed most by Eastern Cooperative Oncology Group (ECOG) 1594, which asked the question of whether any specific platinum doublet was superior to a reference regimen of cisplatin and paclitaxel.[3] A total of 1207 patients with NSCLC were randomized to receive one of four regimens: (1) cisplatin and paclitaxel, (2) cisplatin and gemcitabine, (3) cisplatin and docetaxel, or (4) carboplatin and paclitaxel. Median age was 63, and 63% were male; there was no breakdown by histologic subtype. The overall response rate of 19% and median overall survival (OS) of 7.9 months were not significantly different in any of the four arms. Patients with PS 2 were noted to have a higher rate of serious adverse events and the study was ultimately amended to include only patients with PS 0 to 1. Of note, PS was a significant prognostic factor, with median survival among patients with PS 0 of 10.8 months, PS 1 of 7.1 months, and PS 2 of 3.9 months. ECOG 1594 established platinum-based combination chemotherapy as the first-line standard for the treatment of metastatic disease, with the choice of second agent being based primarily on toxicity profile rather than any efficacy advantage.

More recent studies have shown that further refining NSCLC by histologic subtype is critical to optimal management. Scagliotti and colleagues[4] compared the combination of cisplatin and pemetrexed with cisplatin and gemcitabine in the treatment of advanced NSCLC in a noninferiority phase 3 randomized study. A total of 1725 patients with stage IIIB or IV NSCLC with ECOG PS 0 to 1 were randomly assigned to receive cisplatin with pemetrexed or cisplatin with gemcitabine. OS in the entire population was noninferior for cisplatin/pemetrexed as compared with cisplatin/gemcitabine (median OS, 10.3 months vs 10.3 months; hazard ratio [HR], 0.94; 95% confidence interval [CI], 0.84–1.05). Importantly, a prespecified analysis of OS by histology showed a significant interaction by histology. Among patients with nonsquamous histology (adenocarcinoma and large cell carcinoma), OS was significantly better with treatment with cisplatin/pemetrexed as compared with cisplatin/gemcitabine (median OS, 12.6 months vs 10.9 months in adenocarcinoma,

P = .03; 10.4 months vs 6.7 months in large cell carcinoma, P = .03). However, among patients with squamous histology, survival was better when treated with cisplatin/gemcitabine rather than cisplatin/pemetrexed (median OS, 10.8 months vs 9.4 months; P = .05). Overall safety analysis showed that grade 3 or 4 treatment-related hematologic toxicities and febrile neutropenia were significantly lower for cisplatin/pemetrexed as compared with cisplatin/gemcitabine (neutropenia, 15% vs 27%; anemia, 6% vs 10%; thrombocytopenia, 4% vs 13%; febrile neutropenia (F&N), 1% vs 4%), whereas treatment-related grade 3 to 4 nausea was higher (7% vs 4%). This was the first study that prospectively showed a survival difference among the various chemotherapy combinations by histologic subtype. The current standard of care in lung cancer treatment requires pathologic distinction of the histologic subtype of NSCLC.

Addition of Biologic Agents to Platinum Combinations

Although platinum-based chemotherapy has been the backbone of treatment strategies for first-line treatment, there have been numerous attempts to add biologic agents to this backbone to increase response and OS. Although most of these attempts have been unsuccessful, angiogenesis inhibitors and epidermal growth factor receptor (EGFR) inhibitors have seen success in specific populations and are part of the consideration in the optimal approach in selected patients (**Table 1**).

Table 1
First-line studies with biologic agents

Study	Regimen	N	RR	Median PFS (mo)	Median OS (mo)
ECOG 4599	Carboplatin/paclitaxel	444	15[a]	4.5[a]	10.3[a]
	Carboplatin/paclitaxel/ bevacizumab	434	35	6.2	12.3
AVAIL	Cisplatin/gemcitabine	347	20.1	6.1[a]	13.1
	Cisplatin/gemcitabine/ bevacizumab (7.5)	345	34.1	6.7	13.6
	Cisplatin/gemcitabine (15)	351	30.4	6.5	13.4
POINTBREAK	Carboplatin/pemetrexed/ bevacizumab	472	34.1	6.0[a]	12.6
	Carboplatin/paclitaxel/ bevacizumab	467	33.0	5.6	13.4
FLEX	Cisplatin/vinorelbine	568	29[a]	4.8	10.1[a]
	Cisplatin/vinorelbine/ cetuximab	557	36	4.8	11.3
BMS099	Carboplatin/taxane	338	17.2[a]	4.24	8.38
	Carboplatin/taxane/ cetuximab	338	25.7	4.40	9.69
INSPIRE	Cisplatin/pemetrexed	315	32	5.6	11.5
	Cisplatin/pemetrexed/ necitumumab	318	31	5.6	11.3
SQUIRE	Cisplatin/gemcitabine	548	29	5.5[a]	9.9[a]
	Cisplatin/gemcitabine/ necitumumab	545	31	5.7	11.5

Abbreviations: PFS, progression-free survival; RR, relative risk.
[a] Statistically significant.

Angiogenesis inhibition

In the ECOG 4599, a total of 878 patients with recurrent or advanced NSCLC were randomized to receive first-line treatment with carboplatin and paclitaxel, or carboplatin and paclitaxel plus bevacizumab.[5] Patients with squamous histology were excluded based on previous phase 2 data where squamous patients suffered higher rates of serious hemorrhagic events, including fatal pulmonary hemorrhage. Platinum chemotherapy was given for six cycles, and patients in the bevacizumab arm continued to receive bevacizumab thereafter until disease progression or toxicity. Response rate, progression-free survival (PFS), and OS were all significantly improved with the addition of bevacizumab to platinum chemotherapy (relative risk, 35% vs 15%, $P<.001$; PFS, 6.2 months vs 4.5 months, $P<.001$; OS, 12.3 months vs 10.3 months, $P = .003$). Class effects of angiogenesis inhibition, such as hypertension, proteinuria, and bleeding, were all significantly higher in the bevacizumab-containing arm. In addition, rates of neutropenia, febrile neutropenia, and thrombocytopenia were also higher in the bevacizumab-containing arm.

Key exclusions in the ECOG 4599 study included squamous histology, history of hemoptysis, and the presence of brain metastases. Subsequent to the positive results from ECOG 4599, multiple studies were undertaken to better define a "bevacizumab-eligible" population. BRIDGE was an open-label phase 2 study for patients with squamous lung cancer.[6] Baseline risk factors for pulmonary hemorrhage, such as tumor cavitation or tumor involvement of major blood vessels, and history of hemoptysis or a bleeding diasthesis, were exclusionary. Patients with squamous histology were treated initially with carboplatin/paclitaxel for two cycles, with bevacizumab added with the third cycle. The primary end point of the trial was the incidence of grade 3 or higher pulmonary hemorrhage. One of 31 patients (3.2%) who received bevacizumab had a grade 3 to 4 pulmonary hemorrhage; there was one additional grade 1 pulmonary hemorrhage that occurred on study. A European study in which patients with squamous NSCLC were treated with bevacizumab from cycle 2, after a 3-week course of radiation treatment before start of chemotherapy, was terminated early after 2 of the first 20 patients had grade 3 to 4 pulmonary hemorrhage.[6] Overall, given the potentially catastrophic consequences of pulmonary hemorrhage, treatment of squamous patients with bevacizumab is considered contradindicated and has not been adopted by the oncology community.

Other exclusions to "bevacizumab-eligibility" have been loosened since the original ECOG 4599 study as more data support safety in these populations. PASSPORT was an open-label phase 2 study of bevacizumab in combination with chemotherapy among patients with nonsquamous NSCLC with treated brain metastases.[7] The primary end point was the incidence of symptomatic grade 2 or higher central nervous system hemorrhage. Patients received bevacizumab in conjunction with first- and second-line therapy, and multiple different chemotherapy regimens including platinum combinations or single-agent therapies were allowed. A total of 115 patients were enrolled in this study, among whom 80% had received whole-brain radiotherapy, 19.1% had received radiosurgery alone, and 0.9% had neurosurgery alone. There were no reports of grade 1 to 5 central nervous system hemorrhage, supporting the safety of bevacizumab in treated brain metastases. Indeed, it may be that bevacizumab could be considered even in untreated small asymptomatic brain metastases. BRAIN was a phase 2 study that enrolled patients with nonsquamous NSCLC with untreated asymptomatic brain metastases.[8] Patients were treated with carboplatin and paclitaxel with bevacizumab in the first-line setting or erlotinib with bevacizumab in the second-line setting. Among 91 patients enrolled, there was one grade 1 intracranial hemorrhage observed, suggesting that even in small asymptomatic untreated brain mets, treatment with bevacizumab could potentially be considered.

Specific subsets of patients may accrue more benefit from the addition of bevacizumab to their treatment regimen. In a retrospective analysis of elderly patients in ECOG 4599, with elderly defined as age greater than 70, the addition of bevacizumab to chemotherapy was associated with a higher response rate and PFS, but OS between the two arms was not different (median OS, 11.3 months for the bevacizumab-containing arm, 12.1 months for chemotherapy alone; $P = .4$).[9] Moreover, in the elderly population, the addition of bevacizumab was associated with a significantly higher toxicity rate, with grade 3 to 5 toxicities occurring in 87% of those receiving bevacizumab as compared with 61% of those receiving chemotherapy alone. These results suggest that caution should be applied when considering bevacizumab in elderly patients, because side effects and toxicities may outweigh potential benefits. Finally, an analysis by sex showed that although the improvements in relative risk and PFS were seen in men and women in ECOG 4599, the improvement in OS was seen in men only.[10] Median OS in men was significantly better with bevacizumab compared with chemotherapy alone (11.7 months vs 8.7 months), whereas women had comparable OS regardless of treatment arm (13.1 months with chemotherapy alone, 13.3 months with chemotherapy plus bevacizumab; $P = .87$).

Other platinum doublets besides carboplatin and paclitaxel have been combined with bevacizumab, with varying results. AVAIL was a randomized phase 3 trial investigating cisplatin and gemcitabine as first-line chemotherapy with bevacizumab at 7.5 mg/m^2, bevacizumab at 15 mg/m^2, or placebo.[11,12] The study was originally designed with a primary end point of OS, but after ECOG 4599 was reported, the protocol was amended to a primary end point of PFS. The study was designed to allow comparison of the bevacizumab-containing arms with placebo, but was not powered to compare the two doses of bevacizumab. A total of 1043 patients were randomized to the three arms. Response rates were higher for the bevacizumab-containing arms as compared with placebo, and PFS was significantly prolonged with bevacizumab. Median survival, which was greater than 13 months in all groups, was not significantly different with the addition of bevacizumab. The authors hypothesized that the high degree of subsequent therapies and favorable prognostic factors (younger age, higher proportion of dry stage IIIB, high proportions of adenocarcinoma and never-smokers) may have influenced the OS results.[12]

POINTBREAK was a phase 3 study in first-line stage IIIB or IV nonsquamous NSCLC where patients were randomized to treatment with carboplatin, paclitaxel, and bevacizumab followed by bevacizumab, versus carboplatin, pemetrexed, and bevacizumab followed by pemetrexed and bevacizumab.[13] The study was designed with a primary end point of OS to demonstrate superiority of the pemetrexed-containing arm, bearing in mind that pemetrexed had shown particular activity in the nonsquamous NSCLC population. However, OS was not improved with pemetrexed/carboplatin/bevacizumab as compared with paclitaxel/carboplatin/bevacizumab. Response rates were similar (34.1% vs 33.0%) between the two arms. PFS was improved in the pemetrexed-containing arm (HR, 0.83; median PFS, 6.0 months vs 5.6 months; $P = .012$), but OS, the primary end point, was not different. The toxicity profile differed between the two regimens, with more anemia, thrombocytopenia, and fatigue seen in the pemetrexed-containing arm and more neutropenia, febrile neutropenia, sensory neuropathy, and alopecia in the paclitaxel-containing arm. In a prespecified exploratory analysis of patients who reached the maintenance portion of the trial, median PFS and OS favored the patients who were in the pemetrexed-containing arm rather than paclitaxel (ie, those patients receiving pemetrexed/bevacizumab during maintenance rather than bevacizumab alone): median OS was 17.7 months versus 15.7 months, and median PFS 8.6 months versus 6.9 months. However, because of the design of this study, POINTBREAK cannot directly answer the question of which may be the better maintenance regimen. Given the lack of an OS difference in the study as a whole, it also does not establish carboplatin/pemetrexed as a superior regimen to combine with bevacizumab as compared with carboplatin/paclitaxel.

Overall, these studies show that in a selected group of patients, the addition of bevacizumab to platinum-based first-line chemotherapy has benefit. The trials suggest carboplatin and paclitaxel and carboplatin and pemetrexed are both reasonable regimens to combine with bevacizumab. Although the lack of an OS benefit in AVAIL may be caused by prognostic factors related to the population rather than chemotherapy regimen itself, the net effect has been that platinum/gemcitabine is a potential, but not necessarily favored, choice in combination with bevacizumab. The studies leave open the question of optimal maintenance strategy because this question was not directly tested in any of these studies.

Epidermal growth factor receptor inhibition

A series of studies have evaluated the addition of EGFR monoclonal antibodies to chemotherapy in the first-line setting. Two large studies, FLEX and BMS099, investigated the addition of the EGFR antibody cetuxiumab to chemotherapy. BMS099 was a phase 3 trial that enrolled 676 patients for treatment with carboplatin and taxane versus carboplatin, taxane, and cetuximab.[14] Patients were enrolled regardless of histologic subtype and EGFR expression. The primary end point was PFS. Although response rate was higher with the addition of cetuximab (25.7% vs 17.2%; $P = .007$), there was no significant difference in PFS (HR, 0.902; 95% CI, 0.761–1.069; $P = .236$). Similarly, OS was not significantly different between the two arms (median OS, 9.69 months with cetuximab vs 8.38 months without; HR, 0.89; 95% CI, 0.754–1.051; $P = .169$). Biomarker analysis did not show any specific biomarker (KRAS or EGFR mutation, EGFR immunohistochemistry or fluorescence in situ hybridization) that seemed to predict for efficacy.[15] FLEX was a randomized phase 3 trial where patients with advanced NSCLC whose tumors expressed EGFR were treated with chemotherapy plus cetuximab or chemotherapy alone.[16] The trial included all histologies and PS 0 to 2. A total of 1125 patients were treated with cisplatin and vinorelbine versus cisplatin and vinorelbine with cetuximab, which was continued after chemotherapy until disease progression or unacceptable toxicity. The main cetuximab-related side effects were rash, diarrhea, and infusion reactions, and grade 3 to 4 febrile neutropenia was higher with cetuximab. Response rate was higher in the cetuximab-containing arm (36% vs 29%; $P = .01$). PFS was not different between the two groups (median PFS, 4.8 months in both groups; HR, 0.943; 95% CI, 0.825–1.077). The study did meet its primary end point of improvement in OS (median, 11.3 months vs 10.1 months; $P = .044$). However, despite meeting the primary end point of an OS benefit, FLEX did not lead to the widespread adoption of cetuximab in addition to chemotherapy, perhaps because of the relatively small increment in benefit, and the incongruence between the PFS and OS results.

More recently, the EGFR antibody necitumumab has been investigated in combination with chemotherapy. In the nonsquamous setting, necitumumab does not have any benefit. INSPIRE, a phase 3 trial of cisplatin and pemetrexed with or without necitumumab in the first-line treatment of nonsquamous NSCLC, was stopped early because of toxicity.[17] An imbalance was observed in nonfatal and fatal thromboembolic events and overall number of deaths from all causes, with more adverse events noted in the necitumumab arm.

However, necitumumab does show a significant benefit when used in squamous NSCLC. Indeed, this benefit may have been presaged in prior studies, because analysis of FLEX showed that the OS benefit was most pronounced among patients with squamous histology.[16] SQUIRE was a randomized phase 3 study of necitumumab in the first-line treatment of stage IV squamous NSCLC.[18] Patients with squamous histology with PS 0 to 2 were randomized to receive cisplatin and gemcitabine with or without necitumumab. A total of 1092 patients were enrolled. The primary end point was OS. Although objective responses were similar between the two groups, the disease control rate was higher for the necitumumab group. Both PFS and OS were significantly improved with the addition of necitumumab (median OS, 11.5 months vs 9.9 months; HR, 0.84; 95% CI, 0.74–0.96; $P = .01$). Grade 3 or higher adverse events that were more common with necitumumab included hypomagnesemia and rash. There was a higher rate of venous thromboembolic events in the necitumumab arm, both of any grade (9% vs 5%) and grade 3 or higher (5% vs 3%), but unlike in the nonsquamous setting, the rate of fatal thromboembolic events was not different between the two groups. Evaluation by immunohistochemistry for EGFR protein expression (high expression defined as H-score ≥ 200, low as H-score <200) was performed as a prespecified analysis and was not predictive of differential effect. In November 2015, necitumumab was approved by the Food and Drug Administration for use in combination with cisplatin/gemcitabine chemotherapy for the first-line treatment of metastatic squamous NSCLC.

Maintenance Therapy

First-line treatment of metastatic disease has extended beyond the completion of platinum combination therapy as multiple studies have now shown the benefit of continuing with maintenance therapy (**Table 2**). This has been a paradigm shift in the management of metastatic lung cancer. Whereas before oncologists simply waited for progression before starting second-line therapy, now multiple studies have shown that PFS and OS are improved with various forms of maintenance therapy. Both switch maintenance and continuation maintenance strategies have been tested. Conceptually, switch maintenance refers to the continuation of chemotherapy beyond the completion of the initial platinum combination regimen, with a chemotherapy that was not included in the initial regimen. Continuation maintenance refers to the continuation of chemotherapy beyond the completion of the initial platinum combination regimen, with an agent that comprised a part of that regimen. A cautionary note should be sounded in viewing the survival statistics from the maintenance studies, because patients who progressed on first-line therapy were by design excluded from these studies; patients had to have at least stable disease to be considered eligible, thereby skewing the outcomes toward a more favorable population.

The most convincing data to support maintenance therapy have involved studies that included pemetrexed in the maintenance regimen. As would be expected for pemetrexed, this benefit is most clearly seen in the nonsquamous population, and both switch maintenance and continuation maintenance strategies involving pemetrexed have shown benefit.

Ciuleanu and colleagues[19] conducted a study randomizing 663 patients who had not progressed after four cycles of first-line platinum chemotherapy (platinum with a taxane or gemcitabine) to switch maintenance therapy with pemetrexed or best supportive care. Both PFS and OS were significantly improved in the arm receiving pemetrexed (median PFS, 4.3 months vs 2.6 months, P<.0001; median OS, 13.4 months vs 10.6 months, $P = .012$). A significant treatment by histology interaction was noted, with the nonsquamous rather than squamous patients deriving benefit. In

Table 2
Maintenance studies

Study	Induction Base	Number on Induction Therapy	Number Randomized to Maintenance	Maintenance Arms	From Randomization to Maintenance Phase	
					Median PFS (mo)	Median OS (mo)
PARAMOUNT	Cisplatin/pemetrexed	939	539	Pemetrexed	4.4[d]	13.9[d]
				Placebo	2.8	11.0
AVAPERL	Cisplatin/pemetrexed/ bevacizumab	376	253	Pemetrexed/bevacizumab	7.4[d]	n.r.
				Bev	3.7	12.8
Ciuleanu	Platinum doublet[a]	n.r.	663	Pemetrexed	4.0[d]	13.4[d]
				Placebo	2.0	10.6
Fidias	Carboplatin/gemcitabine	566	309	Docetaxel immediate	5.7[d]	12.3
				Docetaxel delayed	2.7	9.7
Perol	Cisplatin/gemcitabine	834	464	Gemcitabine	3.8[d]	12.1
				Erlotinib	2.9[d]	11.4
				Observation	1.9	10.8
SATURN	Platinum doublet[b]	1949	889	Erlotinib	12.3 wk[d]	12.0[d]
				Placebo	11.1	11.0
ATLAS	Platinum doublet + bevacizumab[c]	1145	743	Bevacizumab/erlotinib	4.8[d]	14.4
				Bevacizumab/placebo	3.7	13.3

Abbreviation: n.r., not reached.

[a] Carboplatin/gemcitabine, cisplatin/gemcitabine, cisplatin/gemcitabine, carboplatin/paclitaxel, cisplatin/paclitaxel, carboplatin/docetaxel, cisplatin/docetaxel.

[b] Platinum doublets, most common carboplatin/gemcitabine, cisplatin/gemcitabine, carbo/paclitaxel.

[c] Most common carboplatin/paclitaxel/bevacizumab, carboplatin/gemcitabine/bevacizumab, carboplatin/docetaxel/bevacizumab, cisplatin/gemcitabine/ bevacizumab.

[d] Statistically significant.

nonsquamous patients, median OS was 15.5 months among those receiving peme-trexed and 10.3 months among those on placebo (HR, 0.70; P = .002). In squamous patients, median OS was 9.9 months for pemetrexed and 10.8 months for placebo (HR, 1.078; P = .678). Although drug-related grade 3 or higher events were higher in the pemetrexed than placebo arm (16% vs 4%), the treatment was overall reason-ably well tolerated and there were no treatment-related deaths.

Other studies have shown that a continuation maintenance strategy with peme-trexed can also have benefit. Paramount was a phase 3 study of continuation mainte-nance therapy with pemetrexed versus placebo after initial treatment with cisplatin/pemetrexed.[20] A total of 939 patients with nonsquamous NSCLC were enrolled and received four cycles of cisplatin/pemetrexed as induction therapy. A total of 539 pa-tients with no disease progression after four cycles of doublet chemotherapy were randomized to receive maintenance pemetrexed or placebo. Median OS was 13.9 months with pemetrexed as compared with 11 months with placebo (P = .0195). Higher rates of grade 3 to 4 anemia, neutropenia, and fatigue were seen in those patients randomized to receive pemetrexed.

How to best manage maintenance therapy in bevacizumab-eligible patients remains an open question. The ECOG 4599, which established the role of bevacizumab in first-line treatment, did not ask a maintenance question because patients received either no bevacizumab, or bevacizumab during first-line treatment that was then mandated to continue as a single agent beyond platinum combination therapy until disease pro-gression or toxicity. With the data showing benefit of pemetrexed in maintenance ther-apy, how best to approach maintenance in these patients remains debated. In the AVAPERL trial, patients with nonsquamous NSCLC who were nonprogressors after four cycles of cisplatin/pemetrexed/bevacizumab went on to randomization between maintenance bevacizumab versus maintenance pemetrexed plus bevacizumab.[21] PFS was significantly improved in the pemetrexed plus bevacizumab arm (median PFS, 3.7 months vs 7.4 months; P<.001), but the study was not powered for OS. Similar to ECOG 4599, AVAPERL presumes that bevacizumab should be continued, rather than questioning its role as a maintenance therapy. Further clarity around this question will likely come with the results of ECOG 5508. In the ECOG 5508, after an induction period with carboplatin, paclitaxel, and bevacizumab, patients are random-ized to one of three arms of maintenance therapy: (1) pemetrexed alone, (2) bevacizu-mab alone, or (3) pemetrexed and bevacizumab. The primary end point is OS, and this study should help better define the optimal maintenance regimen among nonsqua-mous patients who are bevacizumab-eligible.

Multiple studies have also investigated the use of other agents in the maintenance setting. Of these studies, SATURN, which used erlotinib in maintenance, showed an OS benefit.[22] In the SATURN trial, 1949 patients were treated initially with platinum-based chemotherapy. The 889 patients without progression were then randomized to maintenance erlotinib or placebo. Median PFS was significantly improved in the erlotinib maintenance arm (12.3 weeks vs 11.1 weeks; P<.0001), as was OS (12 months vs 11 months; P = .0088). This benefit was seen in adenocarcinoma and squamous cell histologies, and EGFR mutation positive and negative patients. As might be expected, the greatest degree of benefit was seen in the EGFR mutation positive patients.

Other studies have shown a PFS benefit but not a clear OS benefit. Fidias and col-leagues[23] treated patients with induction therapy with carboplatin and gemcitabine, and randomized those with stable disease or better to immediate versus delayed docetaxel. Among the 566 patients enrolled in this study, 398 patients completed car-boplatin and gemcitabine induction therapy. A total of 309 were randomized to immediate versus delayed docetaxel. PFS was significantly improved for immediate docetaxel (5.7 months vs 2.7 months; P = .0001). Median OS was numerically greater, but not statistically significant, for immediately versus delayed therapy (12.3 months vs 9.7 months; P = .853). Perol and colleagues[24] treated 834 patients with induction cisplatin and gemcitabine, and then randomized 464 patients who were not progressing after four cycles to observation, gemcitabine, or erlotinib. Compared with observation, maintenance therapy with gemcitabine or erlotinib significantly improved PFS (3.8 months vs 1.9 months, P<.001 for gemcitabine; 2.9 months vs 1.9 months, P = .003 for erlotinib). However, neither arm led to a statistically significant improvement in OS. In the ATLAS trial, 1145 patients were treated with chemotherapy and bevacizumab for four cycles.[25] A total of 743 patients without disease progression after four cycles were randomized to erlotinib with bevacizumab or placebo with bevacizumab. The addition of erlotinib to bevacizumab increased median PFS (4.8 months vs 3.7 months; P<.001), but there was no statistically significant improvement in OS (14.4 months vs 13.3 months; P = .5341). More grade 3 to 4 adverse events were seen in the erlotinib/bevacizumab arm, particularly rash and diarrhea. These studies, which have shown a PFS but not an OS benefit, contribute to the overall bulk of data demonstrating benefits of maintenance therapy. However, in the absence of a defined OS benefit, adoption of these regimens should be weighed carefully against the additional toxicities that come with maintenance.

In summary, pemetrexed maintenance therapy has shown an OS benefit in nonsquamous patients as both a switch maintenance and continuation maintenance strategy. Debate regarding the optimal maintenance regimen, that is, how best to use pemetrexed and/or bevacizumab in this setting, should be resolved once ECOG 5508 is resulted. Erlotinib is another maintenance strategy that has demonstrated a significant, albeit small, OS benefit, among squamous and nonsquamous patients.

SUMMARY

Major advances in the treatment of metastatic NSCLC have led to significant incremental improvements in patient outcomes. Platinum-based combination therapy remains the cornerstone of first-line therapy. The addition of biologic agents, such as bevacizumab or necitumumab, in selected populations has shown benefit over chemotherapy alone. The advent of maintenance therapy has also improved OS outcomes in selected populations of patients. Ongoing studies will further refine optimal treatment in the first-line setting and further advance first-line treatment options.

ADDENDUM

Keynote-024 and CheckMate-026 are both phase 3 trials comparing PD-1 inhibition to platinum based chemotherapy as first-line therapy. At the time this article went to press the data from these studies have not yet been released. However, based on press releases of study results, it is expected that they will provide important information regarding first line therapy decisions. Keynote-024 was a randomized phase 3 study comparing pembrolizumab to first-line platinum chemotherapy in patients with stage IV NSCLC with high PD-L1 expression, defined as a tumor proportion score of 50% or more (NCT02142738). This trial was stopped by the Data Monitoring Committee (DMC) for superiority of pembrolizumab in progression free and overall survival outcomes. Checkmate-026 was a randomized phase 3 study comparing nivolumab to first-line platinum chemotherapy among patients with stage IV NSCLC with tumor PD-L1 expression of at least 5% (NCT02041533). This study did not meet its primary endpoint of progression-free survival. As data from these studies as well as other ongoing first-line immunotherapy studies become published, we anticipate rapid changes in the paradigm of management of patients in the first-line setting.

REFERENCES

1. American Cancer Society. Cancer facts & figures 2016. Atlanta (GA): American Cancer Society; 2016.
2. Non-small Cell Lung Cancer Collaborative Group. Chemotherapy in non-small cell lung cancer: a meta-analysis using updated data on individual patients from 52 randomised clinical trials. BMJ 1995;311:899.
3. Schiller JH, Harrington D, Belani CP, et al. Comparison of four chemotherapy regimens for advanced non-small cell lung cancer. N Engl J Med 2002;346(2):92–8.
4. Scagliotti GV, Parikh P, von Pawel J, et al. Phase III study comparing cisplatin plus gemcitabine with cisplatin plus pemeterxed in chemotherapy-naive patients with advanced non-small cell lung cancer. J Clin Oncol 2008;26(21):3543–51.
5. Sandler A, Gray R, Perry MC, et al. Paclitaxel-carboplatin alone or with bevacizumab for non-small cell lung cancer. N Engl J Med 2007;355(24):2542–50.
6. Hainsworth JD, Fang L, Huang JE, et al. BRIDGE: An open-label phase II trial evaluating the safety of bevacizumab + carboplatin/paclitaxel as first-line treatment for patients with advanced, previously untreated, squamous non-small cell lung cancer. J Thorac Oncol 2011;6(1):109–14.
7. Socinski MA, Langer CJ, Huang JE, et al. Safety of bevacizumab in patients with non-small cell lung cancer and brain metastases. J Clin Oncol 2009;27(31): 5255–61.
8. Besse B, Le Moulec S, Mazieres J, et al. Bevacizumab in patients with nonsquamous non-small cell lung cancer and asymptomatic, untreated brain metastases (BRAIN): a nonrandomized, phase II study. Clin Cancer Res 2015;21(8): 1896–903.
9. Ramalingam SS, Dahlberg SE, Langer C, et al. Outcomes for elderly, advanced stage non-small cell lung cancer patients treated with bevacizumab in combination with carboplatin and paclitaxel: analysis of Eastern Cooperative Oncology Trial 4599. J Clin Oncol 2008;26(1):60–5.
10. Brahmer JR, Dahlberg SE, Gray RJ, et al. Sex differences in outcome with bevacizumab therapy. J Thorac Oncol 2011;6(1):103–8.
11. Reck M, von Pawel J, Zatloukal P, et al. Phase III trial of cisplatin plus gemcitabine with either placebo or bevacizumab as first-line therapy for non-squamous non-small cell lung cancer: AVAIL. J Clin Oncol 2009;27(8):1227–34.
12. Reck M, von Pawel J, Zatloukal P, et al. Overall survival with cisplatin-gemcitabine and bevacizumab or placebo as first-line therapy for non-squamous non-small cell lung cancer: results from a randomised phase III trial (AVAIL). Ann Oncol 2010;21(9):1804–9.
13. Patel JD, Socinski MA, Garon EB, et al. PointBreak: a randomized phase III study of pemetrexed plus carboplatin and bevacizumab followed by maintenance pemetrexed and bevacizumab versus paclitaxel plus carboplatin and bevacizumab followed by maintenance bevacizumab in patients with Stage IIIB or IV non-squamous non-small cell lung cancer. J Clin Oncol 2013;31(34):4349–57.
14. Lynch TJ, Patel T, Dreisbach L, et al. Cetuximab and first-line taxane/carboplatin chemotherapy in advanced non-small cell lung cancer: results from the randomized multicenter phase III trial BMS099. J Clin Oncol 2010;28(6):911–7.
15. Khambata-Ford S, Harbison CT, Hart LL, et al. Analysis of potential predictive markers of cetuximab benefit in BMS099, a phase II study of cetuximab and

first-line taxane/carboplatin in advanced non-small cell lung cancer. J Clin Oncol 2010;28(6):918–27.

16. Pirker R, Pereira JR, Szczesna A, et al. Cetuximab plus chemotherapy in patients with advanced non-small cell lung cancer (FLEX): an open-label randomised phase III trial. Lancet 2009;373:1525–31.

17. Paz-Ares L, Mezger J, Ciuleanu TE, et al. Necitumumab plus pemetrexed and cisplatin as first-line therapy in patients with stage IV non-squamous non-small cell lung cancer (INSPIRE): an open-label randomised, controlled phase 3 study. Lancet Oncol 2015;16:328–37.

18. Thatcher N, Hirsch FR, Luft AV, et al. Necitumumab plus gemcitabine and cisplatin versus gemcitabine and cisplatin alone as first-line therapy in patients with stage IV squamous non-small cell lung cancer (SQUIRE): an open-label randomised, controlled phase 3 study. Lancet Oncol 2015;16:763–74.

19. Ciuleanu TE, Brodowicz T, Zielinski C, et al. Maintenance pemetrexed plus best supportive care versus placebo plus best supportive care for non-small cell lung cancer: a randomised, double-blind, phase 3 study. Lancet 2009;374: 1432–40.

20. Paz-Ares LG, de Marinis F, Dediu M, et al. PARAMOUNT: final overall survival results of the phase III study of maintenance pemetrexed versus placebo imme-diately after induction treatment with pemetrexed plus cisplatin for advanced non-squamous non-small cell lung cancer. J Clin Oncol 2013;31(23):2895–902.

21. Barlesi F, Scherpereel A, Rittmeyer A, et al. Randomized phase III trial of mainte-nance bevacizumab with or without pemetrexed after first-line induction with bev-acizumab, cisplatin, and pemetrexed in advanced non-squamous non-small cell lung cancer: AVAPERL (MO22089). J Clin Oncol 2013;31(24):3004–11.

22. Cappuzzo F, Ciuleanu TE, Stelmakh L, et al. Erlotinib as maintenance treatment in advanced non-small cell lung cancer: multicentre, randomised, placebo-controlled phase 3 study. Lancet Oncol 2010;11:521–9.

23. Fidias PM, Dahil SR, Lyss AP, et al. Phase III study of immediate compared with delayed docetaxel after front-line therapy with gemcitabine plus carboplatin in advanced non-small cell lung cancer. J Clin Oncol 2009;27(4):591–8.

24. Perol M, Chouaid C, Perol D, et al. Randomized phase III study of gemcitabine or erlotinib maintenance therapy versus observation, with predefined second-line treatment, after cisplatin-gemcitabine induction chemotherapy in advanced non-small cell lung cancer. J Clin Oncol 2012;30(28):3516–24.

25. Johnson BE, Kabbinavar F, Fehrenbacher L, et al. ATLAS: randomized, double-blind, placebo-controlled, phase IIIB trial comparing bevacizumab therapy with or without erlotinib, after completion of chemotherapy, with bevacizumab for first-line treatment of advanced non-small cell lung cancer. J Clin Oncol 2013; 31(31):3926–34.

Second-Line Chemotherapy and Beyond for Non–Small Cell Lung Cancer

 CrossMark

Greg Durm, MD*, Nasser Hanna, MD

KEYWORDS

- Non–small cell lung cancer • Chemotherapy • Second-line treatment • Docetaxel
- Pemetrexed • Erlotinib

KEY POINTS

- Docetaxel, pemetrexed, and erlotinib are approved for the second-line treatment of NSCLC.
- The discovery of targetable mutations, the increasing use of maintenance strategies, and the introduction of immunotherapies has made the choice of second-line agents much more complicated.
- Ramucirumab with docetaxel is the only combination regimen that has shown improved overall survival in the second-line setting.
- Erlotinib is the only agent approved in the third-line setting for EGFR wild-type patients.

FIRST-LINE TREATMENT

In patients without targetable genetic alterations, the standard first-line therapy for advanced (stage IIIB or IV) non–small cell lung cancer (NSCLC) is chemotherapy with a platinum doublet for four to six cycles with or without bevacizumab.[1] Historically, several drugs including paclitaxel, docetaxel, gemcitabine, and vinorelbine were considered acceptable platinum partners in the first-line metastatic setting with essentially no differences in progression-free survival (PFS) or overall survival (OS). More recently, additional agents have been approved in combination with platinum in this setting including pemetrexed and nab-paclitaxel.[1–3] One particular advance in the last decade has been the recognition that histology should be considered in the choice of initial chemotherapy. This was discovered after an additional analysis of two studies showed pemetrexed to be more effective in nonsquamous histologies and less active in squamous tumors.[3–5] Based on these findings, the choice of first-line agents in metastatic NSCLC is now strongly based on presenting histology, and this initial choice affects available second-line options.

Department of Hematology/Oncology, Indiana University Simon Cancer Center, 535 Barnhill Drive, Indianapolis, IN 46202, USA
* Corresponding author.
E-mail address: gdurm@iu.edu

Hematol Oncol Clin N Am 31 (2017) 71–81
http://dx.doi.org/10.1016/j.hoc.2016.08.002
0889-8588/17/© 2016 Elsevier Inc. All rights reserved.

MAINTENANCE THERAPY

Historically, patients treated with first-line platinum doublet chemotherapy who had objective responses or stable disease were placed on surveillance following completion of four to six cycles. However, over the last decade, new data suggests that there is benefit to the addition of maintenance therapy following initial chemotherapy. There are two maintenance strategies including continuation of an agent used in the first-line setting or switching to a previously unused agent (switch maintenance). There are data supporting the use of bevacizumab, pemetrexed, and erlotinib in the maintenance setting either as single agents or in combination.[6-11] Prior maintenance therapy is of particular importance when discussing second-line chemotherapy options because the use of maintenance therapy, particularly when switch maintenance is used, influences the availability of agents in the second-line setting and beyond.

CHEMOTHERAPY AS SECOND-LINE TREATMENT

Historically, nearly all patients received platinum doublet chemotherapy followed by single-agent chemotherapy in the second-line setting. However, with the discovery of targetable mutations, the development of tyrosine kinase inhibitors (TKI), the increasing use of maintenance strategies, and the introduction of immunotherapies to the current list of approved medications, choosing an appropriate second-line therapy has become more complicated. In general, those patients treated with targeted therapies receive a platinum doublet at the time of progression. For those who are wild-type for exploitable mutations, immunotherapy has become an increasingly popular second-line option because of its tolerability and potential for durable responses. However, there remains a role for additional treatments following second-line platinum doublets or immunotherapy, or alternatively, a role for second-line chemotherapy in those with contraindications to immunotherapy. This article discusses the available data for chemotherapy in the second-line treatment of NSCLC and beyond.

CHEMOTHERAPY IN THE SECOND-LINE SETTING AND BEYOND

With the exception of immunotherapy, there are four Food and Drug Administration (FDA)–approved agents for the second- and third-line treatment of advanced or metastatic NSCLC: (1) docetaxel, (2) pemetrexed, (3) erlotinib, and (4) ramucirumab. Docetaxel was the first agent approved for second-line treatment in 1999, and pemetrexed was approved in the second-line setting in 2004. Erlotinib was also approved in 2004 for second- and third-line treatment of advanced NSCLC and is currently the only FDA-approved third-line therapy. Ramucirumab was approved in 2014 in combination with docetaxel following progression on platinum-based chemotherapy.

SINGLE AGENT VERSUS COMBINATION REGIMENS

In the first-line setting, doublet chemotherapy is clearly superior to single-agent treatment in advanced NSCLC. However, it is unclear whether combination therapy in the second-line setting improves outcomes over single-agent chemotherapy. A meta-analysis of six trials compared combination regimens with single-agent therapy in the second-line setting. The combination arm showed a statistically significant improvement in response rate (RR) (15.1% vs 7.3%; $P = .0004$) and median PFS (14 weeks vs 11.7 weeks; $P = .0009$; hazard ratio [HR], 0.79) compared with single-agent therapy. However, there was no difference in median OS between the two groups (37.3 weeks vs 34.7 weeks; HR, 0.92; $P = .32$). The doublet arms had significantly higher rates of grade 3/4 hematologic (41% vs 25%; $P<.0001$) and nonhematologic (28% vs 22%; P = .034) toxicity.[12] Two additional meta-analyses assessing docetaxel alone versus docetaxel-based doublet chemotherapy and pemetrexed alone versus pemetrexed-based doublet chemotherapy demonstrated similar results. Both analyses showed improvements in RR and PFS with doublet chemotherapy but no improvement in OS. The doublet arms showed significant increases in hematologic toxicity for docetaxel and pemetrexed doublets and in nonhematologic toxicity for docetaxel doublets.[13,14] Based on these findings, current second-line treatment approaches use mainly single-agent chemotherapy.

DOCETAXEL

Docetaxel was the first agent approved for the second-line treatment of patients with advanced NSCLC. This approval came based on two phase III clinical trials. In the TAX 317 trial, 104 patients previously treated with at least one platinum-based regimen were randomized to receive either docetaxel (100 mg/m^2 or 75 mg/m^2 every 3 weeks) or best supportive care (BSC) (**Table 1**). The primary end point of the study was OS, and this favored the docetaxel arms with a median OS of 7.0 versus 4.6 months (P = .047). The group treated with 75 mg/m^2 had a numerically better OS than those treated with 100 mg/m^2 (7.5 months vs 5.9 months) and demonstrated a much better toxicity profile.[15] A subsequently published quality of life analysis of this trial demonstrated a significant improvement in pain scores for the docetaxel arms and a trend toward improved overall quality of life.[16]

A second study evaluating docetaxel in the second-line setting following progression on platinum-based chemotherapy was the TAX 320 trial. This trial compared docetaxel at 75 mg/m^2 or 100 mg/m^2 every 3 weeks with a control arm treated with either vinorelbine (30 mg/m^2 on Days 1, 8, and 15) or ifosfamide (2 mg/m^2/d on Days 1–3) repeated every 3 weeks. RR (P = .002) and PFS (P = .005) were better in the docetaxel arms. The median OS was not different among the three groups, although the 1-year OS was 32% in the docetaxel 75 mg/m^2 versus 19% in the control arm (P = .025). The docetaxel 75 mg/m^2 arm again demonstrated much less hematologic and nonhematologic toxicity compared with the 100 mg/m^2 arm.[17] These two trials firmly established docetaxel 75 mg/m^2 as the standard second-line therapy in 1999.

Several studies have compared weekly dosing of docetaxel with treatment every 3 weeks. A meta-analysis, published in 2007, included 865 individual patients and five trials comparing these dosing strategies. Median OS was 27.4 weeks in the every 3 week treatment arm and 26.1 weeks in the weekly arm (P = .24), suggesting no difference in efficacy. There were also no significant differences in the rates of anemia, thrombocytopenia, or nonhematologic toxicity, but there was less febrile neutropenia (P<.00001 for both) in the weekly dosing arm.[18] Weekly dosing with docetaxel is an acceptable treatment alternative for second-line advanced NSCLC, and both treatment schedules are frequently used in practice.

At least three phase III trials have compared alternative chemotherapy agents with docetaxel in the second-line setting. A randomized controlled trial comparing docetaxel with pemetrexed is discussed in more detail later. The first of the other two trials compared docetaxel with vinflunine, a fluorinated vinca alkaloid, in a 1:1 randomization. This study met its noninferiority end point with a median PFS of 2.3 months for both arms. RR stable disease rate and OS were numerically superior in favor of docetaxel but did not reach statistical significance, and the vinflunine arm had higher rates of several hematologic and nonhematologic adverse events.[19] Another study compared docetaxel with oral topotecan following progression on platinum-based

Table 1
Select trials of single-agent and combination chemotherapy in second-line advanced NSCLC

Author	Trial	Treatment	N	RR (%)	PFS or TTP	OS (mo)	1-y Survival (%)
Select cytotoxic chemotherapy trials							
Shepherd et al,[15] 2000	TAX 317	Docetaxel, 100 mg/m²	49	6.3	10.6 wk	5.9	19
		Docetaxel, 75 mg/m²	55	5.5	10.6 wk	7.5	37
		BSC	100	NR	6.7 wk	4.6	19
Fossella et al,[17] 2000	TAX 320	Docetaxel, 100 mg/m²	125	10.8	19%[a]	5.5	21
		Docetaxel, 75 mg/m²	125	6.7	17%[a]	5.7	32
		Vinorelbine/ ifosfamide	123	0.8	8%[a]	5.6	19
Hanna et al,[4] 2004	JMEI	Pemetrexed	265	9.1	2.9	8.3	29.7
		Docetaxel	276	8.8	2.9	7.9	29.7
Di Maio et al,[18] 2007	Meta- analysis	Weekly docetaxel	432	6.7	NR	26.1 wk	27
		Q3 week docetaxel	433	8.1	NR	27.4 wk	24.8
Select trials of combination therapy							
Garon et al,[23] 2014	REVEL	Docetaxel	625	14	3.0	9.1	NR
		Docetaxel + ramucirumab	628	22	4.5	10.5	NR
Reck et al,[22] 2014	LUME- Lung 1	Docetaxel	659	3.3	2.7	9.1 (10.3)[b]	44.7
		Docetaxel + nintedanib	655	4.4	3.4	10.1 (12.6)[b]	52.7
Hanna et al,[26] 2013	LUME- Lung 2	Pemetrexed	360	9	3.6	HR 1.03	NR
		Pemetrexed + nintedanib	353	9	4.4		NR
Herbst et al,[21] 2010	ZODIAC	Docetaxel	697	10	3.2	9.9	41.2
		Docetaxel + vandetanib	694	17	4.0	10.3	44.7
Di Maio et al,[12] 2009	Meta- analysis	Single-agent chemotherapy	428	7.3	11.7 wk	34.7 wk	31.8
		Doublet chemotherapy	419	15.1	14.0 wk	37.3 wk	34.4

Abbreviations: NR, not reported; TTP, time to progression.
[a] Percent survival at 26 weeks.
[b] OS for adenocarcinoma subgroup in parentheses.

therapy. This study also met its primary noninferiority end point; however, PFS at 1-year (25.1% vs 28.7%) and median OS (27.9 weeks vs 30.7 weeks) were both higher in the docetaxel group, although not statistically significant. The docetaxel arm did show a significant improvement in time to progression at 11.3 versus 13.1 weeks ($P = .02$), and grade 3/4 toxicity was similar in the two groups.[20] Vinflunine and topotecan have activity in the second-line setting but neither has shown clear improvement over docetaxel in terms of either efficacy or toxicity. Neither agent is FDA-approved in the United States for the treatment of NSCLC.

Following the approval of docetaxel as a standard second-line option in NSCLC, at least three phase III trials have compared docetaxel with or without a targeted agent. In the ZODIAC trial, 1331 patients with advanced NSCLC were randomized to receive docetaxel plus placebo or docetaxel plus the oral multikinase inhibitor vandetanib, an inhibitor of vascular endothelial growth factor (VEGF) receptor, EGFR, and rearranged during transfection tyrosine kinases. The primary end point was met with a median PFS in the vandetanib group of 4.0 months versus 3.2 months in the placebo group (HR, 0.79; P<.0001), and RR was also improved in the vandetanib group (17% vs 10%; P = .0001). OS was a secondary end point in this study. There was no difference between the two groups with a median OS of 10.3 months in the treatment arm versus 9.9 months in the placebo (HR, 0.95; P = .371).[21] The LUME-Lung 1 trial compared docetaxel plus placebo with docetaxel plus nintedanib, an oral angiokinase inhibitor that blocks VEGFR 1 to 3, fibroblast growth factor receptors 1 to 3, and platelet-derived growth factor receptors α and β. The combination arm met its primary end point of PFS at 3.4 months versus 2.7 months (HR, 0.79; P = .0019). However, it failed to show a difference in OS between the two groups, although in a prespecified sub-group analysis, there was an improvement in OS in patients with adenocarcinoma (12.6 months vs 10.3 months; HR, 0.83; P = .0359).[22] Based on this trial, nintedanib in combination with docetaxel was approved in Europe, but not the United States, for the second-line treatment of patients with NSCLC with adenocarcinoma.

Most recently, the REVEL trial randomized 1253 patients who had progressed after first-line platinum-based therapy to receive docetaxel plus either ramucirumab, an IgG1 monoclonal antibody against VEGF receptor 2, or placebo. The primary end point was OS. This study met its primary end point with a median OS of 10.5 months in the ramucirumab arm versus 9.1 months in the placebo arm (HR, 0.86; P = .023). PFS was also improved in the treatment arm at 4.5 months versus 3 months (HR, 0.76; P<.0001). There were slightly higher rates of grade 3 neutropenia, febrile neutropenia, and leukopenia in the ramucirumab arm and higher grade 3 fatigue and hypertension.[23] Based on this study, the FDA approved ramucirumab in combination with docetaxel for the second-line treatment of NSCLC following progression on platinum-based chemotherapy. Although the OS advantage is modest, this regimen remains a consideration for patients in the second-line setting.

PEMETREXED

Pemetrexed was evaluated in a second-line trial where 571 patients were randomized to receive either docetaxel, 75 mg/m^2, or pemetrexed, 500 mg/m^2, every 3 weeks. This trial had a noninferiority design comparing the OS of the two arms. The study showed no difference in OS between the two groups with a median of 8.3 months in the peme-trexed arm versus 7.9 months in the docetaxel arm (HR, 1.0; P = .226), and the 1-year survival rates were 29.7% in both arms. RRs were also similar with 9.1% and 8.8% in the pemetrexed and docetaxel arms, respectively. There were, however, differences in the toxicity profile of these two drugs. The docetaxel arm had significantly higher rates of hematologic toxicity including neutropenia, febrile neutropenia, infection related to neutropenia, and hospitalizations for neutropenic fever. There were also higher rates of hospitalizations because of other drug-related adverse events, increased use of granulocyte colony–stimulating factor, and alopecia in the docetaxel arm.[4]

Following this study, a reanalysis of the data detected a difference in outcomes be-tween squamous and nonsquamous histologies in patients treated with pemetrexed. Those with nonsquamous NSCLC had superior OS when treated with pemetrexed with a median OS of 9.3 months versus 8.0 months (HR, 0.78; P = .48). Conversely, those with squamous cell carcinoma of the lung did significantly worse when treated with pemetrexed with a median OS of 6.2 months versus 7.4 months (HR, 1.56;

$P = .018$).[5] This differential efficacy according to histology was confirmed in other trials in the first-line and maintenance settings.[3,6] Based on these findings, pemetrexed became a standard second-line treatment option for patients with recurrent, advanced NSCLC with nonsquamous histology and has been FDA-approved since 2004.

Initial studies of pemetrexed showed the maximum tolerated dose to be 500 mg/m^2 to 600 mg/m^2. It was later demonstrated that the addition of vitamin B$_{12}$ and folic acid could ameliorate the hematologic toxicities, and subsequent studies using these vitamins reported maximum tolerated dose of 900 mg/m^2 to 1000 mg/m^2. Therefore, two clinical trials assessed whether higher doses of pemetrexed would improve outcomes in second-line NSCLC. The first was a phase III trial comparing pemetrexed 500 mg/m^2 with 900 mg/m^2 every 3 weeks. This trial was stopped early after an interim analysis showed a low likelihood of improved OS and a numerically higher rate of adverse rates in the 900 mg/m^2 arm.[24] The second trial was a phase II trial from Japan comparing pemetrexed 500 mg/m^2 with 1000 mg/m^2. This trial showed no difference in RR, disease control rate, or median PFS between the two arms, and the 500 mg/m^2 was numerically superior for each of these end points.[25] Based on these trials, 500 mg/m^2 has remained the standard dose of pemetrexed with vitamin B$_{12}$ and folic acid support.

Two large phase III trials have also looked at the combination of pemetrexed with additional agents in the second-line setting in patients with nonsquamous histologies. The LUME-Lung 2 trial compared nintedanib with placebo in combination with pemetrexed with a primary end point of PFS. The study was stopped early for futility following accrual of 713 of a planned 1300 patients based on investigator-assessed PFS. However, a central review of enrolled patients actually reported a statistically significant improvement in median PFS (4.4 months vs 3.6 months; HR, 0.83; $P = .04$) in favor of the combination arm. OS (HR, 1.03) and RR (9%) did not differ between the two arms.[26] A second phase III trial (ZEAL) randomized patients to receive pemetrexed in combination with either vandetanib or placebo. The combination arm failed to improve either PFS (HR, 0.86; $P = .108$) or OS (HR, 0.86; $P = .219$) compared with placebo.[27] Based on these studies, neither nintedanib nor vandetanib are approved for use in combination with pemetrexed.

EPIDERMAL GROWTH FACTOR RECEPTOR TYROSINE KINASE INHIBITORS

Erlotinib was initially approved for the second- and third-line treatment of advanced NSCLC based on the results of the BR.21 trial, which randomized 731 unselected patients to receive erlotinib or BSC following progression on first-line platinum-based chemotherapy. Erlotinib demonstrated improved RR (8.9% vs <1%; $P<.001$), PFS (2.2 months vs 1.8 months; HR, 0.6; $P<.001$), and OS (6.7 months vs 4.7 months; HR, 0.7; $P<.001$) compared with BSC alone (**Table 2**).[28] A subsequent analysis of this trial revealed that patients treated with erlotinib had a longer time to deterioration and improved physical function and quality of life compared with BSC.[29]

Several trials have also compared erlotinib with chemotherapy (either docetaxel or pemetrexed) in either unselected or purely EGFR wild-type (EGFRwt) populations. No major trial in unselected or EGFRwt patients has shown erlotinib to be statistically superior to chemotherapy. The TITAN, HORG, and PROSE trials all failed to demonstrate any difference in RR, PFS, or OS between the two groups.[30–32] There have, however, been two trials that suggest that chemotherapy in the second-line setting may be superior to erlotinib in EGFRwt patients. The TAILOR trial was a comparison of docetaxel versus erlotinib in a purely EGFRwt population. This study demonstrated improved RR

Table 2
Select trials of EGFR TKIs versus chemotherapy trials in EGFR wild-type patients

Author	Trial	Treatment	N	RR (%)	TTP or PFS	OS (mo)	1-y Survival (%)
Shepherd et al,[28] 2005	BR.21	Erlotinib	488	8.9	2.2	6.7	31.2
		BSC	243	<1.0	1.8	4.7	21.5
Karampeazis et al,[31] 2013	HORG	Erlotinib	166	9.0	3.6	8.2	39.5
		Pemetrexed	166	11.4	2.9	10.1	43.6
Garassino et al,[33] 2013	TAILOR	Erlotinib	112	3.0	2.4	5.4	31.8
		Docetaxel	110	15.5	2.9	8.2	39.6
Kawaguchi et al,[34] 2014	DELTA	Erlotinib	150	17	2.0 (1.3)[a]	14.8 (9.0)[a]	NR
		Docetaxel	151	17.9	3.2 (2.9)[a]	12.2 (10.1)[a]	NR
Ciuleanu et al,[30] 2012	TITAN	Erlotinib	203	7.9	6.3 wk	5.3	26
		Pemetrexed or docetaxel	221	6.3	8.6 wk	5.5	24

Abbreviations: NR, not reported; TTP, time to progression.
[a] PFS and OS for subgroup of EGFRwt patients in parentheses.

(15.5% vs 3%; $P = .003$) and PFS (2.9 months vs 2.4 months; HR, 0.71; $P = .02$) favoring the docetaxel arm. It also showed a nonsignificant but numerically superior OS advantage of 2.8 months (8.2 months vs 5.4 months; adjusted HR, 0.73; $P = .05$) for the chemotherapy arm.[33] The DELTA trial compared erlotinib with docetaxel as second- or third-line therapy. In the overall group, there was no difference in RR, PFS, or OS, but in the subgroup of EGFRwt patients, the docetaxel arm had a higher PFS (2.9 months vs 1.3 months; $P = .01$) although no difference in OS (10.1 months vs 9 months; $P = .907$).[34] Lastly, a meta-analysis including six trials with a total of 990 EGFRwt patients demonstrated improved PFS for second-line chemotherapy compared with EGFR-TKIs (HR, 1.37; $P<.00001$) but no difference in OS (HR, 1.02; $P = .81$).[35] Based on these findings, many practitioners prefer chemotherapy over erlotinib for fit patients receiving second-line therapy.

OTHER THERAPEUTIC AGENTS

The utility of other chemotherapeutic agents has been investigated but only in phase I and II trials. These agents include gemcitabine, vinorelbine, paclitaxel, and irinotecan. These trials have demonstrated varying degrees of efficacy and toxicity.[36–40] Gemcitabine is the most studied agent with multiple phase II studies suggesting that it has efficacy in the second-line setting as a single agent[41,42] and in combination.[43]

SUMMARY

The landscape for the second- and third-line treatment of advanced NSCLC has changed dramatically over the last two decades. Immunotherapeutic agents have become a preferred choice following progression on platinum-based first-line chemotherapy. However, there remains a role for cytotoxic chemotherapy and pemetrexed and docetaxel (with or without ramucirumab) are approved for single-agent use in the second-line setting. Furthermore, the EGFR TKI, erlotinib, is approved for either second- or third-line use in unselected patients, although many experts believe it is less effective than chemotherapy in EGFRwt patients. With the discovery of new genetic alterations and the development of novel targeted drugs, the treatment of advanced NSCLC following progression on first-line therapy will likely continue to become more complicated as new treatment algorithms evolve.

REFERENCES

1. Masters GA, Temin S, Azzoli CG, et al. Systemic therapy for stage IV non-small-cell lung cancer: American Society of Clinical Oncology clinical practice guideline update. J Clin Oncol 2015;33(30):3488–515.
2. Socinski MA, Bondarenko I, Karaseva NA, et al. Weekly nab-paclitaxel in combination with carboplatin versus solvent-based paclitaxel plus carboplatin as first-line therapy in patients with advanced non-small-cell lung cancer: final results of a phase III trial. J Clin Oncol 2012;30(17):2055–62.
3. Scagliotti GV, Parikh P, von Pawel J, et al. Phase III study comparing cisplatin plus gemcitabine with cisplatin plus pemetrexed in chemotherapy-naive patients with advanced-stage non-small-cell lung cancer. J Clin Oncol 2008;26(21):3543–51.
4. Hanna N, Shepherd FA, Fossella FV, et al. Randomized phase III trial of pemetrexed versus docetaxel in patients with non-small-cell lung cancer previously treated with chemotherapy. J Clin Oncol 2004;22(9):1589–97.
5. Scagliotti G, Hanna N, Fossella F, et al. The differential efficacy of pemetrexed according to NSCLC histology: a review of two phase III studies. Oncologist 2009; 14(3):253–63.
6. Ciuleanu T, Brodowicz T, Zielinski C, et al. Maintenance pemetrexed plus best supportive care versus placebo plus best supportive care for non-small-cell lung cancer: a randomised, double-blind, phase 3 study. Lancet 2009;374(9699):1432–40.
7. Paz-Ares L, de Marinis F, Dediu M, et al. Maintenance therapy with pemetrexed plus best supportive care versus placebo plus best supportive care after induction therapy with pemetrexed plus cisplatin for advanced non-squamous non-small-cell lung cancer (PARAMOUNT): a double-blind, phase 3, randomised controlled trial. Lancet Oncol 2012;13(3):247–55.
8. Cappuzzo F, Ciuleanu T, Stelmakh L, et al. Erlotinib as maintenance treatment in advanced non-small-cell lung cancer: a multicentre, randomised, placebo-controlled phase 3 study. Lancet Oncol 2010;11(6):521–9.
9. Johnson BE, Kabbinavar F, Fehrenbacher L, et al. ATLAS: randomized, double-blind, placebo-controlled, phase IIIB trial comparing bevacizumab therapy with or without erlotinib, after completion of chemotherapy, with bevacizumab for first-line treatment of advanced non-small-cell lung cancer. J Clin Oncol 2013; 31(31):3926–34.
10. Perol M, Chouaid C, Perol D, et al. Randomized, phase III study of gemcitabine or erlotinib maintenance therapy versus observation, with predefined second-line treatment, after cisplatin-gemcitabine induction chemotherapy in advanced non-small-cell lung cancer. J Clin Oncol 2012;30(28):3516–24.
11. Barlesi F, Scherpereel A, Rittmeyer A, et al. Randomized phase III trial of maintenance bevacizumab with or without pemetrexed after first-line induction with bevacizumab, cisplatin, and pemetrexed in advanced nonsquamous non-small-cell lung cancer: AVAPERL (MO22089). J Clin Oncol 2013;31(24):3004–11.
12. Di Maio M, Chiodini P, Georgoulias V, et al. Meta-analysis of single-agent chemotherapy compared with combination chemotherapy as second-line treatment of advanced non-small-cell lung cancer. J Clin Oncol 2009;27(11):1836–43.
13. Qi WX, Shen Z, Yao Y. Meta-analysis of docetaxel-based doublet versus docetaxel alone as second-line treatment for advanced non-small-cell lung cancer. Cancer Chemother Pharmacol 2012;69(1):99–106.

14. Qi WX, Tang LN, He AN, et al. Effectiveness and safety of pemetrexed-based doublet versus pemetrexed alone as second-line treatment for advanced non-small-cell lung cancer: a systematic review and meta-analysis. J Cancer Res Clin Oncol 2012;138(5):745–51.
15. Shepherd FA, Dancey J, Ramlau R, et al. Prospective randomized trial of docetaxel versus best supportive care in patients with non-small-cell lung cancer previously treated with platinum-based chemotherapy. J Clin Oncol 2000;18(10): 2095–103.
16. Dancey J, Shepherd FA, Gralla RJ, et al. Quality of life assessment of second-line docetaxel versus best supportive care in patients with non-small-cell lung cancer previously treated with platinum-based chemotherapy: results of a prospective, randomized phase III trial. Lung Cancer 2004;43(2):183–94.
17. Fossella FV, DeVore R, Kerr RN, et al. Randomized phase III trial of docetaxel versus vinorelbine or ifosfamide in patients with advanced non-small-cell lung cancer previously treated with platinum-containing chemotherapy regimens. The TAX 320 non-small cell lung cancer study group. J Clin Oncol 2000;18(12): 2354–62.
18. Di Maio M, Perrone F, Chiodini P, et al. Individual patient data meta-analysis of docetaxel administered once every 3 weeks compared with once every week second-line treatment of advanced non-small-cell lung cancer. J Clin Oncol 2007;25(11):1377–82.
19. Krzakowski M, Ramlau R, Jassem J, et al. Phase III trial comparing vinflunine with docetaxel in second-line advanced non-small-cell lung cancer previously treated with platinum-containing chemotherapy. J Clin Oncol 2010;28(13):2167–73.
20. Ramlau R, Gervais R, Krzakowski M, et al. Phase III study comparing oral topotecan to intravenous docetaxel in patients with pretreated advanced non-small-cell lung cancer. J Clin Oncol 2006;24(18):2800–7.
21. Herbst RS, Sun Y, Eberhardt WE, et al. Vandetanib plus docetaxel versus docetaxel as second-line treatment for patients with advanced non-small-cell lung cancer (ZODIAC): a double-blind, randomised, phase 3 trial. Lancet Oncol 2010;11(7):619–26.
22. Reck M, Kaiser R, Mellemgaard A, et al. Docetaxel plus nintedanib versus docetaxel plus placebo in patients with previously treated non-small-cell lung cancer (LUME-Lung 1): a phase 3, double-blind, randomised controlled trial. Lancet Oncol 2014;15(2):143–55.
23. Garon EB, Ciuleanu TE, Arrieta O, et al. Ramucirumab plus docetaxel versus placebo plus docetaxel for second-line treatment of stage IV non-small-cell lung cancer after disease progression on platinum-based therapy (REVEL): a multicentre, double-blind, randomised phase 3 trial. Lancet 2014;384(9944):665–73.
24. Cullen MH, Zatloukal P, Sorenson S, et al. A randomized phase III trial comparing standard and high-dose pemetrexed as second-line treatment in patients with locally advanced or metastatic non-small-cell lung cancer. Ann Oncol 2008; 19(5):939–45.
25. Ichinose Y, Nakagawa K, Tamura T, et al. A randomized phase II study of 500 mg/m2 and 1,000 mg/m2 of pemetrexed in patients (pts) with locally advanced or metastatic non-small cell lung cancer (NSCLC) who had prior chemotherapy. J Clin Oncol 2007;25(18):S7590.
26. Hanna N. Lume-lung 2: a multicenter, randomized, double-blind, phase III study of nintedanib plus pemetrexed versus placebo plus pemetrexed in patients with advanced nonsquamous non-small cell lung cancer (NSCLC) after failure of first-line chemotherapy. 2013;31(suppl;abstr 8034).

27. de Boer RH, Arrieta O, Yang CH, et al. Vandetanib plus pemetrexed for the second-line treatment of advanced non-small-cell lung cancer: a randomized, double-blind phase III trial. J Clin Oncol 2011;29(8):1067–74.
28. Shepherd FA, Rodrigues Pereira J, Ciuleanu T, et al. Erlotinib in previously treated non-small-cell lung cancer. N Engl J Med 2005;353(2):123–32.
29. Bezjak A, Tu D, Seymour L, et al. Symptom improvement in lung cancer patients treated with erlotinib: quality of life analysis of the National Cancer Institute of Canada clinical trials group study BR.21. J Clin Oncol 2006;24(24):3831–7.
30. Ciuleanu T, Stelmakh L, Cicenas S, et al. Efficacy and safety of erlotinib versus chemotherapy in second-line treatment of patients with advanced, non-small-cell lung cancer with poor prognosis (TITAN): a randomised multicentre, open-label, phase 3 study. Lancet Oncol 2012;13(3):300–8.
31. Karampeazis A, Voutsina A, Souglakos J, et al. Pemetrexed versus erlotinib in pretreated patients with advanced non-small cell lung cancer: a Hellenic Oncology Research Group (HORG) randomized phase 3 study. Cancer 2013; 119(15):2754–64.
32. Gregorc V, Novello S, Lazzari C, et al. Predictive value of a proteomic signature in patients with non-small-cell lung cancer treated with second-line erlotinib or chemotherapy (PROSE): a biomarker-stratified, randomised phase 3 trial. Lancet Oncol 2014;15(7):713–21.
33. Garassino MC, Martelli O, Broggini M, et al. Erlotinib versus docetaxel as second-line treatment of patients with advanced non-small-cell lung cancer and wild-type EGFR tumours (TAILOR): a randomised controlled trial. Lancet Oncol 2013; 14(10):981–8.
34. Kawaguchi T, Ando M, Asami K, et al. Randomized phase III trial of erlotinib versus docetaxel as second- or third-line therapy in patients with advanced non-small-cell lung cancer: docetaxel and erlotinib lung cancer trial (DELTA). J Clin Oncol 2014;32(18):1902–8.
35. Zhao N, Zhang XC, Yan HH, et al. Efficacy of epidermal growth factor receptor inhibitors versus chemotherapy as second-line treatment in advanced non-small-cell lung cancer with wild-type EGFR: a meta-analysis of randomized controlled clinical trials. Lung Cancer 2014;85(1):66–73.
36. Kontopodis E, Hatzidaki D, Varthalitis I, et al. A phase II study of metronomic oral vinorelbine administered in the second line and beyond in non-small cell lung cancer (NSCLC): a phase II study of the Hellenic Oncology Research Group. J Chemother 2013;25(1):49–55.
37. Sculier JP, Berghmans T, Lafitte JJ, et al. A phase II study testing paclitaxel as second-line single agent treatment for patients with advanced non-small cell lung cancer failing after a first-line chemotherapy. Lung Cancer 2002;37(1):73–7.
38. Rosati G, Rossi A, Nicolella G, et al. Second-line chemotherapy with paclitaxel, cisplatin and gemcitabine in pre-treated sensitive cisplatin-based patients with advanced non-small cell lung cancer. Anticancer Res 2000;20(3b):2229–33.
39. Nakanishi Y, Takayama K, Takano K, et al. Second-line chemotherapy with weekly cisplatin and irinotecan in patients with refractory lung cancer. Am J Clin Oncol 1999;22(4):399–402.
40. Takiguchi Y, Moriya T, Asaka-Amano Y, et al. Phase II study of weekly irinotecan and cisplatin for refractory or recurrent non-small cell lung cancer. Lung Cancer 2007;58(2):253–9.
41. Crino L, Mosconi AM, Scagliotti G, et al. Gemcitabine as second-line treatment for advanced non-small-cell lung cancer: A phase II trial. J Clin Oncol 1999; 17(7):2081–5.

42. van Putten JW, Baas P, Codrington H, et al. Activity of single-agent gemcitabine as second-line treatment after previous chemotherapy or radiotherapy in advanced non-small-cell lung cancer. Lung Cancer 2001;33(2–3):289–98.

43. Hainsworth JD, Burris HA 3rd, Litchy S, et al. Gemcitabine and vinorelbine in the second-line treatment of nonsmall cell lung carcinoma patients: a Minnie Pearl Cancer Research Network phase II trial. Cancer 2000;88(6):1353–8.

Epidermal Growth Factor Receptor Mutated Advanced Non–Small Cell Lung Cancer: A Changing Treatment Paradigm

CrossMark

Suchita Pakkala, MD*, Suresh S. Ramalingam, MD

KEYWORDS

- Non–small cell lung cancer • Epidermal growth factor receptor (EGFR)
- Tyrosine kinase inhibitors (TKI) • TKI resistance • Osimertinib • Gefitinib • Erlotinib
- Afatinib

KEY POINTS

- Activating mutations in the epidermal growth factor receptor (EGFR) are present in approximately 15% of patients with lung adenocarcinoma in the United States.
- EGFR tyrosine kinase inhibitors (TKIs) are associated with high response rate and progression-free survival for patients with non–small cell lung cancer with this genotype.
- Gefitinib, erlotinib, and afatinib are the 3 approved 1st line TKIs for EGFR mutated non–small cell lung cancer (NSCLC).
- Understanding resistance mechanisms has led to the identification of a secondary mutational target, T790M, in more than half of patients, for which osimertinib, a third-generation TKI, has been developed and approved. Other resistance mechanisms besides T790M seem to be more complex because of tumor heterogeneity and multiple overlapping pathways, requiring better methods for detection and monitoring.
- This article reviews the current treatments, resistance mechanisms, and strategies to overcome resistance.

INTRODUCTION

Discovery of epidermal growth factor receptor (EGFR) sensitizing mutations in 2004 changed the treatment paradigm for advanced non–small cell lung cancer (NSCLC).[1,2] At that time, combination chemotherapy resulted in modest improvements in patient outcomes and had reached a therapeutic plateau with a median survival of approximately 8 to 10 months.[3–5] Although most patients present with advanced stage

---

Department of Hematology and Medical Oncology, Winship Cancer Institute, Emory University School of Medicine, Clifton Rd, Atlanta, GA 30322, USA
* Corresponding author. Winship Cancer Institute, Clifton Rd, Atlanta, GA 30322, USA.
E-mail address: Suchita.pakkala@emoryhealthcare.org

Hematol Oncol Clin N Am 31 (2017) 83–99
http://dx.doi.org/10.1016/j.hoc.2016.08.003
0889-8588/17/© 2016 Elsevier Inc. All rights reserved.

disease, one study of the National Cancer Database showed that 25% of all patients diagnosed with stage IV NSCLC from 2000 to 2008 did not receive any cancer-directed treatment.[6] Many of these patients who are diagnosed at a median age of 70 years have multiple comorbidities or reduced functional status and are not offered therapy because of concerns that they will not tolerate it in light of its limited benefits.

The molecular characterization of NSCLC has provided novel therapeutic targets that are amenable to targeted therapies. The development of EGFR tyrosine kinase inhibitors (TKIs) resulted from the observation that malignant cells overexpress EGFR compared with benign neighboring cells.[7] Activation of EGFR on the cell surface was found to be associated with cell proliferation, angiogenesis, invasion, metastasis, and an ability to escape apoptosis.[8] However, only 10% to 20% of unselected patients responded to EGFR TKIs after chemotherapy in initial studies.[9,10] Of these patients, east Asians, women, and never smokers with adenocarcinoma were more likely to achieve partial response with EGFR inhibitor therapy.[10,11] It was later elucidated that ~80% to 90% of these responses were related to the 2 most common activating mutations: exon 19 deletion (del 19) and exon 21 L858R point mutation, which affect the ATP (Adenosine triphosphate) EGFR binding sites.[12] Although EGFR mutated NSCLCs are exquisitely sensitive to TKIs and have led to improvements in progression-free survival (PFS) compared with standard first-line chemotherapy, patients inevitably progress.[13–19] Several resistance mechanisms have been identified, with the most common being the emergence of secondary T790M mutations and bypass pathways. In an effort to overcome resistance, second-generation/third-generation TKIs have been developed and have led to the US Food and Drug Administration (FDA) approval of the first T790M-targeted TKI, osimertinib. However, as understanding of the complexity of resistance mechanisms improves, so does the need for better techniques to detect clinically relevant targets and to treat them. This article discusses the evidence to support current clinical recommendations for EGFR mutated advanced NSCLC, emerging resistance mechanisms, and strategies to treat them.

CHARACTERISTICS OF EPIDERMAL GROWTH FACTOR RECEPTOR MUTATED SUBSETS

Adenocarcinoma of the lung is the most common subtype, representing about 50% of all NSCLCs. The US Lung Cancer Mutation Consortium showed that 64% of these patients have an oncogenic mutation, most of which are mutually exclusive.[20] EGFR represents the second most common mutation at ~15% after Kirsten rat sarcoma (KRAS), but it is the most clinically relevant because of the availability of FDA-approved targeted drugs.[21] In Asians, EGFR mutations are even more common and represent 30% to 40% of the population.[22,23] EGFR mutated NSCLC represents 40% to 60% of never smokers and 15% to 30% of former or current smokers.[22,24,25] Less than 5% of squamous cell cancers have EGFR mutations, which are more common in adenosquamous carcinomas.[21,26] Therefore, all patients with nonsquamous cancers, and never/light smokers, should have molecular profiling.

EGFR mutations are located in exons 18 to 21, which encode the ATP binding site of the tyrosine kinase domain. At present, 2 reversible ATP competitive TKIs (gefitinib, erlotinib) and 1 irreversible TKI (afatinib) are approved in the first-line setting to treat EGFR mutated NSCLC. However, not all mutations seem to have the same sensitivity to TKIs. Patients with del 19 treated with EGFR TKIs seem to have a better outcome compared with those with exon 21 mutation.[17–19,27–29] Some of the other less common EGFR mutations also seem susceptible to EGFR TKIs. The most prevalent of these rarer mutations include exon 18 (G719X), exon 19 insertions, exon 20 insertions (20 ins), de novo exon 20 T790M, exon 20 Ser768I, exon 21 (L861Q), and combined mutations.[30] In an analysis of 123 Chinese patients with NSCLC and uncommon mutations, it was noted that although TKI therapy prolonged overall survival (OS) in these patients, the PFS and overall response rate (ORR) were highest for del 19 or L858R combinations either with other mutations (9.53 months, 55%) or each other (9.79 months, 71.4%) and poor with 20 ins (2 months, 8.3%) or de novo T790M even if combined with del 19/L858R (1.94 months, 22%). T790M and most of the Exon 20 ins tend to confer resistance with poorer outcomes.[31–33] Although numerous mutations have been identified, the numbers of patients in these reports are too small to make broad statements about efficacy of TKIs for each of them.

EPIDERMAL GROWTH FACTOR RECEPTOR TYROSINE KINASE INHIBITOR MONOTHERAPY AS FIRST-LINE THERAPY

Nine randomized phase III trials have shown that EGFR TKIs surpass standard first-line platinum chemotherapy in objective response rate, PFS, and quality-of-life measures for patients with activating EGFR mutations, but have failed to show a difference in OS (**Table 1**).[13–19,34,35] The lack of OS benefit has been attributed to postprogression therapy with TKIs for patients who receive first-line chemotherapy. In these studies, OS for patients treated with a TKI ranged from 19.3 to 35.5 months. Although most of these trials evaluated patients with del 19 and L858R mutations, the IPASS ((IRESSA (gefitinib) Pan-Asia Study), NEJ002 (North-East Japan Study), LUX-LUNG 3, and LUX-LUNG 6 studies also included patients with uncommon mutations, although the proportion of these was low (~10%).

The IPASS study was the first phase III study to prospectively show the predictive role of EGFR mutations in determining therapeutic outcomes.[13] The trial enrolled 1217 east

Table 1
Phase III trials of EGFR TKIs in first-line therapy

Trial	Patient Population	N	Comparator Arms	RR (%)	PFS (mo)
			Gefitinib vs		
IPASS[13]	East Asian, EGFR mutated subgroup	261	Carboplatin/paclitaxel	71 vs 47	9.5 vs 6.3
First-SIGNAL[14]	Korean, EGFR mutated subgroup	42 (26/16)	Cisplatin/gemcitabine	85 vs 38	8 vs 6.3
WJTOG3405[15]	Japanese, EGFR mutated	172	Cisplatin/docetaxel	62 vs 32	9.2 vs 6.3
NEJ002[16]	Japanese, EGFR mutated	228	Carboplatin/paclitaxel	74 vs 31	10.8 vs 5.4
			Erlotinib vs		
OPTIMAL[17]	Chinese, EGFR mutated	154	Carboplatin/ gemcitabine	83 vs 36	13.1 vs 4.6
EURTAC[18]	European, EGFR mutated	173	Platinum/gemcitabine or docetaxel	63 vs 18	9.7 vs 5.2
ENSURE[19]	East Asian, EGFR mutated	210	Cisplatin/gemcitabine	63 vs 34	11 vs 5.5
			Afatinib vs		
LUX-Lung 3[34]	International, EGFR mutated	345	Cisplatin/pemetrexed	56 vs 23	11.1 vs 6.9
LUX-Lung 6[35]	East Asian, EGFR mutated	364	Cisplatin/gemcitabine	67 vs 23	11 vs 5.6

Abbreviation: N, number of months.

Asian patients who were light/never smokers with adenocarcinoma, 60% of whom had EGFR mutations, and randomized them to gefitinib or carboplatin/paclitaxel. Despite an initial benefit to chemotherapy, the Kaplan-Meier curves crossed and gefitinib significantly improved PFS at 12 months (25% vs 7%). The preplanned subgroup analysis revealed striking differences in the efficacy of gefitinib, with an ORR of 71% in EGFR mutated patients versus 1% in EGFR mutation–negative patients. Among patients with EGFR mutations, 95% had del 19 or L858R, and 4% had other less common mutations. In EGFR mutated patients, gefitinib prolonged PFS (9.6 vs 6.3 months; hazard ratio [HR], 0.48; P<.001), but in wild-type (wt) patients the PFS was inferior compared with chemotherapy (1.5 vs 6.5 months; HR, 2.85; P<.001). In addition, quality of life was significantly better for those who received gefitinib, with the main side effects being rash, diarrhea, and increase in liver transaminase levels compared with more nausea/vomiting, hematologic toxicities, and neuropathy in the carboplatin/paclitaxel group.

Three other east Asian phase III studies of gefitinib compared with chemotherapy showed similar results.[14–16] Though the First-Signal trial (First-line single-agent Iressa (gefitinib) versus gemcitabine and cisplatin trial in never-smokers with adenocarcinoma of the lung) also enrolled patients based on clinical characteristics, both the WJTOG 3405 (West Japan Thoracic Oncology Group) and NEJ02 included only patients with EGFR mutations. The magnitude of benefit in favor of EGFR TKIs was consistently higher regardless of whether cisplatin-based or carboplatin-based regimens were used in the comparator arm.

OPTIMAL (erlotinib vs chemotherapy in the first-line treatment of patients with advanced EGFR mutation-positive) was the first phase III study to evaluate erlotinib versus first-line chemotherapy.[17] One-hundred and fifty-four Chinese patients with either del 19 or L858R mutations were randomized to erlotinib versus carboplatin/gemcitabine and showed a significant improvement in PFS (HR, 0.16; P<.0001) in favor of erlotinib. These results were confirmed in a European patient population (EURTAC [European Tarceva (erlotinib) versus Chemotherapy]) showing that the superiority of TKIs compared with chemotherapy is not exclusive to east Asians. Similar to gefitinib, the most common adverse events (AEs) with erlotinib were rash, diarrhea, and an increase in transaminase levels.

Afatinib, a second-generation TKI, binds covalently to the EGFR and inhibits the receptor irreversibly in addition to targeting the HER2 receptors. Afatinib was compared with platinum-based chemotherapy in 2 large phase III (LUX-LUNG 3 and LUX-LUNG 6) studies of treatment-naive EGFR mutated patients.[34,35] LUX-LUNG 3 was unique in that it was the only phase III trial that compared a TKI with cisplatin/pemetrexed as a comparator arm, a regimen that is considered to be a preferred treatment option for lung adenocarcinoma.[5] At the time, maintenance chemotherapy was not allowed because it was not considered standard of care until after accrual completed. In conjunction, the LUX-LUNG 6 study randomized EGFR mutated Asian patients to afatinib or cisplatin/gemcitabine. Common side effects of afatinib included rash, diarrhea, stomatitis, and paronychia and were generally tolerable, although grade 3/4 toxicities were more frequently reported than with first-generation TKIs. Although both studies affirmed that afatinib was superior to chemotherapy in terms of ORR (56%–67% vs 23%) and PFS (11–11.1 months vs 5.6–6.9 months), there was once again no OS advantage in either study individually or combined. However, the pooled analysis of LUX-LUNG 3 and LUX-LUNG 6 showed a significant improvement in OS with afatinib compared with chemotherapy for the del 19 subgroup.[36] Although it was noted that a lower proportion of patients received subsequent therapies and may have contributed to this finding, no difference in postprogression therapy was observed between the mutation subtypes.

COMPARISON OF EPIDERMAL GROWTH FACTOR RECEPTOR TYROSINE KINASE INHIBITORS

Although direct comparisons of gefitinib, erlotinib, and afatinib in the clinic are limited, 3 meta-analyses suggested that efficacy between these agents were not significantly different.[37–39] Recently, 2 large prospective studies have added some clarity by comparing afatinib with gefitinib in treatment-naive patients and gefitinib with erlotinib as second-line therapy after chemotherapy (**Table 2**).

In an international phase IIB study, 319 EGFR mutated patients were randomized to afatinib or gefitinib and revealed significant improvements in ORR (70% vs 56%; $P = .0083$), time to treatment failure (13.7 vs 11.5 months; $P = .0073$), and PFS (11 vs 10.9 months; HR, 0.73; $P = .017$) in favor of afatinib.[40] Although median PFS was similar, the difference in PFS was more pronounced over time (47.4% vs 41.3% at 12 months and 17.6% vs 7.6% at 24 months) suggesting a more sustained response. These findings persisted irrespective of mutation subtype. Severe AEs (grade $\geq$ 3) were higher with afatinib (31% vs 17%). Diarrhea, rash, and fatigue were the most prominent for those taking afatinib as opposed to increased liver transaminase levels, rash, and interstitial lung disease (ILD) (3%) for those on gefitinib. Although afatinib showed modest improvement in outcomes compared with gefitinib, this was at the expense of increase toxicity.

The phase III study comparing gefitinib with erlotinib was initially designed as a non-inferiority trial for unselected patients in the second-line setting, and hence it did not meet its primary PFS end point (6.5 vs 7.5 months; HR, 1.125; 95% confidence interval [CI], 0.94–1.35) with an OS of 22.8 versus 24.5 months (HR, 1.04; 95% CI, 0.83–1.29).[41] Of the 516 patients enrolled, 401 had EGFR mutations and revealed a similar PFS for the 2 TKIs (8.3 vs 10 months; $P = .424$) in this subgroup. Although patients with del 19 seemed to have a longer PFS compared with patients with L858R, gefitinib and erlotinib proved equally effective in both mutation subtypes. Side effects for both drugs were manageable, but grade 3/4 increases in liver transaminase levels were more frequent with gefitinib as opposed to more frequent grade 3/4 rash with erlotinib. The incidence of ILD was similar (4%). Overall, gefitinib fared better in terms of worst grade per patient toxicity ($P<.01$). In one of the largest studies to date, gefitinib and erlotinib had comparable efficacy with a side effect profile that slightly favored gefitinib. A recent phase II study comparing gefitinib with erlotinib in EGFR mutated patients showed similar results and comparable toxicities between the two agents.[42] However, note that erlotinib significantly prolonged PFS in the subset of patients treated second line or beyond (11.4 vs 7.9 months; HR, 0.58; $P = .015$).

In a pooled analysis of 2 randomized studies, dacomitinib, a second-generation irreversible TKI, was compared with erlotinib in previously treated patients after

Table 2 Comparing EGFR TKIs					
Trial	Patient Population	N	Treatment	RR (%)	PFS (mo)
LUX-Lung 7[40]	Treatment naive, EGFR mutated	319	Afatinib vs gefitinib	70 vs 56	11 vs 10.9
WJOG 5108L[41]	Postchemotherapy, EGFR mutated subgroup	401	Erlotinib vs gefitinib	44 vs 46	10 vs 8.3
ARCHER 1009/ A7471028[43]	Pooled analysis postchemotherapy EGFR mutated subgroups	101	Dacomitinib vs erlotinib	68 vs 65	14.6 vs 9.6

chemotherapy.[43] Among the 101 patients with advanced NSCLC that had a common EGFR sensitizing mutation, PFS for dacomitinib was 14.6 months versus 9.6 months for erlotinib (HR, 0.77; P = .146). ORR was similar (67.9%; CI, 53.7%–80.1% vs 64.6%; CI, 49.5%–77.8%), but seemed to be slightly higher for those patients with del 19 treated with dacomitinib compared with patients with L858R. Dacomitinib had a higher incidence of diarrhea, paronychia, mucositis, and rash. Despite a PFS trend in favor of dacomitinib, further randomized studies are needed to evaluate its role in treatment of EGFR mutated patients. A phase II trial comparing gefitinib with erlotinib, a phase III trial comparing gefitinib with second-generation TKI (dacomitinib), and 2 phase III trials comparing third-generation TKIs (AZD9291, ASP8273) with erlotinib/gefitinib are ongoing.

ACQUIRED RESISTANCE MECHANISMS AND PREDICTIVE BIOMARKERS

Although first-line TKIs have proved effective in blocking an oncogenic addicted driver mutation, progression generally occurs at approximately 1 year in most patients. Escape mechanisms include newly acquired gatekeeper EGFR mutations (T790M), bypass pathways (MET/HER2 [MNNG HOS Transforming gene/human epidermal growth factor receptor] amplification), activation of downstream pathways (PIK3CA [phosphatidylinositol 3'-kinase], BRAF (v-raf murine sarcoma viral oncogene homolog B) mutations), and histologic transformation to small cell.[44–46] Of those who progress on a first-generation TKI, 50% to 60% have an acquired exon 20 T790M mutation that enhances EGFR's affinity for ATP more than TKIs. Although tumorigenesis may develop from an activating mutation, recent evidence suggests that, in contrast, resistance often develops from emerging subclones, which leads to more tumor heterogeneity.[47] As such, EGFR sensitizing mutations have consistently been found across biopsy sites, but detection of T790M seems more discordant.[48] Piotrowska and colleagues[49] found that T790M wt and T790M-positive clones coexisted in a pretreated specimen compared with post–TKI treatment cells that still retained their original EGFR activating mutation despite cell variability in T790M expression. Furthermore, they also noted that those patients who had higher proportions of T790M cells compared with T790Mwt on pretreatment biopsies had a better tumor response to third-generation TKIs. However, others have suggested that, in addition to subclones, drugs can still promote the development of novel T790M mutations.[50] Ultimately, it is likely that multiple mechanisms are at play within an individual, accounting for intertumor and intratumor variability, as seen when autopsy specimens were analyzed.[51]

Tumor heterogeneity can have broad clinical implications for determining the next steps in a patient's treatment and for future clinical trials. With osimertinib, a third-generation TKI now available for T790M mutated patients, it has become standard of care to rebiopsy patients on progression to determine their T790M status. However, it is clear that a single biopsy may not fully reflect the resistance mechanisms at play. Researchers have shown that detection of T790M may vary with sequential biopsies with no clear correlation with TKI therapy and can subsequently be negative despite an initial positive biopsy.[52,53] In other cases, a biopsy may not even be feasible or tissue may be inadequate for testing. Therefore, alternative noninvasive methods are being investigated in the form of circulating cell free DNA (cfDNA) and circulating tumor cells (CTCs).

cfDNA is used to detect cell fragments in the blood and hence it may be more representative of the disease burden as a whole. Recently, the cobas EGFR mutation test v2 was FDA approved to prescreen plasma for exon del 19 and L858R mutations based on the ENSURE trial (First-line erlotinib versus gemcitabine/cisplatin in patients with advanced EGFR mutation-positive), which showed a sensitivity of 77% and specificity of 98% to tissue testing.[54] A meta-analysis of 3110 patients determined that cfDNAs have a high specificity (0.96; CI, 0.93–0.98), but a moderate sensitivity (0.62; CI, 0.51–0.72) for detecting EGFR mutations compared with tissue.[55] Although the false-negative rate improved in patients with advanced-stage disease, it seemed that chemotherapy also affected its accuracy. A separate concurrent analysis of T790M detection in cfDNA, CTCs, and tissue biopsies from 40 patients who had progressed on a prior TKI showed that cfDNA and CTCs each missed 20% to 30% of the mutations.[56] However, both tests combined had an even higher rate of detection than the matched tissue biopsies, implying that multimodality testing may be warranted for a complete assessment. Such clinically relevant pretreatment differences between plasma and tissue detection of T790M were noted in patients treated with a third-generation inhibitor, rociletinib.[57] Fifty-eight percent of patients with wt T790M and 69% of patients with inadequate tissue were found to have cfDNA-positive T790M. In contrast, 19% of patients were found to have positive tissue testing that was not confirmed by cfDNA. Of those patients with urine specimens available, 68% of T790Mwt and 72% of patients with inadequate tissue were found to have urine positive for T790M, whereas 18% of patients had T790M-positive tissue testing that was not confirmed by the urine. Overall, 96% of patients were T790M positive by at least 1 method. Detection by blood or urine was better for stage IV patients who had extrathoracic metastatic disease, although the difference was only statistically significant for plasma testing. Regardless of the method of T790M detection used, the ORR (34% by tissue, and 32% by plasma, 37% by urine), duration of response (DOR) (8.7 by tissue, 7.2 by plasma, 8.7 by urine), and PFS (5 months by tissue, 4.1 months by plasma, 4.3 months by urine) were similar.

Using cfDNA as a method to monitor therapy may be just as important as initial detection of predictive biomarkers. In the FAST-ACT 2 trial (First-line Asian Sequential Tarceva (erlotinib) and Chemotherapy), cfDNA EGFR mutation–positive patients who had undetectable cfDNA mutation level after 3 cycles of chemotherapy combined with erlotinib had an improvement in PFS (12 vs 7.2 months; HR, 0.31; $P<.0001$) and OS (31.9 vs 18.2 months; HR, 0.51; $P = .0066$).[58] Other reports have not only observed similar correlations between response and plasma levels but have also noted early markers of resistance such as T790M before radiologic progression.[49,59,60] One report of cfDNAs from 57 patients revealed that suppression of activating mutations and the increase of T790M mutations correlated with response and progression, respectively.[61] Because these cfDNA platforms are now becoming widely available, its role for patient care needs to be better defined.

MANAGEMENT OF ACQUIRED RESISTANCE

Second-generation TKIs (afatinib, dacomitinib, and neratinib) were initially developed in an attempt to overcome acquired T790M resistance that arose after treatment with first-generation TKIs. Although preclinical data against T790M mutated cell lines were encouraging, dose-limiting toxicities hindered translation of those effects clinically, resulting in poor response rates in T790M-positive patients.[31,62–64]

In contrast, third-generation TKIs (osimertinib, rociletinib, olmutinib, ASP8273, EGF816) have selective activity against T790M. Osimertinib also inhibits the native exon 19 and 21 mutations. It has nearly 300-fold selectivity to the mutated EGFR compared with the wt receptor. Osimertinib received accelerated approval to treat EGFR mutated patients harboring an acquired T790M mutation after initial TKI therapy based on phase I/II data. In a pooled analysis of 411 T790M-positive patients from 2 phase II studies, the ORR was 66% (CI, 61–71), the median PFS was 11 months (CI, 9.6–12.4), the disease control rate (DCR) was 93% (CI, 84–98), and DOR of 15.3 months.[65] The most common AEs were rash (41%), diarrhea (38%), and paronychia (29%). The toxicities were generally mild, with minimal (1%) grade 3 or higher toxicity. In the phase I study, osimertinib induced an ORR of 21% in T790M-negative patients, but the median PFS was fairly short for T790M-negative patients.[66] A randomized phase 3 study that compares osimertinib with platinum-based chemotherapy in patients who develop T790M-mediated acquired resistance to EGFR TKI has completed accrual and the results are awaited. Presently osimertinib is the only approved option for the treatment of acquired resistance mediated by T790M mutation. Although the pivotal study showed objective responses at the lowest dose evaluated (20 mg/d) and good tolerability even at the highest dose evaluated (240 mg/d), the dose of 80 mg/d was chosen for further development based on the most favorable therapeutic index.

Rociletinib initially showed similar encouraging results with an ORR of 59%, but updated pooled analysis revealed a lower ORR of 28% to 34%.[67,68] Based on these findings, the FDA voted against accelerated approval and the drug company decided to halt further drug development. Another third-generation TKI, olmutinib, recently received approval in South Korea based on an ORR of 56% and DCR of 90% in the 71 patients with T790M evaluated after prior TKI.[69] ASP8273 and EGF816 are both being assessed in ongoing phase 1 studies with promising preliminary data.[70,71]

Resistance After Third-generation Tyrosine Kinase Inhibitors

Even before these third-generation inhibitors become widely available, new resistance mechanisms have been identified. As previously described, third-generation TKI-resistant cancers similarly use novel mutations (C797S, L884V, L718Q), alternate pathways (MET/HER2 amplification), and histologic transformation to small cell cancer to circumvent targeted therapies.[49,60,72,73] C797S represents the most frequent secondary resistance mutation and results in a modification in the binding site for these TKIs. However, cfDNA in 43 previously treated patients with T790M detected that multiple mechanisms are at play within an individual in up to 46% of cases.[74] Hence, these resistant cancer cells seem to be temporally adaptive to selective pressures in the form of TKI therapy. Tumor heterogeneity and multiple parallel resistance pathways may explain observations that T790M expression can be lost in the course of third-generation TKI therapy in some patients, but not in others.[75,76] Although in these 2 reported cases suppression of T790M was associated with response, resistance correlated with an increase in T790M levels in conjunction with the original activating mutation in 1 case and an increase in the initial activating mutation without T790M in the other. An MET amplification was identified in the second case, further showing the complexity of resistance and highlighting the challenges in overcoming it.

Tyrosine Kinase Inhibitors Continued Beyond Progression

Optimization of available therapies is a constant goal for patient care. As such, it is a challenge to determine when patients who may be deriving ongoing clinical benefit need to switch to another therapy in the setting of slight radiologic progression. In the case of TKIs, stopping therapy has been linked to tumor regrowth with response on reintroduction, all within 6 weeks, signifying that the cancer remains sensitive to TKIs.[77] In light of this, the ASPIRATION (Asian Pacific trial of Tarceva (erlotinib) as first-line in EGFR mutation Trial) trial sought to prospectively evaluate treatment of erlotinib beyond progression in 207 EGFR mutated patients.[78] Fifty-two percent of patients who progressed were able to continue therapy for a median of 3.1 additional months irrespective of mutational subtype. Patients who responded to erlotinib initially had a longer PFS with continued treatment. Although this is feasible in clinical practice, the study had inherent selection biases because the patients were selected at the investigators' discretion, hence leaving no clear guidelines on which patients may benefit the most from such a strategy. However, a retrospective study of 42 patients with activating mutations revealed that longer time to progression, slower tumor growth, and lack of new lesions outside the thorax were associated with increased time to treatment change.[79] In addition, another study showed that patients who survived 5 years on a TKI therapy were more likely to have del 19, disease limited to the chest, or the absence of brain metastasis.[80] Local therapies have also successfully been used to extend the duration of therapy, as was seen in a data set of patients who progressed with nonleptomeningeal disease and/or less than or equal to 4 extracranial sites.[81] These patients were able to continue therapy for a median of 6.2 months longer. Therefore, it can be reasonable to consider continued therapy beyond progression in select cases.

Despite increasing therapeutic options, the use of chemotherapy in EGFR mutated patients is still relevant for those who are T790M negative or have progressed beyond a second-line TKI. When patients have clear progressive disease, the question then becomes whether to continue a TKI in addition to chemotherapy. This question was addressed in the IMPRESS trial (Iressa (gefitinib) Mutation Positive Multicentre Treatment beyond Progression Study), which randomized patients with NSCLC who progressed after at least 4 months on gefitinib to cisplatin/pemetrexed for 6 cycles with or without continued gefitinib.[82] The study accrued 265 patients internationally and found no difference in DCR (84.2% vs 78.2%; $P = .31$) or median PFS (5.4 vs 5.4 months) for gefitinib versus chemotherapy alone. Preliminary results indicated a trend toward worse OS (14.8 vs 17.2 months) with gefitinib, but this was attributed in part to a higher number of patients with brain metastases, lower rates of complete responses to first-line therapy, and lower exposure to subsequent TKIs and doublet chemotherapy postprogression in the gefitinib arm. However, a subset analysis revealed that the 43% of T790M-negative patients by cfDNA had significant PFS benefit with gefitinib (6.7 vs 5.4 months; HR, 0.67; $P = .07$), indicating a possible role for continuing a TKI in conjunction with the addition of chemotherapy beyond progression.[83]

Combination Therapy

It is becoming increasing clear that drugs such as TKIs that are effective in selectively targeting an oncogenic addicted pathway provide subclones the opportunity to escape inhibition while simultaneously exerting pressure toward alternative pathways. Hence the growing interest in combination therapies to potentially delay resistance. Platinum chemotherapy combined with first-generation TKIs has proved ineffective in unselected treatment-naive patients in the INTACT1, INTACT2 (The Iressa (gefitinib) NSCLC Trial Assessing Combination Treatment), TRIBUTE (Tarceva (erlotinib) Responses in Conjunction with Paclitaxel and Carboplatin), and TALENT trials (Tarceva (erlotinib) Lung Cancer Investigation Trial).[84–87] However, a meta-analysis of 7 randomized trials found that both EGFR mutated (HR, 0.48; $P = .009$) and EGFR mutation–negative (HR, 0.84; $P = .02$) patients had a PFS benefit with a slight benefit noted in the EGFR mutated compared with nonmutated patients ($P = .05$), but no improvement in OS.[88] Although this implies that EGFR mutated patients may delay disease progression, this is often at the cost of added toxicity without a clear improvement in long-term outcomes. So the question remains as to whether combination therapy is better than sequential treatment overall. Subset analysis of the FAST-ACT 2 study of carboplatin/gemcitabine with or without intercalated erlotinib (days 15–28) followed by maintenance erlotinib showed a prolonged median OS (31.4 vs 20.6 months; HR, 0.48; P = .0092) in favor of the combination only for those with EGFR sensitizing mutations.[89] A randomized phase II study supported this strategy of concurrent treatment rather than alternating sequential gefitinib with first-line chemotherapy in EGFR mutated patients. Despite immature data and an equal ORR, OS was 41.9 and 30.7 months (HR, 0.51; P = .042), respectively.[90] In addition, another study randomized 121 patients to either combined carboplatin/pemetrexed plus gefitinib for 6 cycles followed by pemetrexed/gefitinib maintenance, chemotherapy followed by pemetrexed maintenance, or gefitinib alone. ORR and median PFS for the combination were 82.5% and 18.8 months, respectively, compared with 32.5% and 5.75 months for chemotherapy or 65.9% and 12 months for gefitinib alone.[91] Taken together, the value of the addition of chemotherapy with TKIs in the first-line setting is not conclusively proved and it cannot be recommended.

Combinations with antiangiogenesis and dual EGFR inhibition are currently being evaluated in an effort to overcome resistance. Erlotinib and bevacizumab, an angiogenic inhibitor, was active as first-line therapy in a randomized phase 2 study of 154 patients with EGFR mutation resulting in a median PFS of 16 months compared with 9.7 months with erlotinib alone (HR, 0.54; P = .0015).[92] Side effects were as expected, with hypertension and proteinuria being more common in the bevacizumab arm. This regimen was recently approved for first-line therapy for EGFR mutated patients with NSCLC in Europe. A prospective study is presently underway to verify the efficacy of this combination in the United States. In a phase 1b study, afatinib plus the anti-EGFR antibody, cetuximab proved effective in patients with an ORR of 29% and median PFS of 4.7 months regardless of T790M status in previously treated patients who received at least first-generation TKIs.[93] However, 44% developed grade 3/4 AEs and 36% required dose reductions. In addition, preliminary data seem encouraging for TKI-immunotherapy combinations with 60% DCR and some showing durable responses.[94] Although combined MET inhibition is currently in early trials, remarkable responses have been documented in case reports of patients with MET amplification.[95]

FUTURE DIRECTIONS

Although EGFR inhibitors are effective for the treatment of patients with advanced-stage NSCLC, their role in earlier stages of the disease is still unproved. A phase 2 study by the NRG Oncology Group will evaluate the efficacy of erlotinib in patients with stage III locally advanced NSCLC with an EGFR mutation. The ALCHEMIST (The Adjuvant Lung Cancer Enrichment Marker Identification and Sequencing Trials) study is currently evaluating the role of erlotinib in patients with surgically resected early stage NSCLC after adjuvant chemotherapy in the presence of EGFR activating mutation.

In a cohort of 60 EGFR mutated patients treated with front-line osimertinib, 77% achieved a response with a median PFS of 19.3 months and DOR of 16.7 months when taking the 160-mg dose (N = 30).[96] Median PFS and DOR were not yet reached for the patients on the 80-mg dose (N = 30). Of the 5 patients with a de novo T790 mutation, DOR ranged from 12.2 to 20.7 months. Based on these results, osimertinib is being compared with erlotinib/gefitinib in an ongoing phase 3 study. Osimertinib is also being studied as adjuvant therapy in early-stage NSCLC. In addition, several other novel third-generation EGFR TKIs are also under development. Recent reports have already suggested the development of tertiary C797S mutations as a potential mechanism of resistance to third-generation EGFR inhibitors. Strategies to overcome this new mechanism of resistance are being studied. From these developments, it is clear that the EGFR mutated NSCLC landscape is moving ahead rapidly.

SUMMARY

The discovery of EGFR sensitizing mutations has revolutionized treatment of a subset of patients with NSCLC who are now able to take a well-tolerated oral TKI (gefitinib, erlotinib, afatinib) with a significant improvement in PFS compared with chemotherapy. Although afatinib has proved slightly more effective, it also has the most side effects, and gefitinib is generally the best tolerated drug that is approved in the first-line setting. However, resistance occurs in most patients within a year because of secondary mutations such as T790M and alternative activation pathways. Some patients with limited slowly progressive disease may still benefit from continuing the same TKI and locoregional therapies as needed. The recent approval of osimertinib has provided patients with a second-line option against T790M mutated NSCLC. For those who are T790M negative or progress on a third-generation TKI, chemotherapy is still recommended outside a clinical trial. However, as the understanding of resistance evolves so does the awareness of underlying tumor heterogeneity and the need for more representative tumor assessments. Whether cfDNAs will provide a more comprehensive assessment for diagnosis and therapeutic guidance is yet to be seen. In the meantime, repeat tissue testing remains the gold standard and therapies should be directed toward available pathways of resistance whenever possible. As such, clinical trials are currently evaluating combination therapies as a possible option to target multiple resistance pathways. As treatment options improve, further investigation will help define standard guidelines for monitoring disease progression and the use of EGFR-directed therapies.

REFERENCES

1. Lynch TJ, Bell DW, Sordella R, et al. Activating mutations in the epidermal growth factor receptor underlying responsiveness of non–small-cell lung cancer to gefitinib. N Engl J Med 2004;350(21):2129–39.
2. Paez JG, Jänne PA, Lee JC, et al. EGFR mutations in lung cancer: correlation with clinical response to gefitinib therapy. Science 2004;304(5676):1497–500.
3. Schiller JH, Harrington D, Belani CP, et al. Comparison of four chemotherapy regimens for advanced non–small-cell lung cancer. N Engl J Med 2002;346(2):92–8.
4. Scagliotti GV, De Marinis F, Rinaldi M, et al. Phase III randomized trial comparing three platinum-based doublets in advanced non–small-cell lung cancer. J Clin Oncol 2002;20(21):4285–91.
5. Scagliotti GV, Parikh P, von Pawel J, et al. Phase III study comparing cisplatin plus gemcitabine with cisplatin plus pemetrexed in chemotherapy-naive patients with advanced-stage non–small-cell lung cancer. J Clin Oncol 2008;26(21):3543–51.
6. Small AC, Tsao CK, Moshier EL, et al. Prevalence and characteristics of patients with metastatic cancer who receive no anticancer therapy. Cancer 2012;118(23):5947–54.
7. Rusch V, Baselga J, Cordon-Cardo C, et al. Differential expression of the epidermal growth factor receptor and its ligands in primary non-small cell lung cancers and adjacent benign lung. Cancer Res 1993;53(10):2379–85.
8. Mendelsohn J. Blockade of receptors for growth factors: an anticancer therapy — the Fourth Annual Joseph H. Burchenal American Association for Cancer Research Clinical Research Award Lecture. Clin Cancer Res 2000;6(3):747–53.

9. Kris MG, Natale RB, Herbst RS, et al. Efficacy of gefitinib, an inhibitor of the epidermal growth factor receptor tyrosine kinase, in symptomatic patients with non–small cell lung cancer: a randomized trial. JAMA 2003;290(16):2149–58.

10. Fukuoka M, Yano S, Giaccone G, et al. Multi-institutional randomized phase II trial of gefitinib for previously treated patients with advanced non–small-cell lung cancer. J Clin Oncol 2003;21(12):2237–46.

11. Miller VA, Kris MG, Shah N, et al. Bronchioloalveolar pathologic subtype and smoking history predict sensitivity to gefitinib in advanced non–small-cell lung cancer. J Clin Oncol 2004;22(6):1103–9.

12. Sharma SV, Bell DW, Settleman J, et al. Epidermal growth factor receptor mutations in lung cancer. Nat Rev Cancer 2007;7(3):169–81.

13. Mok TS, Wu YL, Thongprasert S, et al. Gefitinib or carboplatin–paclitaxel in pulmonary adenocarcinoma. N Engl J Med 2009;361(10):947–57.

14. Han JY, Park K, Kim SW, et al. First-SIGNAL: First-line Single-agent Iressa versus Gemcitabine and Cisplatin Trial in never-smokers with adenocarcinoma of the lung. J Clin Oncol 2012;30(10):1122–8.

15. Mitsudomi T, Morita S, Yatabe Y, et al. Gefitinib versus cisplatin plus docetaxel in patients with non-small-cell lung cancer harbouring mutations of the epidermal growth factor receptor (WJTOG3405): an open label, randomised phase 3 trial. Lancet Oncol 2010;11(2):121–8.

16. Maemondo M, Inoue A, Kobayashi K, et al. Gefitinib or chemotherapy for non–small-cell lung cancer with mutated EGFR. N Engl J Med 2010;362(25):2380–8.

17. Zhou C, Wu YL, Chen G, et al. Erlotinib versus chemotherapy as first-line treatment for patients with advanced EGFR mutation-positive non-small-cell lung cancer (OPTIMAL, CTONG-0802): a multicentre, open-label, randomised, phase 3 study. Lancet Oncol 2011;12(8):735–42.

18. Rosell R, Carcereny E, Gervais R, et al. Erlotinib versus standard chemotherapy as first-line treatment for European patients with advanced EGFR mutation-positive non-small-cell lung cancer (EURTAC): a multicentre, open-label, randomised phase 3 trial. Lancet Oncol 2012;13(3):239–46.

19. Wu YL, Zhou C, Liam CK, et al. First-line erlotinib versus gemcitabine/cisplatin in patients with advanced EGFR mutation-positive non-small-cell lung cancer: analyses from the phase III, randomized, open-label, ENSURE study. Ann Oncol 2015;26(9):1883–9.

20. Kris MG, Johnson BE, Berry LD, et al. Using multiplexed assays of oncogenic drivers in lung cancers to select targeted drugs. JAMA 2014;311(19):1998–2006.

21. Dearden S, Stevens J, Wu YL, et al. Mutation incidence and coincidence in non small-cell lung cancer: meta-analyses by ethnicity and histology (mutMap). Ann Oncol 2013;24(9):2371–6.

22. Shi Y, Au JS, Thongprasert S, et al. A prospective, molecular epidemiology study of EGFR mutations in Asian patients with advanced non–small-cell lung cancer of adenocarcinoma histology (PIONEER). J Thorac Oncol 2014;9(2):154–62.

23. Han B, Tjulandin S, Hagiwara K, et al. Determining the prevalence of EGFR mutations in Asian and Russian patients (PTS) with advanced non-small-cell lung cancer (ANSCLC) of adenocarcinoma (ADC) and non-ADC histology: IGNITE Study. Ann Oncol 2015;26(Suppl 1):i29–30 [abstract: 9055].

24. Dogan S, Shen R, Ang DC, et al. Molecular epidemiology of EGFR and KRAS mutations in 3,026 lung adenocarcinomas: higher susceptibility of women to smoking-related KRAS-mutant cancers. Clin Cancer Res 2012;18(22):6169–77.

25. Ou SH. Lung cancer in never-smokers. Does smoking history matter in the era of molecular diagnostics and targeted therapy? J Clin Pathol 2013;66(10):839–46.

26. Toyooka S, Yatabo Y, Tokumo M, et al. Mutations of epidermal growth factor receptor and K-ras genes in adenosquamous carcinoma of the lung. Int J Cancer 2006;118(6):1588–90.
27. Riely GJ, Pao W, Pham D, et al. Clinical course of patients with non–small cell lung cancer and epidermal growth factor receptor exon 19 and exon 21 mutations treated with gefitinib or erlotinib. Clin Cancer Res 2006;12(3):839–44.
28. Jackman DM, Yeap BY, Sequist LV, et al. Exon 19 deletion mutations of epidermal growth factor receptor are associated with prolonged survival in non–small cell lung cancer patients treated with gefitinib or erlotinib. Clin Cancer Res 2006; 12(13):3908–14.
29. Lee CK, Wu YL, Ding PN, et al. Impact of specific epidermal growth factor receptor (EGFR) mutations and clinical characteristics on outcomes after treatment with EGFR tyrosine kinase inhibitors versus chemotherapy in EGFR-mutant lung cancer: a meta-analysis. J Clin Oncol 2015;33(17):1958–65.
30. Xu J, Jin B, Chu T, et al. EGFR tyrosine kinase inhibitor (TKI) in patients with advanced non-small cell lung cancer (NSCLC) harboring uncommon EGFR mutations: a real-world study in China. Lung Cancer 2016;96:87–92.
31. Yang JC, Sequist LV, Geater SL, et al. Clinical activity of afatinib in patients with advanced non-small-cell lung cancer harbouring uncommon EGFR mutations: a combined post-hoc analysis of LUX-Lung 2, LUX-Lung 3, and LUX-Lung 6. Lancet Oncol 2015;16(7):830–8.
32. Yasuda H, Park E, Yun CH, et al. Structural, biochemical, and clinical characterization of epidermal growth factor receptor (EGFR) exon 20 insertion mutations in lung cancer. Sci Transl Med 2013;5(216):216ra177.
33. Klughammer B, Brugger W, Cappuzzo F, et al. Examining treatment outcomes with erlotinib in patients with advanced non–small cell lung cancer whose tumors harbor uncommon EGFR mutations. J Thorac Oncol 2016;11(4):545–55.
34. Sequist LV, Yang JC, Yamamoto N, et al. Phase III study of afatinib or cisplatin plus pemetrexed in patients with metastatic lung adenocarcinoma with EGFR mutations. J Clin Oncol 2013;31(27):3327–34.
35. Wu YL, Zhou C, Hu CP, et al. Afatinib versus cisplatin plus gemcitabine for first-line treatment of Asian patients with advanced non-small-cell lung cancer harbouring EGFR mutations (LUX-Lung 6): an open-label, randomised phase 3 trial. Lancet Oncol 2014;15(2):213–22.
36. Yang JC, Wu YL, Schuler M, et al. Afatinib versus cisplatin-based chemotherapy for EGFR mutation-positive lung adenocarcinoma (LUX-Lung 3 and LUX-Lung 6): analysis of overall survival data from two randomised, phase 3 trials. Lancet Oncol 2015;16(2):141–51.
37. Haaland B, Tan PS, de Castro G Jr, et al. Meta-analysis of first-line therapies in advanced non-small-cell lung cancer harboring EGFR-activating mutations. J Thorac Oncol 2014;9(6):805–11.
38. Haspinger ER, Agustoni F, Torri V, et al. Is there evidence for different effects among EGFR-TKIs? Systematic review and meta-analysis of EGFR tyrosine kinase inhibitors (TKIs) versus chemotherapy as first-line treatment for patients harboring EGFR mutations. Crit Rev Oncol Hematol 2015;94(2):213–27.
39. Popat S, Mok T, Yang JC, et al. Afatinib in the treatment of EGFR mutation-positive NSCLC - a network meta-analysis. Lung Cancer 2014;85(2):230–8.
40. Park K, Tan EH, O'Byrne K, et al. Afatinib versus gefitinib as first-line treatment of patients with EGFR mutation-positive non-small-cell lung cancer (LUX-Lung 7): a phase 2B, open-label, randomised controlled trial. Lancet Oncol 2016;17(5): 577–89.

41. Urata Y, Katakami N, Morita S, et al. Randomized phase III study comparing gefitinib with erlotinib in patients with previously treated advanced lung adenocarcinoma: WJOG 5108L. J Clin Oncol 2016;34(27):3248–57.
42. Yang JJ, Zhou Q, Yan H, et al. A randomized controlled trial of erlotinib versus gefitinib in advanced non-small cell lung cancer harboring EGFR mutations (CTONG0901). J Thorac Oncol 2015;9(S2).
43. Ramalingam SS, O'Byrne K, Boyer M, et al. Dacomitinib versus erlotinib in patients with EGFR-mutated advanced nonsmall-cell lung cancer (NSCLC): pooled subset analyses from two randomized trials. Ann Oncol 2016;27(3):423–9.
44. Sequist LV, Waltman BA, Dias-Santagata D, et al. Genotypic and histological evolution of lung cancers acquiring resistance to EGFR inhibitors. Sci Transl Med 2011;3(75):75ra26.
45. Yu HA, Arcila ME, Rekhtman N, et al. Analysis of tumor specimens at the time of acquired resistance to EGFR-TKI therapy in 155 patients with EGFR-mutant lung cancers. Clin Cancer Res 2013;19(8):2240–7.
46. Ohashi K, Sequist LV, Arcila ME, et al. Lung cancers with acquired resistance to EGFR inhibitors occasionally harbor BRAF gene mutations but lack mutations in KRAS, NRAS, or MEK1. Proc Natl Acad Sci U S A 2012;109(31):E2127–33.
47. Vignot S, Frampton GM, Soria JC, et al. Next-generation sequencing reveals high concordance of recurrent somatic alterations between primary tumor and metastases from patients with non-small-cell lung cancer. J Clin Oncol 2013;31:2167–72.
48. Sherwood J, Dearden S, Ratcliffe M, et al. Mutation status concordance between primary lesions and metastatic sites of advanced non-small-cell lung cancer and the impact of mutation testing methodologies: a literature review. J Exp Clin Cancer Res 2015;34(1):1–18.
49. Piotrowska Z, Niederst MJ, Karlovich CA, et al. Heterogeneity underlies the emergence of EGFRT790 wild-type clones following treatment of T790M-positive cancers with a third-generation EGFR inhibitor. Cancer Discov 2015;5(7):713–22.
50. Hata AN, Niederst MJ, Archibald HL, et al. Tumor cells can follow distinct evolutionary paths to become resistant to epidermal growth factor receptor inhibition. Nat Med 2016;22(3):262–9.
51. Suda K, Murakami I, Katayama T, et al. Reciprocal and complementary role of MET amplification and EGFR T790M mutation in acquired resistance to kinase inhibitors in lung cancer. Clin Cancer Res 2010;16(22):5489–98.
52. Piotrowska Z, Niederst MJ, Mino-Kenudso M, et al. Variation in mechanisms of acquired resistance among EGFR-mutant NSCLC patients with more than 1 postresistant biopsy. Int J Radiat Oncol Biol Phys 2014;90(5):S6–7.
53. Kuiper JL, Heideman DA, Thunnissen E, et al. Incidence of T790M mutation in (sequential) rebiopsies in EGFR-mutated NSCLC-patients. Lung Cancer 2014; 85(1):19–24.
54. cobas EGFR mutation test v2. Approved drugs. Available at: http://www.fda.gov/Drugs/InformationOnDrugs/ApprovedDrugs/ucm504540.htm. Accessed July 31, 2016.
55. Qiu M, Wang J, Xu Y, et al. Circulating tumor DNA is effective for the detection of EGFR mutation in non-small cell lung cancer: a meta-ANALYSIS. Cancer Epidemiol Biomarkers Prev 2015;24(1):206–12.
56. Sundaresan TK, Sequist LV, Heymach JV, et al. Detection of T790M, the acquired resistance EGFR mutation, by tumor biopsy versus noninvasive blood-based analyses. Clin Cancer Res 2016;22(5):1103–10.
57. Wakelee HA, Gadgeel SM, Goldman JW, et al. Epidermal growth factor receptor (EGFR) genotyping of matched urine, plasma and tumor tissue from non-small

cell lung cancer (NSCLC) patients (pts) treated with rociletinib. J Clin Oncol 2016; 34(15 Suppl).

58. Mok T, Wu YL, Lee JS, et al. Detection and dynamic changes of EGFR mutations from circulating tumor DNA as a predictor of survival outcomes in NSCLC patients treated with first-line intercalated erlotinib and chemotherapy. Clin Cancer Res 2015;21(14):3196–203.

59. Oxnard GR, Paweletz CP, Kuang Y, et al. Noninvasive detection of response and resistance in EGFR-mutant lung cancer using quantitative next-generation genotyping of cell-free plasma DNA. Clin Cancer Res 2014;20(6):1698–705.

60. Thress KS, Paweletz CP, Felip E, et al. Acquired EGFR C797S mutation mediates resistance to AZD9291 in non-small cell lung cancer harboring EGFR T790M. Nat Med 2015;21(6):560–2.

61. Uchida J, Imamura F, Kukita Y, et al. Dynamics of circulating tumor DNA represented by the activating and resistant mutations in epidermal growth factor receptor tyrosine kinase inhibitor treatment. Cancer Sci 2016;107(3):353–8.

62. Katakami N, Atagi S, Goto K, et al. LUX-Lung 4: a phase II trial of afatinib in patients with advanced non–small-cell lung cancer who progressed during prior treatment with erlotinib, gefitinib, or both. J Clin Oncol 2013;31(27):3335–41.

63. Reckamp KL, Giaccone G, Camidge DR, et al. A phase 2 trial of dacomitinib (PF-00299804), an oral, irreversible pan-HER (human epidermal growth factor receptor) inhibitor, in patients with advanced non–small cell lung cancer after failure of prior chemotherapy and erlotinib. Cancer 2014;120(8):1145–54.

64. Sequist LV, Besse B, Lynch TJ, et al. Neratinib, an irreversible Pan-ErbB receptor tyrosine kinase inhibitor: results of a phase II trial in patients with advanced non-small-cell lung cancer. J Clin Oncol 2010;28(18):3076–83.

65. Yang JC, Ramalingam S, Janne PA, et al. Osimertinib (AZD 9291) in pre-treated pts with T790M-positive advanced NSCLC: updated phase 1 (p1) and pooled phase 2 (p2) results. in 2016 European Lung Cancer Conference. Geneva (Switzerland), 2016.

66. Jänne PA, Yang JC, Kim DW, et al. AZD9291 in EGFR inhibitor–resistant non–small-cell lung cancer. N Engl J Med 2015;372(18):1689–99.

67. Sequist LV, Soria JC, Goldman JW, et al. Rociletinib in EGFR-mutated non–small-cell lung cancer. N Engl J Med 2015;372(18):1700–9.

68. Dhingra K. Rociletinib: has the TIGER lost a few of its stripes? Ann Oncol 2016; 27(6):1161–4.

69. Park K, Lee JS, Lee KH, et al. BI 1482694 (HM61713), an EGFR mutant-specific inhibitor, in T790M+ NSCLC: efficacy and safety at the RP2D. J Clin Oncol 2016; 34(Suppl) [abstract: 9055].

70. Yu HA, Oxnard GR, Spira AI, et al. Phase I dose escalation study of ASP8273, a mutant-selective irreversible EGFR inhibitor, in subjects with EGFR mutation positive NSCLC. J Clin Oncol 2015;33(15 Suppl).

71. Daniel Shao-Weng Tan TS, Leighl NB, Riley GJ, et al. First-in-human phase I study of EGF816, a third generation, mutant-selective EGFR tyrosine kinase inhibitor, in advanced non-small cell lung cancer (NSCLC) harboring T790M. J Clin Oncol 2015;33(Suppl) [abstract: 8013].

72. Ercan D, Choi HG, Yun CH, et al. EGFR mutations and resistance to irreversible pyrimidine-based EGFR inhibitors. Clin Cancer Res 2015;21(17):3913–23.

73. Planchard D, Loriot Y, André F, et al. EGFR-independent mechanisms of acquired resistance to AZD9291 in EGFR T790M-positive NSCLC patients. Ann Oncol 2015;26(10):2073–8.

74. Chabon JJ, Simmons AD, Lovejoy AF, et al. Circulating tumour DNA profiling reveals heterogeneity of EGFR inhibitor resistance mechanisms in lung cancer patients. Nat Commun 2016;7:11815.

75. Kim TM, Song A, Kim DW, et al. Mechanisms of acquired resistance to AZD9291: a mutation-selective, irreversible EGFR inhibitor. J Thorac Oncol 2015;10(12): 1736–44.

76. Chia PL, Do H, Morey A, et al. Temporal changes of EGFR mutations and T790M levels in tumour and plasma DNA following AZD9291 treatment. Lung Cancer 2016;98:29–32.

77. Riely GJ, Kris MG, Zhao B, et al. Prospective assessment of discontinuation and reinitiation of erlotinib or gefitinib in patients with acquired resistance to erlotinib or gefitinib followed by the addition of everolimus. Clin Cancer Res 2007;13(17): 5150–5.

78. Park K, Yu CJ, Kim SW, et al. First-line erlotinib therapy until and beyond response evaluation criteria in solid tumors progression in Asian patients with epidermal growth factor receptor mutation–positive non–small-cell lung cancer: the ASPIRATION study. JAMA Oncol 2016;2(3):305–12.

79. Lo PC, Dahlberg SE, Nishino M, et al. Delay of treatment change after objective progression on first-line erlotinib in epidermal growth factor receptor-mutant lung cancer. Cancer 2015;121(15):2570–7.

80. Lin JJ, Cardarella S, Lydon CA, et al. Five-year survival in EGFR-mutant metastatic lung adenocarcinoma treated with EGFR-TKIs. J Thorac Oncol 2016;11(4): 556–65.

81. Weickhardt AJ, Scheier B, Burke JM, et al. Local ablative therapy of oligoprogressive disease prolongs disease control by tyrosine kinase inhibitors in oncogene addicted non-small cell lung cancer. J Thorac Oncol 2012;7(12):1807–14.

82. Soria JC, Wu YL, Nakagawa K, et al. Gefitinib plus chemotherapy versus placebo plus chemotherapy in EGFR-mutation-positive non-small-cell lung cancer after progression on first-line gefitinib (IMPRESS): a phase 3 randomised trial. Lancet Oncol 2015;16(8):990–8.

83. Soria J, Kim S, Wu Y, et al. Gefitinib/chemotherapy vs chemotherapy in EGFR mutation-positive NSCLC resistant to first-line gefitinib: IMPRESS T790M subgroup analysis in WLCL. 2015. Denver (CO).

84. Giaccone G, Herbst RS, Manegold C, et al. Gefitinib in combination with gemcitabine and cisplatin in advanced non–small-cell lung cancer: a phase III trial— INTACT 1. J Clin Oncol 2004;22(5):777–84.

85. Herbst RS, Giaccone G, Schiller JH, et al. Gefitinib in combination with paclitaxel and carboplatin in advanced non–small-cell lung cancer: a phase III trial— INTACT 2. J Clin Oncol 2004;22(5):785–94.

86. Herbst RS, Prager D, Hermann R, et al. TRIBUTE: a phase III trial of erlotinib hydrochloride (OSI-774) combined with carboplatin and paclitaxel chemotherapy in advanced non–small-cell lung cancer. J Clin Oncol 2005;23(25):5892–9.

87. Gatzemeier U, Pluzanska A, Szczesna A, et al. Phase III study of erlotinib in combination with cisplatin and gemcitabine in advanced non–small-cell lung cancer: the Tarceva Lung Cancer Investigation Trial. J Clin Oncol 2007;25(12):1545–52.

88. OuYang PY, Su Z, Mao YP, et al. Combination of EGFR-TKIs and chemotherapy as first-line therapy for advanced NSCLC: a meta-analysis. PLoS One 2013; 8(11):e79000.

89. Wu YL, Lee JS, Thongprasert S, et al. Intercalated combination of chemotherapy and erlotinib for patients with advanced stage non-small-cell lung cancer (FASTACT-2): a randomised, double-blind trial. Lancet Oncol 2013;14(8):777–86.

90. Sugawara S, Oizumi S, Minato K, et al. Randomized phase II study of concurrent versus sequential alternating gefitinib and chemotherapy in previously untreated non-small cell lung cancer with sensitive EGFR mutations: NEJ005/TCOG0902. Ann Oncol 2015;26(5):888–94.

91. Han B, Jin B, Zhang Y, et al. 1310: combination of chemotherapy and gefitinib as first-line treatment of patients with advanced lung adenocarcinoma and sensitive EGFR mutations: a randomised controlled trial. J Thorac Oncol 2016;11(4 Suppl): S113–4.

92. Seto T, Kato T, Nishio M, et al. Erlotinib alone or with bevacizumab as first-line therapy in patients with advanced non-squamous non-small-cell lung cancer harbouring EGFR mutations (JO25567): an open-label, randomised, multicentre, phase 2 study. Lancet Oncol 2014;15(11):1236–44.

93. Janjigian YY, Smit EF, Groen HJ, et al. Dual inhibition of EGFR with afatinib and cetuximab in kinase inhibitor–resistant EGFR-mutant lung cancer with and without T790M mutations. Cancer Discov 2014;4(9):1036–45.

94. Rizvi NA, Man Chow LQ, Borghaei H, et al. Safety and response with nivolumab (anti-PD-1; BMS-936558, ONO-4538) plus erlotinib in patients (pts) with epidermal growth factor receptor mutant (EGFR MT) advanced NSCLC. J Clin Oncol 2014;32(5 Suppl) [abstract: 8022].

95. Gainor JF, Niederst MJ, Lennerz JK, et al. Dramatic response to combination erlotinib and crizotinib in a patient with advanced, EGFR-mutant lung cancer harboring De Novo MET amplification. J Thorac Oncol 2016;11(7):e83–5.

96. Ramalingam S, Yang JC, Lee CK, et al. Osimertinib as first-line treatment for EGFR mutation-positive advanced NSCLC: updated efficacy and safety results from two phase I expansion cohorts. in European Lung Cancer Conference. Geneva (Switzerland). JTO 2016;11(4):S152.

Diagnosis and Treatment of Anaplastic Lymphoma Kinase–Positive Non–Small Cell Lung Cancer

CrossMark

Kathryn C. Arbour, MD[a], Gregory J. Riely, MD, PhD[b],*

KEYWORDS

- EML4-ALK rearrangement • Non–small cell lung cancer (NSCLC)
- Anaplastic lymphoma kinase inhibitors (ALK inhibitors) • Crizotinib • Ceritinb
- Alectinib

KEY POINTS

- Anaplastic lymphoma kinase (ALK) rearrangements occur in approximately 5% of patients diagnosed with non–small cell lung cancer, are more frequently found in patients with no significant smoking history, and can be identified with routine testing (fluorescence in situ hybridization, immunohistochemistry, or next-generation sequencing).
- Crizotinib, the first-available ALK inhibitor, is superior to chemotherapy as both initial treatment and for patients who have progressed following platinum-doublet therapy.
- Resistance to crizotinib develops after a median of 8 to 11 months with numerous resistance mechanisms identified.
- Ceritinib and alectinib are second-generation ALK inhibitors that have been approved for patients who have become resistant to or are intolerant of crizotinib.
- Additional ALK inhibitors are currently in clinical development.

INTRODUCTION

Fusions of the echinoderm microtubule-associated protein-like 4 (EML4) gene and the anaplastic lymphoma kinase (ALK) gene were first identified as a likely molecular driver in patients with non–small cell lung cancer (NSCLC) in 2007.[1] These rearrangements are observed in approximately 5% of NSCLC. At the time of the discovery of EML4-ALK fusions, crizotinib, a MET and ALK inhibitor, was already being evaluated, and following a confirmatory phase II trial, crizotinib received accelerated approval for patients with ALK-positive NSCLC in 2011. Subsequent clinical trials demonstrated its

a Department of Medicine, Memorial Sloan Kettering Cancer Center, 300 East 66th Street, New York, NY 10065, USA; b Department of Medicine, Memorial Sloan Kettering Cancer Center, Weill Cornell Medical College, New York, NY, USA
* Corresponding author.
E-mail address: rielyg@mskcc.org

Hematol Oncol Clin N Am 31 (2017) 101–111
http://dx.doi.org/10.1016/j.hoc.2016.08.012
0889-8588/17/© 2016 Elsevier Inc. All rights reserved.

superiority to first- and second-line chemotherapy. Additional ALK inhibitors (such as alectinib and ceritinib) have become crucial therapies as patients often develop resistance to first-line therapy within 1 year of treatment. Numerous ALK-dependent and ALK-independent mechanisms of resistance have been identified. These individual mechanisms of resistance may have important implications for treatment strategies.

PATIENT EVALUATION
Clinical and Radiographic Characteristics

ALK rearrangements occur in approximately 5% of patients with NSCLC.[1] Although initially identified as EML4-ALK,[2,3] fusions with a variety of other genes have been reported, all leading to dysregulated overexpression of ALK. Patients with ALK-positive tumors tend to be younger and more likely to be never or light smokers,[3,4] with ALK rearrangements occurring in 12% of never-smokers compared with only 2% of former or current smokers.[5] ALK rearrangements almost never co-occur with activating mutations in EGFR or KRAS.[6] As compared with patients with *EGFR*-mutant NSCLC, patients with ALK-positive tumors are more likely to be men,[7] and radiographically, are associated with larger-volume, multifocal thoracic lymphadenopathy.[8]

Methods for Identifying Patients with Anaplastic Lymphoma Kinase–Positive Lung Cancers

ALK-positive tumors represent a subset of adenocarcinomas and may be more likely to exhibit certain histopathological features such as solid growth pattern and signet-ring cell cytomorphology or mucinous cribriform pattern[9,10]; however, these characteristics are neither sensitive nor specific for ALK rearrangements. Specific testing for the molecular patterns of ALK gene fusion or the resultant ALK protein overexpression is required for diagnosis of ALK-positive NSCLC.

During initial evaluation of crizotinib, the ALK break-apart test was used to identify ALK-positive patients. This test uses fluorescence in situ hybridization (FISH), capitalizes on disruption of the ALK gene, and was the first test to be US Food and Drug Administration (FDA) approved. Although the FISH test can identify many ALK rearrangements, routine next-generation sequencing (NGS) can identify ALK rearrangements not previously identified and those with complex fusion partners,[11–13] thus identifying more patients that would be appropriate for ALK-directed therapy. Furthermore, routine NGS can identify co-occurring mutations, which may provide additional clinical value.[14]

Because ALK is rarely expressed at significant levels in normal lung tissue and ALK gene rearrangements lead to ALK overexpression, tests looking for ALK protein can also be clinically useful. Immunohistochemical detection of ALK protein has been shown to reliably detect ALK-positive NSCLCs, and there are currently 2 FDA-approved commercial assays for this use.[15,16] The convenience and widespread availability of immunohistochemistry (IHC) in most pathology laboratories make IHC an appealing method for detection of ALK in routine care.

PHARMACOLOGIC TREATMENT OPTIONS
Crizotinib

Crizotinib is a potent, orally available, ATP-competitive, small-molecule inhibitor of ALK and Met receptor tyrosine kinases that entered initial clinical trials in 2006 before the discovery of ALK rearrangements in NSCLC. In the initial phase I trial, the ALK-positive cohort had a response rate (RR) of 61%.[17] The most frequently occurring treatment-related adverse events were visual disturbance, gastrointestinal events (nausea, diarrhea, vomiting, and constipation), and peripheral edema. Of note, although visual disturbances were common, occurring in 60% of patients, they were not associated with abnormalities on ophthalmologic examination and did not lead to frequent drug discontinuation.[18]

Subsequently, crizotinib was evaluated in randomized clinical trials in 2 clinical contexts (**Table 1**). In patients previously treated with platinum doublet chemotherapy, crizotinib was superior to chemotherapy (either pemetrexed or docetaxel), with an improvement in median progression-free survival (PFS) to 7.7 months as compared with 3.0 months for patients receiving chemotherapy.[19] Similarly, crizotinib treatment was associated with an improved RR of 65% compared with only 20% in patients who received chemotherapy. Crizotinib also demonstrated superiority to first-line chemotherapy in a randomized phase III study comparing crizotinib to platinum-pemetrexed as initial therapy. Patients receiving crizotinib had an improved median PFS (10.9 months vs 7.0 months).[20]

Identification of Crizotinib Resistance

Clinically apparent drug resistance occurs after a median of 8 to 11 months of crizotinib treatment through a variety of mechanisms. Broadly, these include alterations of ALK (second-site mutations, alternative splicing, or gene amplification) and reactivation of signaling through alternate pathways. These patterns of resistance stand in contrast to EGFR mutant NSCLC, where resistance to EGFR inhibitors is associated with the EGFR T790M mutation in most patients.[21]

A variety of mutations in the ALK kinase domain have been identified in patients at the time of progression on crizotinib (see **Table 3**). One of the most frequently identified mutations, L1196M substitution,[22] occurs at the conserved gatekeeper site within the kinase domain and is analogous to EGFR T790M mutation. Even mutations at non-active sites can affect interactions between drug and ALK, as was demonstrated in the case of the C1156Y substitution.[23] Further adding to the complexity, multiple separate secondary mutations have been identified in individual crizotinib-resistant patients demonstrating either tumor heterogeneity or multiple cooperative mutations.[24] Given the diversity of point mutations that occur as resistance mechanisms to ALK inhibition, it will become important to perform repeat biopsyies at the time of progression, potentially yielding information that may help guide further treatment decisions.

Table 1
Summary of landmark crizotinib clinical trials

Authors	Study Arms	N	ORR (%)	Median PFS (mo)	Conclusion
Camidge et al,[17] 2012	Crizotinib phase I study	143	60.8	9.7	Crizotinib was well tolerated and demonstrated efficacy
Shaw et al,[19] 2013	Crizotinib Chemotherapy (Docetaxel or Pemetrexed)	173 174	65 20	7.7 3.0	Crizotinib is superior to chemotherapy in the 2nd-line setting
Solomon et al,[20] 2014	Crizotinib Cisplatin or Carboplatin + Pemetrexed	172 171	74 45	10.9 7.0	Crizotinib is superior to chemotherapy in the 1st-line setting

In most patients with progression on crizotinib, no ALK-resistance mutations are identified,[24] and therefore, other mechanisms of resistance are likely to be present. One such mechanism is the activation of other pathways such as EGFR and KIT. Although EGFR and ALK mutations are thought to be mutually exclusive,[6] in crizotinib-resistant cell lines, increased EFGR activation due to increased EGFR ligand levels has been demonstrated.[24–26] Crizotinib resistance caused by amplification of the KIT gene has also been reported, and treatment with imatinib, a small molecule inhibitor of KIT, reversed the resistance phenotype in vitro.[24]

In resistance, changes in ALK copy number (ALK amplification or loss) have been observed in patients,[27,28] consistent with prior data from cell lines.[29] Although there have also been reports of loss of ALK positivity upon rebiopsy, it remains unclear if this reflects a true loss of an ALK-gene fusion or false negative testing.[27,30]

Second-Generation Anaplastic Lymphoma Kinase Inhibitors: Ceritinib and Alectinib

Ceritinib is a more potent and specific ALK inhibitor that has demonstrated ability to overcome crizotinib-resistance mutations in vitro.[31–33] A phase I/II study, including patients who had received crizotinib previously, reported a median PFS of 7.0 months and an RR of 56%. Responses were seen in patients who were found to have a variety of crizotinib-resistance mutations and in patients in whom no resistance mutation was identified.[32] On the basis of this clinical activity in patients with ALK-positive lung cancer who had become resistant to crizotinib, ceritinib received accelerated FDA approval in April 2014.

Similarly, alectinib is a potent and specific ALK inhibitor that has in vitro activity against a variety of ALK mutations that are observed in patients with resistance to crizotinib. After an initial phase I trial in ALK inhibitor–naive patients, investigators conducted global phase I clinical trials that included patients who had progressed or were intolerant to crizotinib, demonstrating an RR of 55%.[34] This RR was confirmed in another phase II study (RR 52%) with patients experiencing a median PFS of 8.1 months. Based on these

Table 2
Recommended dosing and side effect profiles of US Food and Drug Administration–approved anaplastic lymphoma kinase inhibitors

Drug	Starting Dose	Common Toxicities (Any Grade)	Most Common Grade 3 or 4 Treatment Adverse Events	Reference
Crizotinib	250 mg bid	Vision disorder (60%) Diarrhea (60%) Nausea (55%) Vomiting (47%)	Elevated aspartate aminotransferase (AST)/alanine aminotransferase (ALT) (16%) Dyspnea (4%) Neutropenia (13%)	Camidge et al,[17] 2012
Ceritinib	750 mg once a day	Nausea (82%) Diarrhea (75%) Vomiting (65%) Fatigue (47%) ALT elevation (35%)	ALT increase (21%) AST increase (11%) Diarrhea (7%) Lipase increase (7%)	Shaw et al,[32] 2014
Alectinib	600 mg bid	Constipation (36%) Fatigue (33%) Myalgia (24%) Peripheral edema (23%)	CPK increase (8%) ALT increase (6%) AST increase (5%)	Shaw et al,[42] 2016

data, alectinib received an accelerated approval by the FDA in December 2015 for patients resistant to or intolerant of crizotinib. **Table 2** summarizes the currently FDA-approved ALK inhibitors and the associated toxicity profiles that have been reported for each agent.

Identification of individual ALK-resistance mutations may have important implications for treatment as these resistance mutations can confer variable sensitivity to second-generation inhibitors. For example, cell lines expressing the I1171T secondary mutation were found to be sensitive to ceritinib[33] but resistant to alectinib,[35] whereas the F1174C mutation appears to confer resistance to ceritinib[33] but sensitivity to alectinib.[36] Notably, the ALK secondary mutation G1202R appears to confer resistance to both ceritinib and alectinib[37] (and therefore all currently FDA-approved ALK inhibitors), representing a particular challenge. Lorlatinib, a newer ALK inhibitor currently in clinical development, may have efficacy in patients with this mutation. The sensitivity of such mutations to currently FDA-approved ALK inhibitors is summarized in **Table 3**.

Resistance Patterns to Second-Generation Inhibitors

Only 20% of patients who become resistant to crizotinib will have an ALK-resistance mutation identified.[38] However, this rate appears to be higher following treatment with newer ALK inhibitors. A recent analysis identified resistance mutations in 54% of patients who progressed following ceritinib therapy and 53% following alectinib therapy. The most frequent resistance mutation identified following treatment with a second-generation inhibitor was G1202R. The proportion of patients without identifiable resistance mutations following progression on a second-generation inhibitor continues to be substantial, suggesting that additional mechanisms beyond ALK point mutations are driving resistance for some patients.

Special Considerations for Patients with Central Nervous System Disease

The management of brain metastases and leptomeningeal disease is an important consideration in the treatment of ALK-positive NSCLC, because 26% of patients have brain metastases at the time of presentation.[20] A pooled analysis of patients

Table 3
Summary of the reported sensitivity and resistance of second-generation anaplastic lymphoma kinase inhibitors to known crizotinib-resistance mutations

ALK Secondary Mutation	Reported Sensitive Inhibitors	Reported Resistant Inhibitors
1151Tins	Alectinib[36]	Ceritinib[53]
L1152R	Alectinib[36,54]	Ceritinib[54]
C1156Y	Alectinib[36]	Ceritinib[53]
I1171T	Ceritinib[33]	Alectinib[35]
F1174L/V/C	Alectinib[36]	Ceritinib[33]
L1196M	Ceritinib[33] Alectinib[36]	
G1202R		Ceritinib[33] Alectinib[36]
S1206Y	Ceritinib[33]	
F1245C	Ceritinib[55]	
G12569A	Ceritinib[33] Alectinib[56]	

from clinical trials demonstrated modest central nervous system (CNS) responses to crizotinib therapy in patients with untreated brain metastases. However, in patients with CNS disease at the start of therapy, it remained the most common site of progression of disease,[39] raising the concern that CNS penetration of the drug is low.[40] Ceritinib and alectinib appear to have improved CNS activity. Ceritinib demonstrated a CNS RR of 45% in patients with measurable CNS disease.[41] Alectinib has also demonstrated high CNS RRs in both the phase I (52%)[34] and the phase II trials (75%), including 25% of patients who achieved a complete CNS response.[42] Additional reports have also described significant clinical and radiographic improvements in leptomeningeal disease with alectinib treatment.[43]

Optimal Sequence of Therapy

With 3 ALK inhibitors currently approved by the FDA, the appropriate sequence of the use of these agents is unclear. It has been traditionally posited that one could extend overall survival using them in sequence (crizotinib followed by a second-generation ALK inhibitor as opposed to second-generation ALK inhibitor as initial therapy). To explore this question, investigators compared alectinib with crizotinib as initial therapy, with preliminary presentation of the data suggesting that initial alectinib is associated with a markedly improved median PFS, which was longer than historical experience with crizotinib followed by a second-generation inhibitor and a more favorable toxicity profile.[44] The authors look forward to final results of the trial and results from a global trial with the same comparator arms. If these data are supported by the ongoing global study, they may lead to a paradigm shift in the treatment of ALK-positive NSCLC. Multiple promising ALK inhibitors are also currently in clinical development and are summarized in **Table 4**.

Potential Role of Adjuvant Treatment with Anaplastic Lymphoma Kinase–Tyrosine Kinase Inhibitors

Historically, effective agents for metastatic cancer have been tested in the early stage setting to assess whether these can improve the cure rate compared with today's multimodality therapy. All clinical trials with ALK inhibitors have treated only patients with metastatic disease. A large phase III prospective clinical trial, Adjuvant Lung Cancer Enrichment Marker Identification and Sequencing Trials (ALCHEMIST Treatment Trial), is currently enrolling patients and looking to address this question. Patients with ALK rearrangements will be randomly assigned to receive the drug crizotinib or placebo for 2 years. The primary outcome measure of the ALCHEMIST treatment trial

Table 4
Selected anaplastic lymphoma kinase tyrosine-kinase inhibitors currently in clinical development

Clinical Trial	Drug	Status of Relevant Trials
NCT02737501	Brigatinib	• Phase I/II completed • Phase III study of brigatinib vs crizotinib in TKI-naive patients currently ongoing
NCT01970865	Lorlatinib	• Phase I completed • Phase II ongoing
NCT01625234	X-396	• Phase I completed • Phase II ongoing

is overall survival and disease-free survival, with toxicity as secondary outcomes, and is expected to be completed in 2022.[45]

Non–Tyrosine Kinase Inhibitor Therapy: Role of Chemotherapy and Immunotherapy

In addition to molecularly targeted therapy, there is still an important role for cytotoxic chemotherapy in the treatment of ALK-positive NSCLC. Multiple series have identified a longer PFS with pemetrexed-based treatment regimens (monotherapy or combination therapy) in ALK-positive crizotinib-naive tumors compared with ALK negative tumors.[46] In the pivotal phase II study comparing crizotinib to single-agent chemotherapy, pemetrexed monotherapy demonstrated a 29% overall response rate (ORR) compared with 7% with docetaxel monotherapy.[19] The place of pemetrexed in the sequence of ALK-positive treatment still needs to be further elucidated, because small retrospective studies comparing the outcomes of patients who received pemetrexed before or after crizotinib have suggested it may be less effective following crizotinib.[47]

Although immune checkpoint blockade has been a major advance in the treatment of NCSLC, its role for patients with ALK-positive tumors is less clear. Preclinical data suggested that overexpression of ALK fusion protein increased PD-L1 expression, raising the possibility that PD-L1 antibodies may be effective in the treatment of ALK-positive NSCLC.[48,49] Retrospective data, however, indicate that patients with ALK rearrangements have lower RRs to PD-1/PD-L1 inhibitors compared with patients with ALK-negative tumors.[50]

ROLE OF NONPHARMACOLOGIC THERAPY IN THE MANAGEMENT OF ANAPLASTIC LYMPHOMA KINASE–POSITIVE NON–SMALL CELL LUNG CANCER

Data regarding the appropriate role of surgery and/or radiation for patients with ALK-positive disease is limited, in part because routine testing for ALK rearrangements is not often performed in early stage disease. For patients with metastatic disease, radiation therapy can play an important role particularly when progression occurs at a limited number of sites (oligoprogressive) as opposed to widespread disease. A retrospective analysis reviewed outcomes of patients who developed oligoprogressive disease while on therapy with an ALK inhibitor (including patients with isolated CNS progression) and were treated with local ablative therapy and subsequently resumed the same ALK tyrosine kinase inhibitor (TKI). The median PFS observed after local therapy was 6.2 months, essentially extending the time on an individual therapy from 9.0 months to 15.2 months.[51] These results are similar to prior published experience of local therapy for *EGFR*-mutant NSCLC.[52] For patients with oligoprogressive disease, this strategy could meaningfully extend courses of treatment, thus providing clinical benefit. Although these data are promising, further prospective clinical studies are warranted to validate this approach.

SUMMARY

ALK-positive NSCLC is a distinct subset of lung cancer with a different natural history and response to therapies. Routine testing for ALK rearrangements should be performed in all patients with newly diagnosed NSCLC. Efforts to identify mechanisms of resistance to ALK inhibitors have demonstrated a multitude of point mutations (demonstrating variable sensitivity to second-generation inhibitors) as well as alternative signaling pathways that likely contribute to cancer growth. As the duration of response to each ALK-directed TKI is limited, future clinical trials will need to not just focus on the development of more potent ALK inhibitors but also formally assess the effectiveness of other strategies such as immunotherapy.

REFERENCES

1. Soda M, Choi YL, Enomoto M, et al. Identification of the transforming EML4–ALK fusion gene in non-small-cell lung cancer. Nature 2007;448(7153):561–6.
2. Rikova K, Guo A, Zeng Q, et al. Global Survey of phosphotyrosine signaling identifies oncogenic kinases in lung cancer. Cell 2007;131(6):1190–203.
3. Rodig SJ, Mino-Kenudson M, Dacic S, et al. Unique clinicopathologic features characterize ALK-rearranged lung adenocarcinoma in the western population. Clin Cancer Res 2009;15(16):5216–23.
4. Wong DW-S, Leung EL-H, So KK-T, et al. The EML4-ALK fusion gene is involved in various histologic types of lung cancers from nonsmokers with wild-type EGFR and KRAS. Cancer 2009;115(8):1723–33.
5. Paik PK, Johnson ML, D'Angelo SP, et al. Driver mutations determine survival in smokers and never-smokers with stage IIIB/IV lung adenocarcinomas. Cancer 2012;118(23):5840–7.
6. Gainor JF, Varghese AM, Ou S-HI, et al. ALK rearrangements are mutually exclusive with mutations in EGFR or KRAS: an analysis of 1,683 patients with non–small cell lung cancer. Clin Cancer Res 2013;19(15):4273–81.
7. Shaw AT, Yeap BY, Mino-Kenudson M, et al. Clinical features and outcome of patients with non–small-cell lung cancer who harbor EML4-ALK. J Clin Oncol 2009; 27(26):4247–53.
8. Halpenny DF, Riely GJ, Hayes S, et al. Are there imaging characteristics associated with lung adenocarcinomas harboring ALK rearrangements? Lung Cancer 2014;86(2):190–4.
9. Popat S, Gonzalez D, Min T, et al. ALK translocation is associated with ALK immunoreactivity and extensive signet-ring morphology in primary lung adenocarcinoma. Lung Cancer 2012;75(3):300–5.
10. Yoshida A, Tsuta K, Nakamura H, et al. Comprehensive histologic analysis of ALK-rearranged lung carcinomas. Am J Surg Pathol 2011;35(8):1226–34.
11. Drilon A, Wang L, Arcila ME, et al. Broad, hybrid capture–based next-generation sequencing identifies actionable genomic alterations in lung adenocarcinomas otherwise negative for such alterations by other genomic testing approaches. Clin Cancer Res 2015;21(16):3631–9.
12. Arcila ME, Yu HA, Drilon AE, et al. Comprehensive assessment of targetable alterations in lung adenocarcinoma samples with limited material using MSK-IMPACT, a clinical, hybrid capture-based, next-generation sequencing (NGS) assay. Journal of Clinical Oncology 2015;33(15_suppl):e22160. ASCO Meet Abstr.
13. Peled N, Palmer G, Hirsch FR, et al. Next-generation sequencing identifies and immunohistochemistry confirms a novel crizotinib-sensitive ALK rearrangement in a patient with metastatic non–small-cell lung cancer. J Thorac Oncol 2012; 7(9):e14–6.
14. Chaft JE, Arcila ME, Paik PK, et al. Coexistence of PIK3CA and other oncogene mutations in lung adenocarcinoma-rationale for comprehensive mutation profiling. Mol Cancer Ther 2012;11(2):485–91.
15. Mino-Kenudson M, Chirieac LR, Law K, et al. A novel, highly sensitive antibody allows for the routine detection of ALK-rearranged lung adenocarcinomas by standard immunohistochemistry. Clin Cancer Res 2010;16(5):1561–71.

16. Marchetti A, Lorito AD, Pace MV, et al. ALK protein analysis by IHC staining after recent regulatory changes: a comparison of two widely used approaches, revision of the literature, and a new testing algorithm. J Thorac Oncol 2016;11(4):487–95.
17. Camidge DR, Bang Y-J, Kwak EL, et al. Activity and safety of crizotinib in patients with ALK-positive non-small-cell lung cancer: updated results from a phase 1 study. Lancet Oncol 2012;13(10):1011–9.
18. Kwak EL, Bang Y-J, Camidge DR, et al. Anaplastic lymphoma kinase inhibition in non–small-cell lung cancer. N Engl J Med 2010;363(18):1693–703.
19. Shaw AT, Kim D-W, Nakagawa K, et al. Crizotinib versus chemotherapy in advanced ALK-positive lung cancer. N Engl J Med 2013;368(25):2385–94.
20. Solomon BJ, Mok T, Kim D-W, et al. First-line crizotinib versus chemotherapy in ALK-positive lung cancer. N Engl J Med 2014;371(23):2167–77.
21. Pao W, Miller VA, Politi KA, et al. Acquired resistance of lung adenocarcinomas to gefitinib or erlotinib is associated with a second mutation in the EGFR kinase domain. PLoS Med 2005;2(3):e73.
22. Choi YL, Soda M, Yamashita Y, et al. EML4-ALK mutations in lung cancer that confer resistance to ALK inhibitors. N Engl J Med 2010;363(18):1734–9.
23. Sun H-Y, Ji F-Q. A molecular dynamics investigation on the crizotinib resistance mechanism of C1156Y mutation in ALK. Biochem Biophys Res Commun 2012;423(2):319–24.
24. Katayama R, Shaw AT, Khan TM, et al. Mechanisms of acquired crizotinib resistance in ALK-rearranged lung cancers. Sci Transl Med 2012;4(120):120.
25. Sasaki T, Koivunen J, Ogino A, et al. A novel ALK secondary mutation and EGFR signaling cause resistance to ALK kinase inhibitors. Cancer Res 2011;71(18):6051–60.
26. Yamada T, Takeuchi S, Nakade J, et al. Paracrine receptor activation by microenvironment triggers bypass survival signals and ALK inhibitor resistance in EML4-ALK lung cancer cells. Clin Cancer Res 2012;18(13):3592–602.
27. Doebele RC, Pilling AB, Aisner DL, et al. Mechanisms of resistance to crizotinib in patients with ALK gene rearranged non-small cell lung cancer. Clin Cancer Res 2012;18(5):1472–82.
28. Kim S, Kim TM, Kim D-W, et al. Heterogeneity of genetic changes associated with acquired crizotinib resistance in ALK-rearranged lung cancer. J Thorac Oncol 2013;8(4):415–22.
29. Katayama R, Khan TM, Benes C, et al. Therapeutic strategies to overcome crizotinib resistance in non-small cell lung cancers harboring the fusion oncogene EML4-ALK. Proc Natl Acad Sci U S A 2011;108(18):7535–40.
30. Giri S, Patel JK, Mahadevan D. Novel mutations in a patient with ALK-rearranged lung cancer. N Engl J Med 2014;371(17):1655–6.
31. Marsilje TH, Pei W, Chen B, et al. Synthesis, structure–activity relationships, and in vivo efficacy of the novel potent and selective anaplastic lymphoma kinase (ALK) inhibitor 5-chloro-N2-(2-isopropoxy-5-methyl-4-(piperidin-4-yl)phenyl)-N4-(2-(isopropylsulfonyl)phenyl)pyrimidine-2,4-diamine (LDK378) currently in phase 1 and phase 2 clinical trials. J Med Chem 2013;56(14):5675–90.
32. Shaw AT, Kim D-W, Mehra R, et al. Ceritinib in ALK-rearranged non–small-cell lung cancer. N Engl J Med 2014;370(13):1189–97.
33. Friboulet L, Li N, Katayama R, et al. The ALK inhibitor ceritinib overcomes crizotinib resistance in non–small cell lung cancer. Cancer Discov 2014;4(6):662–73.
34. Gadgeel SM, Gandhi L, Riely GJ, et al. Safety and activity of alectinib against systemic disease and brain metastases in patients with crizotinib-resistant ALK-

rearranged non-small-cell lung cancer (AF-002JG): results from the dose-finding portion of a phase 1/2 study. Lancet Oncol 2014;15(10):1119–28.

35. Toyokawa G, Hirai F, Inamasu E, et al. Secondary mutations at I1171 in the ALK gene confer resistance to both Crizotinib and Alectinib. J Thorac Oncol 2014; 9(12):e86–7.

36. Kodama T, Tsukaguchi T, Yoshida M, et al. Selective ALK inhibitor alectinib with potent antitumor activity in models of crizotinib resistance. Cancer Lett 2014; 351(2):215–21.

37. Ou S-H, Milliken JC, Azada MC, et al. ALK F1174V mutation confers sensitivity while ALK I1171 mutation confers resistance to alectinib. The importance of serial biopsy post progression. Lung Cancer 2016;91:70–2.

38. Gainor JF, Dardaei L, Yoda S, et al. Molecular mechanisms of resistance to first- and second-generation ALK inhibitors in ALK-rearranged lung cancer. Cancer Discov 2016. http://dx.doi.org/10.1158/2159-8290.CD-16-0596.

39. Costa DB, Shaw AT, Ou S-HI, et al. Clinical experience with crizotinib in patients with advanced ALK-rearranged non-small-cell lung cancer and brain metastases. J Clin Oncol 2015;33(17):1881–8.

40. Costa DB, Kobayashi S, Pandya SS, et al. CSF concentration of the anaplastic lymphoma kinase inhibitor crizotinib. J Clin Oncol 2011;29(15):e443–5.

41. Crinò L, Ahn M-J, Marinis FD, et al. Multicenter phase II study of whole-body and intracranial activity with ceritinib in patients with ALK-rearranged non–small-cell lung cancer previously treated with chemotherapy and crizotinib: results from ASCEND-2. J Clin Oncol 2016. http://dx.doi.org/10.1200/JCO.2015.65.5936.

42. Shaw AT, Gandhi L, Gadgeel S, et al. Alectinib in ALK-positive, crizotinib-resistant, non-small-cell lung cancer: a single-group, multicentre, phase 2 trial. Lancet Oncol 2016. http://dx.doi.org/10.1016/S1470-2045(15)00488-X.

43. Gainor JF, Sherman CA, Willoughby K, et al. Alectinib salvages CNS relapses in ALK-positive lung cancer patients previously treated with crizotinib and ceritinib. J Thorac Oncol 2015;10(2):232–6.

44. Alectinib (ALC) versus crizotinib (CRZ) in ALK-inhibitor naive ALK-positive non-small cell lung cancer (ALK+ NSCLC): primary results from the J-ALEX study. J Clin Oncol. Available at: http://meetinglibrary.asco.org/content/167434-176. Accessed June 27, 2016.

45. Crizotinib in treating patients with stage IB-IIIA non-small cell lung cancer that has been removed by surgery and ALK fusion mutations (An ALCHEMIST treatment trial)—full text view. ClinicalTrials.gov. Available at: https://clinicaltrials.gov/ct2/show/study/NCT02201992. Accessed July 5, 2016.

46. Lee J-O, Kim TM, Lee S-H, et al. Anaplastic lymphoma kinase translocation: a predictive biomarker of pemetrexed in patients with non-small cell lung cancer. J Thorac Oncol 2011;6(9):1474–80.

47. Berge EM, Lu X, Maxson D, et al. Clinical benefit from pemetrexed before and after crizotinib exposure and from crizotinib before and after pemetrexed exposure in patients with anaplastic lymphoma kinase-positive non–small-cell lung cancer. Clin Lung Cancer 2013;14(6):636–43.

48. Hong S, Chen N, Fang W, et al. Upregulation of PD-L1 by EML4-ALK fusion protein mediates the immune escape in ALK positive NSCLC: implication for optional anti-PD-1/PD-L1 immune therapy for ALK-TKIs sensitive and resistant NSCLC patients. Oncoimmunology 2016;5(3):e1094598.

49. Koh J, Jang J-Y, Keam B, et al. EML4-ALK enhances programmed cell death-ligand 1 expression in pulmonary adenocarcinoma via hypoxia-inducible factor (HIF)-1α and STAT3. Oncoimmunology 2016;5(3):e1108514.

50. Gainor JF, Shaw AT, Sequist LV, et al. EGFR mutations and ALK rearrangements are associated with low response rates to PD-1 pathway blockade in non-small cell lung cancer (NSCLC): a retrospective analysis. Clin Cancer Res 2016. http://dx.doi.org/10.1158/1078-0432.CCR-15-3101.
51. Weickhardt AJ, Scheier B, Burke JM, et al. Local ablative therapy of oligoprogressive disease prolongs disease control by tyrosine kinase inhibitors in oncogene-addicted non–small-cell lung cancer. J Thorac Oncol 2012;7(12):1807–14.
52. Yu HA, Sima CS, Huang J, et al. Local therapy with continued EGFR tyrosine kinase inhibitor therapy as a treatment strategy in EGFR-mutant advanced lung cancers that have developed acquired resistance to EGFR tyrosine kinase inhibitors. J Thorac Oncol 2013;8(3):346–51.
53. Gainor JF, Tan DSW, Pas TD, et al. Progression-free and overall survival in ALK-positive NSCLC patients treated with sequential crizotinib and ceritinib. Clin Cancer Res 2015. http://dx.doi.org/10.1158/1078-0432.CCR-14-3009.
54. Tchekmedyian N, Ali SM, Miller VA, et al. Acquired ALK L1152R mutation confers resistance to ceritinib and predicts response to alectinib. J Thorac Oncol 2016;11(7):e87–8.
55. Kodityal S, Elvin JA, Squillace R, et al. A novel acquired ALK F1245C mutation confers resistance to crizotinib in ALK-positive NSCLC but is sensitive to ceritinib. Lung Cancer 2016;92:19–21.
56. Yoshimura Y, Kurasawa M, Yorozu K, et al. Antitumor activity of alectinib, a selective ALK inhibitor, in an ALK-positive NSCLC cell line harboring G1269A mutation. Cancer Chemother Pharmacol 2016;77(3):623–8.

New Targets in Non–Small Cell Lung Cancer

Soo J. Park, MD, Soham More, Ayesha Murtuza, MD, Brian D. Woodward, Hatim Husain, MD*

KEYWORDS

- NSCLC • ROS1 • RET • NTRK • MET • BRAF • KRAS • Driver mutations

KEY POINTS

- With the implementation of genomic technologies into clinical practice, we have examples of the benefit of targeted therapy for oncogene-addicted cancer and identified unique molecular dependencies in non–small cell lung cancer.
- The clinical success of tyrosine kinase inhibitors against epidermal growth factor receptor and anaplastic lymphoma kinase activation has shifted treatment to emphasize the genomically defined subsets of lung cancer and genotype-directed therapy.
- Continued advances in our understanding of lung cancer biology have validated numerous oncogenic driver genes and have led to the rapid development of targeted agents.
- The current available data on ROS1, RET, NTRK, MET, BRAF, and KRAS aberrations in non–small cell lung cancer are presented.
- The current state of available trials in this space, mechanism of action of the oncogene, mechanisms of resistance to therapy are presented.

INTRODUCTION

Lung cancer remains the leading cause of cancer-related deaths worldwide.[1,2] Historically, the treatment of advanced epidermal growth factor receptor (EGFR) and anaplastic lymphoma kinase (ALK) wild-type non–small cell lung cancer (NSCLC) has relied on platinum-based chemotherapy with a median overall survival (OS) of approximately 1 year.[2,3] Within the last several years, immune checkpoint inhibitors have demonstrated efficacy in both squamous and nonsquamous histologies and are now approved agents for second-line treatment, largely based on improved OS.[4,5]

Conflicts of Interest: Dr S.J. Park and Dr A. Murtuza have no conflicts to disclose. Dr H. Husain participates is a consultant for Bristol Myers Squibb and has received research funds from Trovagene Inc.

Division of Hematology and Oncology, Moores Cancer Center, University of California, San Diego, La Jolla, CA 92093, USA

* Corresponding author. Moores Cancer Center, University of California, San Diego, 3855 Health Sciences Drive, #0987, La Jolla, CA 92093.

E-mail address: hhusain@ucsd.edu

Hematol Oncol Clin N Am 31 (2017) 113–129
http://dx.doi.org/10.1016/j.hoc.2016.08.010
0889-8588/17/

hemonc.theclinics.com

The past decade has seen a paradigm shift in the treatment of NSCLC based on the implementation of broad-based genomics to identify driver mutations and drug development against these targets. Across genotypes, the use of targeted agents for the treatment of patients with EGFR and ALK-mutated NSCLC has improved response rates, time to disease progression, and OS when compared with conventional systemic therapy.[6,7] More than 60% of patients with lung adenocarcinoma have a presumably mutually exclusive oncogenic driver.[3] This article reviews driver mutations, including ROS1 fusions, RET fusions, NTRK1 fusions, c-MET amplification, exon 14 skipping mutations, BRAF mutations, and KRAS mutations, their downstream signaling (**Table 1**; **Fig. 1**), and the current clinical trials that are exploring compounds against these pathways.

Table 1
Genetic alterations and their frequency in lung adenocarcinoma

Target	Alteration	Frequency (%)
ROS1	ROS1 fusion	2
RET	RET fusion	1
NTRK1	NTRK1 fusion	3.3
c-MET	Amplification	2–4
	Exon 14 skipping mutation	3–4
BRAF	V600E mutation	1–4
KRAS	Mutations in codons 12, 13, and 61	15–25

THE ONCOGENIC ROS1 FUSION

ROS1 is a receptor tyrosine kinase (RTK) that belongs to the same insulin receptor superfamily as ALK. The function of ROS1 remains largely unknown, although some studies have suggested that this oncogene may play a role in epithelial cell differentiation.[8] Further progress in the characterization of ROS1 has been difficult owing to the absence of an identified ligand.[9] Expression of the ROS1 fusion protein results in constitutive kinase activity and activation of cellular pathways involved in cell growth and proliferation. Chromosomal rearrangements involving the *ROS1* gene were described originally in glioblastoma cell lines and have since been reported in cholangiocarcinoma and NSCLC.[10–12]

ROS1 gene fusions are found in approximately 2% of NSCLC and have been associated with a younger age of onset and a nonsmoking history, and seem to be mutually exclusive with other oncogenic driver genes.[13] Such demographic characteristics are similar to the clinical profile of patients with ALK-rearranged NSCLC and may be owing in part to the high level of homology between the kinase domains.[14,15] Crizotinib, a small molecule multikinase inhibitor originally developed as a MET kinase inhibitor and approved by the US Food and Drug Administration (FDA) for the treatment of ALK-rearranged NSCLC, was shown to have potent inhibitory activity against ROS1.[13] Results from the expansion cohort of the PROFILE 1001 (A Study Of Oral PF-02341066, A c-Met/Hepatocyte Growth Factor Tyrosine Kinase Inhibitor, In Patients With Advanced Cancer) trial showed that 72% of the participants experienced a complete or partial response in tumor burden, an effect that lead to a median duration of response of 17.6 months.[16] These findings led to recent FDA approval of crizotinib for patients with ROS1-rearranged NSCLC. Other trials with crizotinib are ongoing (**Table 2**). Ceritinib, ASP3026, and AP26113 exhibit activity against ROS1

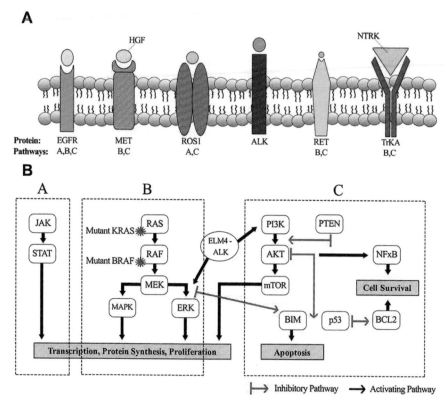

Fig. 1. The EGFR, MET, ROS1, ALK, RET, and NTRK oncogenes and their major signaling networks. (*A*) Presented are the oncogenes EGFR, MET, ROS1, ALK, RET, and NTRK and some of their ligands (ie, HGF for MET and neurotrophins for TRK receptors). (*B*) The signaling networks for each pathway are matched with receptor (ie, EGFR signals through A, B, and C and MET signals through B and C).

tyrosine kinase, whereas alectinib does not. ROS1-specific agents have not yet entered clinical trials.

Parallel to experiences seen with EGFR and ALK inhibition, acquired resistance to targeted therapy remains inevitable and has also been described in ROS1-rearranged patients.[17,18] The secondary G2032R mutation seems to be a dominant

Table 2			
Clinical trials of drugs targeting ROS1			
Drug Class and Target	**Investigational Agent**	**Trial ID Number**	**Phase**
ROS1	Lorlatinib (PF-06463922)	NCT01970865	I/II
	Ceritinib (LDK378, SIGNATURE study)	NCT02186821	II
	Cabozantinib	NCT01639508	II
	Entrectinib (RXDX-101, STARTRK-1 study)	NCT02097810	I
	Entrectinib (RXDX-101, STARTRK-2 study)	NCT02568267	II
	Crizotinib (METROS study – Pretreated, metastatic)	NCT02499614	II
	Crizotinib (EUCROSS study – First line Europe)	NCT02183870	II
	Crizotinib (AcSè study – Safety Study)	NCT02034981	II

resistance mutation and responsible for crizotinib resistance through impaired drug binding.[19,20] Several second-generation ALK inhibitors that were originally developed to address ALK resistance mutations have failed to inhibit crizotinib-resistant ROS1.[21] Multikinase inhibitors with exquisite inhibition potency when compared with crizotinib are currently being investigated for sensitivity to G2032R mutants and include lorlatinib, entrectinib, and ceritinib (see **Table 2**). Lorlatinib, a selective ALK and ROS1 inhibitor noted to have nanomolar potency, was well-tolerated and demonstrated durable clinical responses in an ongoing phase I study (NCT01970865).[22]

Reactivation of key downstream signaling pathways is another mechanism underlying resistance to targeted therapeutics. Increased EGFR phosphorylation and pathway activation have been reported in crizotinib-resistant NSCLC tumor samples and cell lines.[23] RAS mutations have also been shown to mediate crizotinib resistance in ROS1-rearranged patients.[24] These observations suggest that activation of bypass signaling from the original oncogenic driver to other known drivers. Preclinical studies support combinatorial treatment strategies to overcome acquired resistance mechanisms.

THE ONCOGENIC RET FUSION

The *RET* gene encodes a RET family RTK for members of the glial cell line-derived neurotrophic factor family of ligands. RET protein dimerization results in autophosphorylation to activate multiple signal transduction pathways involved in cell motility, proliferation, differentiation, and neuronal nagivation.[25] *RET* gene rearrangements and point mutations lead to gain of function signaling and subsequent tumorigenesis. Germline and somatic mutations in the *RET* oncogene are best known to cause the multiple endocrine neoplasia type 2 syndrome (MEN2), nearly all inherited cases of medullary thyroid cancer, and up to 50% of sporadic thyroid cancer cases.[26,27]

RET fusions were initially identified in lung cancer in 2012 and have since been reported to occur in 1% of NSCLC with adenocarcinoma as the predominant histology.[28,29] Studies have shown that RET fusions may be associated with a never smoker status and are mutually exclusive with known driver oncogenes.[28–31] The *KIF5B-RET* fusion is the most common alteration and accounts for approximately 90% of the rearrangements with fusion partners *CCDC6* and *NCOA4* representing the remaining 10%.[28–33]

Although RET-specific inhibitors have not yet been developed, there are numerous clinical trials looking at the efficacy of multikinase inhibitors for advanced NSCLC harboring *RET* rearrangements (**Table 3**). Treatment with sunitinib and vandetanib has been reported to induce prolonged antitumor activity in several case reports of

Table 3 Clinical trials of drugs targeting RET			
Drug Class and Target	**Investigational Agent**	**Trial ID Number**	**Phase**
RET	Lenvatinib (E7080)	NCT01877083	II
	Apatinib	NCT02540824	II
	Vandetanib (LURET study)	NCT01823068	II
	Ponatinib	NCT01813734	II
	Cabozantinib	NCT01639508	II
	Pazopanib	NCT02193152	0
	Nintedanib	NCT02299141	0
	Ponatinib	NCT01935336	II
	Vandetanib + Everolimus	NCT01582191	I

patients with *RET* fusion–positive lung cancer.[34–36] The drug vandetanib is FDA approved for the treatment of medullary thyroid cancer and showed early results in the phase II LURET (Vandetanib in Advanced NSCLC With RET Rearrangement) study of 17 NSCLC patients with an objective response rate (ORR) of 53% and disease control rate (DCR) of 88% and a median progression-free survival (PFS) of 4.7 months.[37] Treatment response was much higher in patients with the *CCDC6-RET* fusion subtype with an ORR and median PFS of 83% and 8.3 months, respectively. The ORR and median PFS was only 20% and 2.9 months for those with *KIF5B-RET* fusion.[37] Results from a different phase II trial of vandetanib in 18 patients with RET-rearranged lung cancer did not show the robust responses seen in the LURET study (NCT01823068).[38] Three patients were reported to have a partial remission, 8 were reported to have stable disease, and the remaining 7 patients had disease progression.[38] Interim results of a phase II trial of cabozantinib in patients with *RET*-rearranged lung cancers presented last year reported an ORR of 38% (NCT01639508).[39] These findings have suggested that a proportion of tumors may harbor intrinsic resistance mechanisms to *RET* inhibition or there may be different efficacy based on different fusion partners. Recent molecular studies performed on pre-treatment and post-treatment tumor biopsies from patients treated with cabozantinib have identified MDM2 amplification as a potential mechanism of primary or acquired resistance.[40] Cell lines and xenografts with acquired MDM2 amplification have demonstrated significant tumor growth suppression in response to MDM2 inhibition.

The rapid emergence of resistance to RET inhibition underscores the need for combinatorial treatment strategies. In vitro studies after treatment with vandetanib, everolimus, or in combination were performed on 2 cell lines expressing the *CCDC6-RET* fusion subtype. Vandetanib was shown to abrogate signaling through the MAPK pathway with effects on effectors of the mammalian target of rapamycin (MTOR). A phase I study of vandetanib in combination with everolimus was shown to be safe and tolerable with significant activity in RET-rearranged lung cancers (NCT01582191).[41] Of the 6 patients who harbor *RET* fusions by next-generation sequencing, 5 achieved a partial response, including 1 patient who progressed on cabozantinib. Significant antitumor activity in the central nervous system was seen with the combination.[41]

Analysis of a global registry of *RET*-rearranged NSCLC included 41 patients who received RET inhibitor therapy off protocol and reported a median PFS of 2.9 months and an OS of 6.8 months with distributions of patients including the major RET fusion partners.[42] For 35 patients who had serial imaging evaluated by Response Evaluation Criteria In Solid Tumors (RECIST) criteria, the ORR was 23% and DCR was 57%. This proportion is lower than that observed with targeted therapy for EGFR-mutant and ALK-rearranged NSCLC. These results emphasize the need for an improved understanding of the intrinsic tumor biology in this genotype.

THE ONCOGENIC NTRK1 FUSION

NTRK1 is an RTK that belongs to the tropomyosin-related kinases superfamily. Tropomyosin-related kinase signaling is normally involved in the regulation of neural development and maintenance of neural networks.[43,44] Ligand binding to NTRKs leads to the activation of multiple signaling pathways through mitogen-activated protein kinase (MAPK), phospholipase C-γ, and phospoinositide 3-kinase to mediate cell differentiation and survival.[45] The *NTRK1* gene encodes the high-affinity nerve growth factor receptor (TrkA). Fusions involving the *NTRK1* gene result in expression of TrkA fusion proteins with constitutive activity or overexpressed kinase function, hence conferring oncogenic potential.[46] *NTRK1* gene rearrangements were first reported in colorectal cancer several decades ago and have now been reported in other solid tumor malignancies, including sarcomas.[46–50]

Oncogenic *NTRK1* fusions have been identified in 3.3% of lung cancer cases with adenocarcinoma histology that is negative for other common driver mutations.[46] Two different gene fusions have been previously described and are characterized by rearrangements between the *myosin phosphatase Rho-interacting protein* gene (*MPRIP-NTRK1*) and *CD74* gene (*CD74-NTRK1*).[46] Both in-frame gene fusion events have been detected in female never smokers. Additional NTRK1 gene rearrangements have been reported in other studies as well.[51,52] These mutations play an important role in tumorigenesis and drug development has moved quickly against these therapeutic targets.

Numerous phase I trials are in progress with inhibitors targeted toward specific kinases that are active against NTRK (**Table 4**). Entrectinib is a highly potent, selective, orally bioavailable small molecule inhibitor of TrkA, TrkB, TrkC, ROS1, and ALK that has achieved rapid and durable responses across a wide range of advanced malignancies.[53] A phase I dose escalation study of entrectinib (STARTRK-1 [Study of Oral RXDX-101 in Adult Patients With Locally Advanced or Metastatic Cancer Targeting NTRK1, NTRK2, NTRK3, ROS1, or ALK Molecular Alterations] study) demonstrated significant antitumor activity in a patient with metastatic NSCLC harboring a *SQSTM1-NTRK1* gene rearrangement with RECIST-defined partial response and complete response of all brain metastases (NCT02097810).[53] The patient has been on study for more than 12 months with no evidence of progressive disease. Entrectinib was granted FDA Orphan Drug Designation for the treatment of TrkA-, TrkB-, and TrkC-positive NSCLC and colorectal cancers.[54]

A number of phase II trials with entrectinib and other novel NTRK inhibitors are underway with compounds including LOXO-101, entrectinib, and cabozantinib (see **Table 4**). Two phase II basket studies (NAVIGATE LOXO-101 [Study of LOXO-101 in Subjects With NTRK Fusion Positive Solid Tumors] and STARTRK-2 [Basket Study of Entrectinib (RXDX-101) for the Treatment of Patients With Solid Tumors Harboring NTRK1/2/3, ROS1, or ALK Gene Rearrangements (Fusions)] entrectinib) are currently recruiting patients who have advanced solid tumors harboring NTRK fusions (NCT02576431 and NCT02568267). Efficacy data are eagerly awaited to determine

Table 4			
Clinical trials of drugs targeting NTRK1			
Drug Class and Target	**Investigational Agent**	**Trial ID Number**	**Phase**
NTRK1	LOXO-101	NCT02122913	I
	LOXO-101 (NAVIGATE study)	NCT02576431	II
	Entrectinib (RXDX-101, STARTRK-1 study)	NCT02097810	I
	Entrectinib (RXDX-101, STARTRK-2 study)	NCT02568267	II
	Cabozantinib	NCT01639508	II
	Sitravatinib (MGCD516)	NCT02219711	I
	TSR-011	NCT02048488	I/IIa
	Altiratinib (DCC-2701)	NCT02228811	I
	DS-6051b	NCT02279433	I
	PLX7486	NCT01804530	I

Abbreviations: NAVIGATE, Study of LOXO-101 in Subjects With NTRK Fusion Positive Solid Tumors; STARTRK, Study of Oral RXDX-101 in Adult Patients With Locally Advanced or Metastatic Cancer Targeting NTRK1, NTRK2, NTRK3, ROS1, or ALK Molecular Alterations.

whether results seen from the phase I studies can be confirmed in a larger cohort of patients. These findings highlight the clinical utility of molecular testing to identify patients with a subset of lung cancers sensitive to NTRK inhibition. Other agents in earlier stages of development include TSR-011, sitravatinib, altiratinib, DS-6051b, and PLX7486 (see **Table 4**).

AMPLIFICATION AND MUTATION IN C-MET

c-MET is an RTK in the MET/RON family whose only known ligand is hepatocyte growth factor. Ligand binding promotes MET dimerization and phosphorylation to recruit signaling protein complexes including SRC, GRB2, SHC, and the p85 regulatory unit of the phospoinositide 3-kinase, which are required for the activation of several downstream signaling cascades.[55] The presence of hepatocyte growth factor also leads to MET receptor internalization and downregulation whereby they are either recycled to the cell surface or degraded within lysosomes.[56] Degradation of the MET receptor depends on ubiquitination by the Cbl family of ubiquitin–protein ligases.[57] A receptor mutation at tyrosine 1003 (Y1003) abrogates MET ubiquitination and results in elevated MET protein levels and increased protein stability.[57,58] This specific uncoupling leads to oncogenic activation by sustained activation of the RAS–MAPK pathway.[57,59]

Abnormal c-MET signaling has been implicated in a wide variety of malignances, including renal cell carcinoma and lung cancer.[60–62] Germline mutations in *MET* occur in all cases of hereditary papillary renal cell carcinoma and are also found in 10% to 15% of sporadic cases.[63–65] Two main mechanisms of aberrant *MET* activation have been reported in lung cancer, including *MET* gene amplification and *MET* exon 14 skip mutations. *MET* gene amplification has been reported to occur in 2% to 4% of NSCLC.[2,66,67] *MET* exon 14 skipping mutations have been found in 3% to 4% of lung adenocarcinoma with and without gene amplification.[68] Increased *MET* expression has been associated with aggressive tumor biology and is a negative prognostic factor.[69–72] The high frequency of MET overexpression in NSCLC has generated significant clinical interest in this pathway for potential druggable targets.

Acquired *MET* amplification has been associated with secondary resistance across anti-EGFR tyrosine kinase inhibitors.[73,74] This phenomenon may occur in up to 20% of treated patients and has also been reported to cause resistance to selective ALK inhibition.[74–76] Clinical trials investigating treatment with dual EGFR and MET inhibition are underway using compounds including crizotinib, glesatinib, capmatinib, emibetuzumab, and cabozantinib (**Table 5**). Onartuzumab, an anti-MET monoclonal antibody, did not improve efficacy endpoints when combined with erlotinib in a phase III study and was stopped early for futility.[77] More recently, results from a phase II trial combining emibetuzumab (LY2875358), a humanized immunoglobulin G4 bivalent monoclonal MET antibody blocking ligand-dependent and ligand-independent hepatocyte growth factor/MET signaling, with erlotinib found that dual inhibition was unable to overcome acquired resistance to erlotinib in patients with advanced NSCLC. There are, however, subsets of patients with response and ongoing work is focused on defining biomarkers and the mechanisms of those patients with response.[78]

There have been several phase II studies demonstrating increased efficacy with combined targeted therapy in patients with acquired MET amplification in resistant EGFR mutant lung cancer. A study combining the selective c-MET inhibitor capmatinib with EGFR tyrosine kinase inhibitors showed encouraging clinical activity with a disease control rate (partial response + stable disease) of 80% and an ORR of 30% in patients with gene copy number of 6 or greater.[79] The combination of tepotinib, a

Table 5
Clinical trials of drugs targeting c-MET

Drug Class and Target	Investigational Agent	Trial ID Number	Phase
c-MET	Crizotinib (PROFILE 1001 study)	NCT00585195	I
	Glesatinib (MGCD265, AMETHYST study)	NCT02544633	II
	Glesatinib (MGCD265)	NCT00697632	I
	Capmatinib (INC280)	NCT01324479	I
	Capmatinib (INC280 + erlotinib)	NCT01911507	I
	Capmatinib (second/third line)	NCT02414139	II
	Cabozantinib	NCT01639508	II
	SAR125844	NCT02435121	II
	Altiratinib (DCC-2701)	NCT02228811	I
	Foretinib (GSK1363089)	NCT00742131	I
c-MET + EGFR TKI	Capmatinib (INC280) + gefitinib	NCT01610336	II
	Emibetuzumab (LY2875358) + erlotinib	NCT01900652	II
	Tepotinib + gefitinib	NCT01982955	I/II

Abbreviations: AMETHYST, Phase 2 Study of MGCD265 in Patients With Non-Small Cell Lung Cancer With Activating Genetic Alterations in MET; EGFR, epidermal growth factor receptor; PROFILE, A Study Of Oral PF-02341066, A c-Met/Hepatocyte Growth Factor Tyrosine Kinase Inhibitor, In Patients With Advanced Cancer; TKI, tyrosine kinase inhibitor.

selective and potent small molecule inhibitor of the c-MET oncogene, and gefitinib showed efficacy with partial response and stable disease in those patients with high gene copy numbers and higher protein expression via immunohistochemistry particularly with IHC 3+ tumors.[80] These findings support the belief that clinical response to MET inhibition may be associated with higher levels of amplification and protein expression, and studies of combinational therapy warrant further investigation.

Multiple MET inhibitors are in early clinical development as monotherapy (see **Table 5**). Crizotinib, initially developed as a c-MET inhibitor and now approved as an ALK or ROS1-positive NSCLC, has shown antitumor activity in a phase I trial of patients with advanced NSCLC harboring *MET* exon 14 alterations.[81] Results from a phase I study of capmatinib demonstrated promising clinical activity, most notably in a subset of patients defined to have high c-MET expression.[82] Glesatinib is an oral, potent, small molecule inhibitor of MET and Axl has demonstrated robust tumor regression in NSCLC xenograft models of *MET* exon 14 skip mutation and confirmed partial responses in the phase I setting (NCT00697632).[83] A phase II trial of this drug has been accruing nationally (AMEHYST study [Phase 2 Study of MGCD265 in Patients With Non-Small Cell Lung Cancer With Activating Genetic Alterations in MET], NCT02544633).[84]

BRAF MUTATIONS IN LUNG ADENOCARCINOMA

BRAF is a serine–threonine protein kinase that belongs to the RAF family and plays a central role in the regulation of the MAPK pathway. BRAF signals through MEK to activate ERK and its downstream effectors regulate cell differentiation, proliferation, growth, and apoptosis.[85] Activating mutations in the *BRAF* gene result in constitutive activation of MEK/ERK signaling, allowing autonomous cell growth.[86] Mutations in BRAF are found in approximately 30% of human cancers and as a class were originally identified in malignant melanomas.[87,88] BRAF mutations in lung cancer can be either V600E or non-V600E with prevalences of approximately 50% each. The most common non-V600E mutations include G469A, T599_V600insT, D594N, and V600_K601delinsE mutations.[86,88,89]

Somatic mutations in BRAF have been found in 1% to 4% of all NSCLC and more commonly occur in current or former smokers.[89] These mutations are typically mutually exclusive of other driver mutations and confer a shorter OS.[87,90,91] Recent clinical trial results indicate that targeted therapy for mutant *BRAF* is a promising strategy. A phase II basket study of vemurafenib monotherapy in BRAF V600E mutation-positive nonmelanoma cancers included 20 patients with NSCLC.[92] This study demonstrated superior results for the NSCLC cohort with an ORR of 42% and a median PFS of 7.3 months. Another phase II study looking into the efficacy of dabrafenib monotherapy in both previously treated and untreated patients with metastatic BRAF V600E-positive NSCLC. An ORR of 33% and a median PFS of 5.5 months was seen as second-line therapy. Four of the 6 previously untreated patients had objective responses.[93]

Efforts to overcome or prevent resistance to BRAF inhibition while improving efficacy over BRAF inhibitor monotherapy led to a phase II trial of dual MAPK pathway inhibition for patients with metastatic BRAF V600E-mutant NSCLC after failure of prior platinum-based therapy.[94] Patients were treated with dabrafenib in combination with the MEK inhibitor trametinib. This study had robust results with an ORR of 63% and a disease control rate of 79%. The median PFS was 9.7 months. Combination therapy was associated with a manageable adverse effect profile and demonstrated clinically meaningful antitumor activity when compared indirectly with dabrafenib monotherapy.[94]

Next-generation small molecule inhibitors of BRAF are also being actively studied (**Table 6**). It is hoped that these agents can minimize paradoxic reactivation of the MAPK pathway to yield both improved safety and efficacy over first-generation RAF inhibitors.[95–98] PLX8394 and LY3009120 are being developed as second-generation, orally bioavailable BRAF inhibitors that seem to suppress mutant BRAF without MAPK activation.[95,99,100] In a phase I/IIa study, PLX8394 is being studied in the relapsed and refractory setting for advanced, unresectable solid tumors harboring the BRAF mutation (NCT02428712). A phase I study of LY3009120 is being conducted in patients with advanced or metastatic *BRAF* mutated cancer including NSCLC to determine safety, tolerability, pharmacokinetics, and overall response rates (NCT02014116).

KRAS

KRAS is 1 of 3 oncogenes within the RAS subfamily that encodes for membrane-bound GTPase to regulate signal transduction. Activating mutations within the *KRAS* gene result in constitutive activation of GTPase function to cause sustained cell proliferation and survival through the MAPK, phospoinositide 3-kinase, and Janus kinase/signal transducers and activators of transcription (JAK/STAT) signaling pathways.[101] Mutations in the KRAS gene are among the most commonly encountered in lung cancer and can be found in up to 25% of patients with adenocarcinoma histology.[2,102] The vast majority of these mutations involve codons 12 and 13 and

Table 6			
Clinical trials of drugs targeting BRAF			
Drug Class and Target	**Investigational Agent**	**Trial ID Number**	**Phase**
BRAF	PLX8394	NCT02428712	I/IIa
	LY3009120	NCT02014116	I
	Dabrafenib + trametinib	NCT01336634	II

are mutually exclusive with EGFR or ALK alterations.[102] KRAS mutations are frequently associated with a history of smoking, although they are sometimes seen in never smokers, and are predictive of resistance to treatment with erlotinib or gefitinib.[102–104] Smoking causes specific C > G transitions that are specific within the KRAS locus.

Although targeted therapy is available for other molecular subsets of lung cancer, no specific agents have yet been developed successfully for KRAS mutants. This is largely owing to the high affinity of the KRAS oncogene for its substrate and the absence of known allosteric regulatory sites.[105] Because direct inhibition of KRAS has proven clinically challenging, most current efforts to date have focused on targeting downstream effectors in the MAPK pathway. Selumetinib, an orally available selective MEK inhibitor, was shown to have antitumor activity in preclinical and early phase studies and suggested a nonstatistically significant trend toward improvement in OS when combined with docetaxel in a phase II trial of KRAS mutant NSCLC.[106] Results from this trial did demonstrate increased response rates and PFS; however, the trial had a greater number of adverse events including neutropenia. A phase III trial to confirm these findings is underway (NCT01933932) evaluating selumetinib in combination with docetaxel in patients receiving second-line treatment for KRAS-positive NSCLC. MEK inhibition remains an active area of therapeutic investigation and has become the backbone for many other combinational therapies (**Table 7**).

Studies are now looking at combinatorial approaches for KRAS mutant lung cancer to further investigate and attempt to exploit synthetically lethal dependencies and synergism. Preclinical studies have shown the synthetic lethal interaction of combined Bcl-XL and MEK inhibition as well as interactions between KRAS and CDK4 promote tumor regression and apoptosis in KRAS mutant cancer models.[107,108] A phase I study combining trametinib with navitoclax, a Bcl-2 inhibitor, is currently recruiting (NCT02079740). Selective CDK4/6 inhibitors, abemaciclib and palbociclib are in clinical trials across tumor types, and a first-in-human phase I study of abemaciclib in 5 tumor types including KRAS-mutant NSCLC demonstrated early clinical activity.[109] A phase III study is underway of abemaciclib in previously treated KRAS

Table 7
Clinical trials of drugs targeting KRAS

Drug Class and Target	Investigational Agent	Trial ID Number	Phase
KRAS	Trametinib + docetaxel	NCT01362296	II
	Trametinib + docetaxel	NCT02642042	II
	Trametinib + everolimus	NCT00955773	I
	Trametinib + navitoclax	NCT02079740	I/II
	Trametinib + second agent	NCT01192165	I
	Abemaciclib (LY2835219, JUNIPER study)	NCT02152631	III
	CB-839	NCT02071862	I
	Antroquinonol	NCT02047344	II
	Binimetinib (MEK162) + erlotinib	NCT01859026	I
	Selumetinib (AZD6244)	NCT01306045	II
	Trametinib + momelotinib	NCT02258607	I
	Selumetinib + docetaxel	NCT01933932	III
	Palbociclib + PD-0325901	NCT02022982	I/II
	Selumetinib + vistusertib (TORCMEK study)	NCT02583542	I/II

Abbreviations: JUNIPER, A Study of Abemaciclib (LY2835219) in Participants With Previously Treated KRAS Mutated Lung Cancer; TORCMEK, A Study of AZD2014 in Combination With Selumetinib in Patients With Advanced Cancers.

mutated lung cancer (JUNIPER [A Study of Abemaciclib (LY2835219) in Participants With Previously Treated KRAS Mutated Lung Cancer] study, NCT02152631). Combination therapy between palbociclib and PD-0325901, a MEK inhibitor, is being investigated in a phase I/II study (NCT02022982). Momelotinib, a JAK/TANK-binding kinase 1 inhibitor, disrupts KRAS-linked cytokine production to decrease tumorigenesis in murine models.[110] Synergy has been observed when combining momelotinib with MEK inhibition, and this concept is currently being tested in a phase I trial (NCT02258607). Mutations in both KRAS and p53 seem to be associated with increased glycolytic activity as a result of metabolic reprogramming in KRAS mutants.[111] Targeting cellular metabolism through glutaminase inhibition is another novel therapeutic approach for which a phase I trial is being conducted across multiple solid tumor types, including *KRAS* mutant NSCLC (NCT02071862).

SUMMARY

Targeted therapy for advanced NSCLC has now broadened from EGFR and ALK to include additional oncogenic targets. Although many of these mutations affect a relatively smaller proportion of patients with NSCLC, the fact that NSCLC is such a prevalent disease makes the proportion of patients who have specific oncogenic drivers an important focus. Genetic classification has become a standard component in clinical decision making; better outcomes have been reported in patients with clearly defined molecular alterations treated with specific targeted therapy. Acquired resistance has been seen and will require an increased understanding of gene function and novel treatment approaches to combat resistance. The implementation of new technologies in the clinic including larger scale genomic efforts with repeat tissue biopsies and circulating tumor DNA analyses has enabled patient identification and may continue to expand our ability to monitor patients for resistance on genomically defined targeted therapies.

REFERENCES

1. Siegel RL, Miller KD, Jemal A. Cancer statistics, 2015. CA Cancer J Clin 2015; 65:5–29.
2. Kris MG, Johnson BE, Berry LD, et al. Using multiplexed assays of oncogenic drivers in lung cancers to select targeted drugs. JAMA 2014;311(19): 1998–2006.
3. Scagliotti GV, Parikh P, von Pawel J, et al. Phase III study comparing cisplatin plus gemcitabine with cisplatin plus pemetrexed in chemotherapy-naïve patients with advanced-stage non-small-cell lung cancer. J Clin Oncol 2008; 26(21):3543–51.
4. Brahmer J, Reckamp KL, Baas P, et al. Nivolumab versus docetaxel in advanced squamous-cell non-small-cell lung cancer. N Engl J Med 2015; 373(2):123–35.
5. Paz-Ares L, Horn L, Borghaei H, et al. Phase III, randomized trial (CheckMate 057) of nivolumab (NIVO) versus docetaxel (DOC) in advanced non-squamous cell (non-SQ) non-small cell lung cancer (NSCLC). J Clin Oncol 2015;33(suppl) [abstract: LBA109].
6. Mok TS, Wu Y-L, Thongprasert S, et al. Gefitinib or carboplatin-paclitaxel in pulmonary adenocarcinoma. N Engl J Med 2009;361(10):947–57.
7. Kwak EL, Bang YJ, Camidge DR, et al. Anaplastic lymphoma kinase inhibition in non-small-cell lung cancer. N Engl J Med 2012;363(18):1693–703.

8. Acquaviva J, Wong R, Charest A. The multifaceted roles of the receptor tyrosine kinase ROS in development and cancer. Biochim Biophys Acta 2009;1795(1): 37–52.

9. Sonnenberg-Riethmacher E, Walter B, Riethmacher D, et al. The c-ros tyrosine kinase receptor controls regionalization and differentiation of epithelial cells in the epididymis. Genes Dev 1996;10(10):1184–93.

10. Charest A, Lane K, McMahon K, et al. Fusion of FIG to the receptor tyrosine kinase ROS in a glioblastoma with an interstitial del(6)(q21q21). Genes Chromosomes Cancer 2003;37(1):58–71.

11. Rikova K, Guo A, Zeng Q, et al. Global survey of phosphotyrosine signaling identifies oncogenic kinases in lung cancer. Cell 2007;131(6):1190–203.

12. Gu TL, Deng X, Huang F, et al. Survey of tyrosine kinase signaling reveals ROS kinase fusions in human cholangiocarcinoma. PLoS One 2011;6(1): e15640.

13. Bergethon K, Shaw AT, Ou SH, et al. ROS1 rearrangements define a unique molecular class of lung cancers. J Clin Oncol 2012;30(8):863–70.

14. Shaw AT, Yeap BY, Mino-Kenudson M, et al. Clinical features and outcome of patients with non-small-cell lung cancer who harbor EML4-ALK. J Clin Oncol 2009; 27(26):4247–53.

15. Ou SH, Tan J, Yen Y, et al. ROS1 as a 'druggable' receptor tyrosine kinase: lessons learned from inhibiting the ALK pathway. Expert Rev Anticancer Ther 2012; 12(4):447–56.

16. Shaw AT, Ou SH, Bang YJ, et al. Crizotinib in ROS1-rearranged non-small-cell lung cancer. N Engl J Med 2014;371(21):1963–71.

17. Engelman JA, Settleman J. Acquired resistance tyrosine kinase inhibitors during cancer therapy. Curr Opin Genet Dev 2008;18(1):73–9.

18. Song A, Kim TM, Kim DW, et al. Molecular changes associated with acquired resistance to crizotinib in ROS1-rearranged non-small cell lung cancer. Clin Cancer Res 2015;21(10):2379–87.

19. Gainor JF, Friboulet L, Yoda S, et al. Frequency and spectrum of ROS1 resistance mutations in ROS-1 positive lung cancer patients progressing on crizotinib. J Clin Oncol 2016;34(suppl) [abstract: 9072].

20. Sun H, Li Y, Tian S, et al. P-loop conformation governed crizotinib resistance in G2032R-mutated ROS1 tyrosine kinase: clues from free energy landscape. PLoS Comput Biol 2014;10(7):e1003729.

21. Ye M, Zhang X, Li N, et al. ALK and ROS1 as targeted therapy paradigms and clinical implications to overcome crizotinib resistance. Oncotarget 2016;7(11): 12289–304.

22. Solomon BJ, Bauer TM, Felip E, et al. Safety and efficacy of lorlatinib (PF-06463922) from the dose-escalation component of a study in patients with advanced ALK+ or ROS1+ non-small cell lung cancer (NSCLC). J Clin Oncol 2016;34(suppl) [abstract: 9009].

23. Davies KD, Mahale S, Astling DP, et al. Resistance to ROS1 inhibition mediated by EGFR pathway activation in non-small cell lung cancer. PLoS One 2013; 8(12):e82236.

24. Cargnelutti M, Corso S, Pergolizzi M, et al. Activation of RAS family members confers resistance to ROS1 targeting drugs. Oncotarget 2015;6(7):5182–94.

25. Eng C. RET proto-oncogene in the development of human cancer. J Clin Oncol 1999;17(1):380–93.

26. Phay JE, Shah MH. Targeting RET receptor tyrosine kinase activation in cancer. Clin Cancer Res 2010;16(24):5936–41.

27. Blaugrund JE, Johns MM Jr, Eby YJ, et al. RET proto-oncogene mutations in in-herited and sporadic medullary thyroid cancer. Hum Mol Genet 1994;3(10): 1895–7.
28. Takeuchi K, Soda M, Togashi Y, et al. RET, ROS1, and ALK fusions in lung can-cer. Nat Med 2012;18(3):378–81.
29. Lipson D, Capelletti M, Yelensky R, et al. Identification of new ALK and RET gene fusions from colorectal and lung cancer biopsies. Nat Med 2012;18(3): 382–4.
30. Ju YS, Lee WC, Shin JY, et al. A transforming KIF5B and RET gene fusion in lung adenocarcinoma revealed from whole-genome and transcriptome sequencing. Genome Res 2012;22(3):436–45.
31. Wang R, Hu H, Pan Y, et al. RET fusions define a unique molecular and clinico-pathologic subtype of non-small-cell lung cancer. J Clin Oncol 2012;30(35): 4352–9.
32. Kohno T, Ichikawa H, Totoki Y, et al. KIF5B-RET fusions in lung adenocarcinoma. Nat Med 2012;18(3):375–7.
33. Suehara Y, Arcila M, Wang L, et al. Identification of KIF5B-RET and GOPC-ROS1 fusions in lung adenocarcinomas through a comprehensive mRNA-based screen for tyrosine kinase fusions. Clin Cancer Res 2012;18(24):6599–608.
34. Lee J-K, Kim S, Shin J-Y, et al. Activity of sunitinib for lung adenocarcinoma with RET rearrangement. Cancer Res 2015;75(15 Suppl) [abstract: nr 2416].
35. Wu H, Shih JY, Yang JC. Rapid response to sunitinib in a patient with lung adenocarcinoma harboring KIF5B-RET fusion gene. J Thorac Oncol 2015; 10(9):e95–6.
36. Falchook GS, Ordonez NG, Bastida CC, et al. Effect of the RET inhibitor vande-tanib in a patient with RET fusion-positive metastatic non-small-cell lung cancer. J Clin Oncol 2016;34(15):e141–4.
37. Seto T, Yoh K, Satouchi M, et al. A phase II open-label single-arm study of van-detanib in patients with advanced RET-rearranged non-small cell lung cancer (NSCLC): LURET study. J Clin Oncol 2016;34(suppl) [abstract: 9012].
38. Lee S-H, Lee J-K, Ahn M-J, et al. A phase II study of vandetanib in patients with non-small cell lung cancer harboring RET rearrangement. J Clin Oncol 2016; 34(suppl) [abstract: 9013].
39. Drilon AE, Sima CS, Somwar R, et al. Phase II study of cabozantinib for patients with advanced RET-rearranged lung cancers. J Clin Oncol 2015;33(suppl) [ab-stract: 8007].
40. Somwar R, Smith R, Hayashi T, et al. MDM2 amplification (Amp) to mediate ca-bozantinib resistance in patients (Pts) with advanced RET-rearranged lung can-cers. J Clin Oncol 2016;34(suppl) [abstract: 9068].
41. Cascone T, Subbiah V, Hess KR, et al. Significant systemic and CNS activity of RET inhibitor vandetanib combined with mTOR inhibitor everolimus in patients with advanced NSCLC with RET fusion. J Clin Oncol 2016;34(suppl) [abstract: 9069].
42. Gautschi O, Wolf J, Milia J, et al. Targeting RET in patients with RET-rearranged lung cancers: results from a global registry. J Clin Oncol 2016;34(suppl) [abstract: 9014].
43. Nakagawara A. Trk receptor tyrosine kinases: a bridge between cancer and neural development. Cancer Lett 2001;169(2):107–14.
44. Chao MV. Neurotrophins and their receptors: a convergence point for many signaling pathways. Nat Rev Neurosci 2003;4(4):299–309.

45. Alberti L, Carniti C, Miranda C, et al. RET and NTRK1 proto-oncogenes in human diseases. J Cell Physiol 2003;195(2):168–86.
46. Vaishnavi A, Capelletti M, Le AT, et al. Oncogenic and drug-sensitive NTRK1 rearrangements in lung cancer. Nat Med 2013;19(11):1469–72.
47. Martin-Zanca D, Hughes SH, Barbacid M. A human oncogene formed by the fusion of truncated tropomyosin and protein tyrosine kinase sequences. Nature 1986;319(6056):743–8.
48. Greco A, Miranda C, Pierotti MA. Rearrangements of NTRK1 gene in papillary thyroid carcinoma. Mol Cell Endocrinol 2012;321(1):44–9.
49. Kim J, Lee Y, Cho HJ, et al. NTRK1 fusion in glioblastoma multiforme. PLoS One 2014;9(3):e91940.
50. Ross JS, Wang K, Gay L, et al. New routes to targeted therapy of intrahepatic cholangiocarcinomas revealed by next-generation sequencing. Oncologist 2014;19(3):235–42.
51. Stransky N, Cerami E, Schalm S, et al. The landscape of kinase fusions in cancer. Nat Commun 2014;5:4846.
52. Creancier L, Vandenberghe I, Gomes B, et al. Chromosomal rearrangements involving the NTRK1 gene in colorectal carcinoma. Cancer Lett 2015;365(1):107–11.
53. Siena S, Drilon AE, Ou SH, et al. Entrectinib (RXDX-101), an oral pan-Trk, ROS1, and ALK inhibitor in patients with advanced solid tumors harboring gene rearrangements. Eur J Cancer 2015;51(3 Suppl):S724–5.
54. Rolfo C, Ruiz R, Giovannetti E, et al. Entrectinib: a potent new TRK, ROS1, and ALK inhibitor. Expert Opin Investig Drugs 2015;24(11):1493–500.
55. Peruzzi B, Bottaro DP. Targeting the c-MET signaling pathway in cancer. Clin Cancer Res 2006 Jun 15;12(12):3657–60.
56. Teis D, Huber LA. The odd couple: signal transduction and endocytosis. Cell Mol Life Sci 2003;60(10):2020–33.
57. Peschard P, Fournier TM, Lamorte L, et al. Mutation of the c-Cbl TKB domain binding site on the Met receptor tyrosine kinase converts it into a transforming protein. Mol Cell 2001;8(5):995–1004.
58. Abella JV, Peschard P, Naujokas MA, et al. Met/Hepatocyte growth factor receptor ubiquitination suppresses transformation and is required for Hrs phosphorylation. Mol Cell Biol 2005;25(21):9632–45.
59. Peschard P, Ishiyama N, Lin T, et al. A conserved DpYR motif in the juxtamembrane domain of the Met receptor family forms an atypical c-Cbl/Cbl-b tyrosine kinase binding domain binding site required for suppression of oncogenic activation. J Biol Chem 2004;279(28):29565–71.
60. Birchmeier C, Birchmeier W, Gherardi E, et al. Met, metastasis, motility and more. Nat Rev Mol Cell Biol 2003;4(12):915–25.
61. Corso S, Comoglio PM, Giordano S. Cancer therapy: can the challenge be MET? Trends Mol Med 2005;11(6):284–92.
62. Christensen JG, Burrows J, Salgia R. c-MET as a target for human cancer and characterization of inhibitors for therapeutic intervention. Cancer Lett 2005;225(1):1–26.
63. Schmidt L, Duh FM, Chen F, et al. Germline and somatic mutations in the tyrosine kinase domain of the MET proto-oncogene in papillary renal carcinomas. Nat Genet 1997;16(1):68–73.
64. Schmidt L, Junker K, Nakaigawa N, et al. Novel mutations of the MET proto-oncogene in papillary renal carcinomas. Oncogene 1999;18(14):2343–50.

65. Dharmawardana PG, Giubellino A, Bottaro DP. Hereditary papillary renal carcinoma type I. Curr Mol Med 2004;4(8):855–68.
66. Cappuzzo F, Janne PA, Skokan M, et al. MET increased gene copy number and primary resistance to gefitinib therapy in non-small-cell lung cancer patients. Ann Oncol 2009;20(2):298–304.
67. Onozato R, Kosaka T, Kuwano H, et al. Activation of MET by gene amplification or by splice mutations deleting the juxtamembrane domain in primary resected lung cancers. J Thorac Oncol 2009;4(1):5–11.
68. Awad MM, Oxnard GR, Jackman DM, et al. MET exon 14 mutations in non-small-cell lung cancer are associated with advanced age and stage-dependent MET genomic amplification and c-Met overexpression. J Clin Oncol 2016;34(7): 721–30.
69. Benedettini E, Sholl LM, Peyton M, et al. Met activation in non-small cell lung cancer is associated with de novo resistance to EGFR inhibitors and the development of brain metastasis. Am J Pathol 2010;177(1):415–23.
70. Ichimura E, Maeshima A, Nakajima T, et al. Expression of c-met/HGF receptor in human non-small cell lung carcinomas in vitro and in vivo and its prognostic significance. Jpn J Cancer Res 1996;87(10):1063–9.
71. Olivero M, Rizzo M, Madeddu R, et al. Overexpression and activation of hepatocyte growth factor/scatter factor in human non-small-cell lung carcinomas. Br J Cancer 1996;74(12):1862–8.
72. Siegfried JM, Weissfeld LA, Luketich JD, et al. The clinical significance of hepatocyte growth factor for non-small cell lung cancer. Ann Thorac Surg 1998;66(6): 1915–8.
73. Nguyen KS, Kobayashi S, Costa DB. Acquired resistance to epidermal growth factor receptor tyrosine kinase inhibitors in non-small-cell lung cancers dependent on the epidermal growth factor receptor pathway. Clin Lung Cancer 2009; 10(4):281–9.
74. Engelman JA, Zejnullahu K, Mitsudomi T, et al. MET amplification leads to gefitinib resistance in lung cancer by activating ERBB3 signaling. Science 2007; 316(5827):1039–43.
75. Turke AB, Zejnullahu K, Wu YL, et al. Preexistence and clonal selection of MET amplification in EGFR mutant NSCLC. Cancer Cell 2010;17(1):77–88.
76. Sequist LV, Waltman BA, Dias-Santagata D, et al. Genotypic and histological evolution of lung cancers acquiring resistance to EGFR inhibitors. Sci Transl Med 2011;3(75):75ra26.
77. Spigel DR, Edelman MJ, O'Byrne K, et al. Onartuzumab plus erlotinib versus erlotinib in previously treated stage IIIB or IV NSCLC: results from the pivotal phase III randomized, multicenter, placebo-controlled METLung (OAM4971g) global trial. J Clin Oncol 2014;32(5suppl) [abstract: 8000].
78. Camidge DR, Moran T, Demedts I, et al. A randomized, open-label, phase 2 study of emibetuzumab plus erlotinib (LY+E) and emibetuzumab monotherapy (LY) in patients with acquired resistance to erlotinib and MET diagnostic positive (MET Dx+) metastatic NSCLC. J Clin Oncol 2016;34(suppl) [abstract: 9070].
79. Wu Y-L, Kim D-W, Felip E, et al. Phase (Ph) II safety and efficacy results of a single-arm ph ib/II study of capmatinib (INC280) + gefitinib in patients (pts) with EGFR-mutated (mut), cMET-positive (cMET+) non-small cell lung cancer (NSCLC). J Clin Oncol 2016;34(suppl) [abstract: 9020].
80. Wu Y-L, Soo RA, Kim D-W, et al. Tolerability, efficacy and recommended phase II dose (RP2D) of tepotinib plus gefitinib in Asian patients with

c-Met-positive/EGFR-mutant NSCLC: Phase Ib data. J Clin Oncol 2016; 34(suppl) [abstract: e20501].

81. Drilon AE, Camidge DR, Ou SH, et al. Efficacy and safety of crizotinib in patients (pts) with advanced *MET* exon 14-altered non-small cell lung cancer (NSCLC). J Clin Oncol 2016;34(suppl) [abstract: 108].

82. Schuler MH, Berardi R, Lim W-T, et al. Phase (Ph) I study of the safety and efficacy of the cMET inhibitor capmatinib (INC280) in patients (pts) with advanced cMET+ non-small cell lung cancer (NSCLC). J Clin Oncol 2016;34(suppl) [abstract: 9067].

83. Kollmannsberger CK, Sharma S, Shapiro G, et al. Phase I study of receptor tyrosine kinase (RTK) inhibitor, MGCD265, in patients (pts) with advanced solid tumors. J Clin Oncol 2015;33(suppl) [abstract: 2589].

84. Rybkin II, Kio EA, Masood A, et al. Amethyst NSCLC trial: Phase 2, parallel-arm study of receptor tyrosine kinase (RTK) inhibitor, MGCD265, in patients (pts) with advanced or metastatic non-small cell lung cancer (NSCLC) with activating genetic alterations in mesenchymal-epithelial transition factor (MET). J Clin Oncol 2016;34(suppl) [abstract: TPS9099].

85. Cantwell-Dorris ER, O'Leary JJ, Sheils OM. BRAFV600E: implications for carcinogenesis and molecular therapy. Mol Cancer Ther 2011;10(3):385–94.

86. Cardarella S, Ogino A, Nishino M, et al. Clinical, pathologic, and biologic features associated with BRAF mutations in non-small cell lung cancer. Clin Cancer Res 2013;19(16):4532–40.

87. Garnett MJ, Marais R. Guilty as charged: B-RAF is a human oncogene. Cancer Cell 2004;6(4):313–9.

88. Davies H, Bignell GR, Cox C, et al. Mutations of the BRAF gene in human cancer. Nature 2002;417(6892):949–54.

89. Paik PK, Arcila ME, Fara M, et al. Clinical characteristics of patients with lung adenocarcinomas harboring BRAF mutations. J Clin Oncol 2011;29(15): 2046–51.

90. Tang KT, Lee CH. BRAF mutation in papillary thyroid carcinoma: pathologic role and clinical implications. J Chin Med Assoc 2010;73(3):113–28.

91. Houben R, Becker JC, Kappel A, et al. Constitutive activation of the Ras-Raf signaling pathway in metastatic melanoma is associated with poor prognosis. J Carcinog 2004;3(1):6.

92. Hyman DM, Puzanov I, Subbiah V, et al. Vemurafenib in multiple nonmelanoma cancers with BRAF V600 mutations. N Engl J Med 2015;373(8):726–36.

93. Planchard D, Kim TM, Mazieres J, et al. Dabrafenib in patients with BRAF(V600E)-positive advanced non-small-cell lung cancer: a single-arm, multicenter, open-label, phase 2 trial. Lancet Oncol 2016;17(5):642–50.

94. Planchard D, Besse B, Groen HJM, et al. An open-label phase II trial of dabrafenib (D) in combination with trametinib (T) in patients (pts) with previously treated BRAF V600E-mutant advanced non-small cell lung cancer (NSCLC; BRF113928). J Clin Oncol 2016;34(suppl) [abstract: 107].

95. Zhang C, Spevak W, Zhang Y, et al. RAF inhibitors that evade paradoxical MAPK pathway activation. Nature 2015;526(7574):583–6.

96. Heidorn SJ, Milagre C, Whittaker S, et al. Kinase-dead BRAF and oncogenic RAS cooperate to drive tumor progression through CRAF. Cell 2010;140(2): 209–21.

97. Poulikakos PI, Zhang C, Bollag G, et al. RAF inhibitors transactivate RAF dimers and ERK signaling in cells with wild-type BRAF. Nature 2010;464(7287):427–30.

98. Hatzivassiliou G, Song K, Yen I, et al. RAF inhibitors prime wild-type RAF to activate MAPK pathway and enhance growth. Nature 2010;464(7287):431–5.

99. Chen SH, Zhang Y, Van Horn RD, et al. Oncogenic BRAF deletions that function as homodimers and are sensitive to inhibition by RAF dimer inhibitor LY3009120. Cancer Discov 2016;6(3):300–15.

100. Peng SB, Henry JR, Kaufman MD, et al. Inhibition of RAF isoforms and active dimers by LY3009120 leads to anti-tumor activities in RAS or BRAF mutant cancers. Cancer Cell 2015;28(3):384–98.

101. Pylayeva-Gupta Y, Grabocka E, Bar-Sagi D. RAS oncogenes: weaving a tumorigenic web. Nat Rev Cancer 2011;11(11):761–74.

102. Zhu Z, Golay HG, Barbie DA. Targeting pathways downstream of KRAS in lung adenocarcinoma. Pharmacogenomics 2014;15(11):1507–18.

103. Riely GJ, Marks J, Pao W. KRAS mutations in non-small cell lung cancer. Proc Am Thorac Soc 2009;6(2):201–5.

104. Riely GJ, Ladanyi M. KRAS mutations: an old oncogene becomes a new predictive biomarker. J Mol Diagn 2008;10(6):493–5.

105. Ostrem JM, Peters U, Sos ML, et al. K-Ras(G12C) inhibitors allosterically control GTP affinity and effector interactions. Nature 2013;503(7477):548–51.

106. Janne PA, Shaw AT, Pereira JR, et al. Selumetinib plus docetaxel for KRAS-mutant advanced non-small cell lung cancer: a randomized, multicenter, placebo-controlled, phase 2 study. Lancet Oncol 2013;14(1):38–47.

107. Corcoran RB, Cheng KA, Hata AN, et al. Synthetic lethal interaction of combined BCL-XL and MEK inhibition promotes tumor regression in KRAS mutant cancer models. Cancer Cell 2013;23(1):121–8.

108. Puyol M, Martin A, Dubus P, et al. A synthetic lethal interaction between K-Ras oncogenes and Cdk4 unveils a therapeutic strategy for non-small cell lung carcinoma. Cancer Cell 2010;18(1):63–73.

109. Shapiro G, Rosen LS, Tolcher AW, et al. A first-in-human phase I study of the CDK4/6 inhibitor, LY2835219, for patients with advanced cancer. J Clin Oncol 2013;31(suppl) [abstract: 2500].

110. Zhu Z, Aref AR, Cohoon TJ, et al. Inhibition of KRAS-driven tumorigenicity by interruption of an autocrine cytokine circuit. Cancer Discov 2014;4(4):452–65.

111. Kim S-H, Karo A, Basu S, et al. KRAS and P53 mutations and FDG-PET as a measure of glycolytic activity in metastatic non-small cell lung cancer patients. J Clin Oncol 2016;34(suppl) [abstract: 9086].

Immunotherapy in Lung Cancer

Lingling Du, MD[a], Roy S. Herbst, MD, PhD[b], Daniel Morgensztern, MD[a],*

KEYWORDS

- Non–small cell lung cancer • Vaccines • Immune checkpoint inhibitors • PD-L1

KEY POINTS

- Immunotherapy provides a significant benefit in a small percentage of patients.
- Vaccines against non–small cell lung cancer have not been effective.
- Nivolumab and pembrolizumab are approved for previously treated patients with non–small cell lung cancer.

INTRODUCTION

Lung cancer is the leading cause of cancer-related mortality in the United States.[1] Non–small cell lung cancer (NSCLC) comprises approximately 85% of all lung cancer cases.[2] Among patients with NSCLC, approximately 40% present with stage IV disease.[3] Although targeted therapy has been associated with a significant benefit in patients harboring aberrations in epidermal growth factor receptor (*EGFR*), anaplastic lymphoma kinase (*ALK*), or *ROS1*,[4–6] these gene abnormalities are present in a small percentage of patients. For most patients, chemotherapy, with or without antibodies against vascular endothelial growth factor, remains the mainstay of treatment.[7]

Immunotherapy represents a new approach to the treatment of patients with NSCLC, with several vaccines and checkpoint inhibitors currently being investigated.

VACCINES

NSCLC vaccines may be broadly divided into tumor cell (TC) vaccines, which could be from either autologous or allogeneic TCs, and antigen-based vaccines.[8] Vaccines are usually administered with adjuvants, which stimulate the immune response without having intrinsic antigen effect.[9] Low-dose cyclophosphamide, with the intention of

[a] Division of Oncology, Washington University School of Medicine, 660 South Euclid Avenue, Box 8056, St Louis, MO 63110, USA; [b] Thoracic Oncology Research Program, Yale Comprehensive Cancer Center, Yale School of Medicine, 333 Cedar Street, WWW221, New Haven, CT 06520-8028, USA
* Corresponding author.
E-mail address: dmorgens@dom.wustl.edu

Hematol Oncol Clin N Am 31 (2017) 131–141
http://dx.doi.org/10.1016/j.hoc.2016.08.004
hemonc.theclinics.com

decreasing the number and activity of regulatory T cells, is commonly used before the vaccine administration. Vaccines have been evaluated in multiple NSCLC settings including adjuvant, locally advanced, and metastatic (**Table 1**).

Adjuvant Setting

The melanoma-associated antigen-A3 (MAGE-A3) protein, encoded by the *MAGE-A3* gene, is a tumor-specific antigen not expressed in normal adult tissues except for testis and placenta, which do not present the antigen because of the lack of HLA molecules. The MAGE-A3 vaccine is composed of the MAGE-A3 protein plus an adjuvant. In a phase 2 trial, 182 patients with completely resected MAGE-A3-positive stage IB-II NSCLC were randomized (2:1) to receive MAGE-A3 in combination with the immunostimulant AS02B or placebo.[10] The primary end point was disease-free interval. MAGE-A3 vaccine was administered intramuscularly at 0.5 mL with treatments every 3 weeks for five doses followed by every 3 months for eight doses. The study was conducted between 2002 and 2004, before adjuvant chemotherapy became the standard of care. After a median postresection time of 44 months, 35% of patients in the vaccine group and 43% of patients in the placebo group developed recurrence. There were no significant differences in disease-free interval (hazard ratio [HR], 0.75; 95% confidence interval [CI], 0.46–1.23; $P = .2$), disease-free survival (DFS; HR, 0.76; 95% CI, 0.48–1.21; $P = .248$), or overall survival (OS; HR, 0.81; 95% CI, 0.47–1.40; $P = .454$) between the two arms. Nevertheless, the trend toward positive DFS in the vaccine group and the development of the more potent immunostimulant AS15, led to the initiation of the randomized phase III MAGRIT trial, which screened 13,849 patients with completely resected NSCLC stage IB-III for MAGE-A3.[11] Among the 12,820 patients who had a valid sample, 4210 (33%) had MAGE-A3 positive tumors and 2312 met the eligibility criteria for the study. Patients were randomized 2:1 to the vaccine in combination with the immunostimulant AS15 or placebo. The primary objective was DFS. The vaccine schedule was identical to the phase 2 trial, with 13 doses over a period of 27 months. In the overall population, the median DFS for the vaccine and control

Table 1
Randomized clinical trials with cancer vaccines

Vaccine	Setting	N	PFS (m)	OS (m)	OS, HR vs Control (95% CI), P Value
Adjuvant					
MAGE-A3[11]	IB-IIIA	2312	DFS: 60.5 vs 57.9	NR	DFS 1.02 (0.89–1.18), $P = .74$
Maintenance					
Tecemotide[12]	Stage III	65	Not reported	NR vs 13.3	0.52 (0.26–1.05), $P = .06$
Tecemotide[13]	Stage III concurrent CRT	806	Not reported	30.8 vs 20.6	0.78 (0.64–0.95), $P = .016$
Lucanix[15]	Stage III-IV	532	4.3 vs 4.0	20.3 vs 17.8	0.94 (0.73–1.20), $P = .59$
First line					
TG4010[19]	Stage IV	222	5.9 vs 5.1	12.7 vs 10.6	0.78 (0.57–1.06), $P = .055$

Abbreviations: CI, confidence interval; CRT, chemoradiotherapy; DFS, disease-free survival; HR, hazard ratio; NR, not reached; OS, overall survival; PFS, progression-free survival.

groups were 60.5 months and 57.9 months, respectively (HR, 1.02; 95% CI, 0.89–1.18; P = .74). In a subset analysis according to use of adjuvant chemotherapy, MAGE-A3 vaccine was not associated with median DFS improvement in patients who received chemotherapy (HR, 1.10; 95% CI, 0.90–1.34; P = .36) or not (HR, 0.97; 95% CI, 0.80–1.18; P = .76). Based on the MAGRIT results, the development of MAGE-A3 vaccine for NSCLC has been stopped.

Maintenance Therapy

Tecemotide (liposomal BLP-25) is a peptide vaccine targeting MUC1, which is overexpressed and aberrantly glycosylated in NSCLC, making it a target for immunotherapy. In a phase IIB study, 171 patients with advanced NSCLC without disease progression after first-line treatment were randomized to tecemotide plus best supportive care or best supportive care alone.[12] Tecemotide was preceded by one dose of cyclophosphamide, 300 mg/m^2, 3 days before the vaccine. Although the median OS was higher in the vaccine group, it did not reach statistical significance (17.4 vs 13.0 months; HR, 0.745; 95% CI, 0.533–1.042). Nevertheless, when stratified by stage, tecemotide was associated with improved median OS in patients with stage III (median OS not reached vs 13.3 months; HR, 0.52; 95% CI, 0.26–1.05; P = .06) but not for stage IV (15.1 months vs 12.9 months; HR, 0.90; 95% CI, 0.58–0.141; P = .6). To further investigate the role of tecemotide in patients with stage III NSCLC, the larger phase 3 START trial was conducted.[13] A total of 1513 patients were randomly assigned (2:1) to receive tecemotide or placebo, with 1239 patients included in the final analysis. For the total population, tecemotide did not significantly improve OS compared with placebo (median OS, 25.6 months vs 22.3 months; HR, 0.88; 95% CI, 0.75–1.03; P = .123). However, for the 806 patients who previously received concurrent chemoradiotherapy, tecemotide was associated with an increased median OS compared with placebo (30.8 months vs 20.6 months; HR, 0.78; 95% CI, 0.64–0.95; P =.016). However, the subsequent trial START2, which randomized patients to tecemotide or placebo after concurrent chemoradiotherapy, was terminated in September 2014 following the results from the INSPIRE study conducted in Japan, which had a similar design and showed no benefit from tecemotide following chemoradiotherapy in patients with stage III NSCLC.

Belagenpumatucel-L (Lucanix) is a tumor vaccine consisting of four allogeneic NSCLC cell lines modified with transforming growth factor-β_2-antisense plasmid.[14] In a phase III trial, 532 patients with stage III or IV NSCLC without progression after platinum-based chemotherapy were randomly assigned to maintenance belagenpumatucel-L or placebo.[15] The vaccine was well tolerated with injection site reactions and fatigue being the most common adverse events. Nevertheless, it was not associated with a significant improvement in the median progression-free survival (PFS; 4.3 months vs 4.0 months; HR, 0.99; 95% CI, 0.82–1.20; P = .947) or median OS (20.3 months vs 17.8 months; HR, 0.94; 95% CI, 0.73–1.20; P = .594).

Racotumomab-alum is a tumor vaccine targeting the NeuGGM3 tumor-associated ganglioside. In a phase 2 study, 176 patients with advanced NSCLC who received front-line chemotherapy and achieved at least stable disease (SD) were randomly assigned to racotumomab-alum or placebo.[16] Patients in the racotumomab-alum group had better median PFS (5.3 months vs 3.9 months; HR, 0.73; 95% CI, 0.53–0.99; P = .039) and OS (8.2 months vs 6.8 months; HR, 0.63; 95% CI, 0.46–0.87; P = .004) compared with placebo.

Vx-001 is an HLA-A*0201-restricted vaccine targeting the human telomerase reverse transcriptase tumor antigen. In a phase 2 study, 46 HLA-A*0201-positive patients with advanced NSCLC and residual or progressive disease after first-line treatment were treated with six doses of Vx-001.[17] The overall response rate (ORR) and SD rate were 7% and 28%, respectively, with median PFS of 3.8 months and median OS of 19 months. Patients who mounted immune responses (defined as the number of interferon-γ-spots-forming-cells from blood mononuclear cells significantly increased after vaccination compared with the background) had a significantly prolonged median OS compared with those who did not (40.0 months vs 9.2 months; $P = .02$). Vaccination was well tolerated. Common adverse events were mild and included injection-site reaction, anemia, fatigue, and nausea.

First-line Therapy

TG4010 is a vaccine composed of the modified vaccinia virus Ankara containing the sequence for interleukin 2 and MUC-1, which is a tumor-specific antigen overexpressed in many epithelial tumors including lung cancer.[18] The TIME is a phase 2b/3 trial examining the addition of TG4010 immunotherapy to chemotherapy in patients with previously untreated advanced NSCLC and MUC1 expression in greater than or equal to 50% of the TCs.[19] In the phase 2b part, 222 patients were randomly assigned to receive TG4010 versus placebo in addition to chemotherapy with a platinum-based doublet. The primary end point was PFS. For the total population, the median PFS for the TG4010 and the placebo arms were 5.9 months and 5.1 months, respectively (HR, 0.74; 95% CI, 0.55–0.98; $P = .019$). The median OS, however, despite numerically superior in patients treated with TG4010, did not reach statistical significance (12.7 months vs 10.6 months; HR, 0.78; 95% CI, 0.57–1.06; $P = .055$). The most common adverse event with TG4010 was grade 1 or 2 injection-site reactions. There were no grade 3 or 4 adverse events associated with TG4010 only. The phase 3 part of the TIME study is ongoing.

Previously Treated Patients

A phase 2 study evaluated a tumor vaccine composed of a granulocyte-macrophage colony-stimulating factor–producing and CD40L-expressing bystander cell line and allogeneic TCs.[20] Twenty-four patients were enrolled with a median of four previous lines of systemic treatment. No objective responses were observed. Median PFS and OS were 1.7 and 7.9 months, respectively. Common adverse events included headache and injection site reaction.

GVAX is a tumor vaccine consisting of autologous TCs mixed with an allogeneic cell line secreting granulocyte-macrophage colony-stimulating factor. In a phase 1/2 trial, 86 patients with advanced NSCLC had tumor harvested for vaccine preparation, and 49 patients eventually received the vaccine treatment.[21] A total of 76% of patients had received at least one line of chemotherapy before the vaccination. No objective responses were observed but SD for greater than or equal to 12 weeks was observed in 14% of patients. Median PFS and OS were 4.4 and 7.0 months, respectively. The most common adverse events were injection site reactions, fatigue, dyspnea, nausea, and fever.

CHECKPOINT INHIBITORS

Immune checkpoints are inhibitory pathways that modulate the duration and amplitude of the immune responses in the peripheral tissues to maintain self-tolerance and minimize collateral tissue damage.[22] One of the most studied immune checkpoints is the programmed death-ligand 1 (PD-L1)/programmed cell death protein 1 (PD-1) pathway. PD-L1 (also called B7-H1 or CD274) is a transmembrane glycoprotein that may be expressed on TCs and tumor infiltrating immune cells (ICs). Binding of PD-1 to PD-L1 causes T-cell inhibition and downregulation of the T-cell response.[8]

Early Phase Clinical Studies with Immune Checkpoint Inhibitors

Nivolumab is a fully humanized IgG4 antibody against PD-1. In a small phase 1 study, 39 patients with advanced refractory solid tumors were treated with nivolumab, which was well tolerated with no maximum tolerated dose reached.[23] There were six patients with NSCLC among the total of 39 patients. Nivolumab was well tolerated at all dose levels. One out of six patients with NSCLC had a mixed response. In a larger phase 1 trial, the CheckMate 003, a total of 296 patients with melanoma, NSCLC, prostate cancer, renal cancer, or colorectal cancer were treated with nivolumab at the doses of 1, 3, or 10 mg/kg every 2 weeks for up to 96 weeks.[24] The updated report included 129 patients with previously treated NSCLC, of which 54% had received three or more prior systemic therapy regimens.[25] The treatment was well tolerated, with the maximum tolerated dose not reached at the highest planned dose of 10 mg/kg. The most common adverse events were fatigue (24%), decreased appetite (12%), and diarrhea (10%). Four patients (3%) developed grade 3 or higher treatment-related pneumonitis resulting in three deaths. The ORR for the dose levels of 1, 3, 10 mg/kg were 3.0%, 24.3%, and 20.3%, respectively. The median PFS for all patients was 2.3 months. The 3-year OS survivals for the cohorts of 1, 3, and 10 mg/kg were 15%, 27%, and 14%, respectively. There were no significant differences in ORR, PFS, or OS according to histology subtypes. The dose of 3 mg/kg every 2 weeks was selected for phase 3 studies.

Pembrolizumab is a fully humanized IgG4 antibody against PD-1. The Keynote 001 trial was a phase 1 study examining the safety profile of pembrolizumab in advanced NSCLC.[26] A total of 495 patients receiving pembrolizumab were assigned to a training or validation groups. Pembrolizumab was given at 2 mg/kg or 10 mg/kg every 3 weeks, or 10 mg/kg every 2 weeks. Fatigue, pruritus, and decreased appetite were the most common side effects. Severe pneumonitis occurred in 1.8% of patients, including one death. The ORR for all patients, previously untreated, and previously treated patients was 19.4%, 24.8%, and 18.0%, respectively, without differences according to dose, regimen, or histology. The median PFS for all patients, treatment-naive and previously treated, was 3.7 months, 6.0 months, and 3.0 months, respectively. The median OS for all patients, previously untreated, and previously treated patients was 12.0, 16.2, and 9.3 months, respectively. Using a training group of 182 patients, a proportion score (PS), defined as the percentage of TCs positive for membranous PD-L1 expression of at least 50%, was selected as the cutoff level and subsequently tested in the validation group. In patients with a PS of greater than or equal to 50%, the ORR for all patients, those previously treated, and those who were treatment-naive were 45.2%, 43.9%, and 50.0%, respectively. In this group, the median PFS for all patients, previously treated, and previously untreated patients was 6.3, 6.1, and 12.5 months, respectively, with median OS not reached in any of the groups. The median PFS and OS in patients with a PS of greater than or equal to 50% were longer compared with those with a PS of 1% to 49% or less than 1%.

Atezolizumab (MPDL3280A) is a fully humanized monoclonal antibody against PD-L1. In a phase 1 study, 277 patients with advanced cancer were treated with atezolizumab given intravenously every 3 weeks.[27] In patients with NSCLC, the ORR and 24-week PFS were 21% and 45%, respectively. The response to atezolizumab was associated with PD-L1 expressions on tumor-infiltrating ICs ($P = .015$) but not on the TCs ($P = .920$). Treatment was well tolerated up to the maximum dose of 20 mg/kg. The most common toxicities included fatigue (24.2%), decreased appetite (11.9%), nausea (11.6%), and pyrexia (11.6%). Severe adverse events occurred in 12.6% of patients, with fatigue being the most frequent (1.8%). One percent of patients had immune-associated severe adverse events.

Randomized Clinical Trials with Immune Checkpoint Inhibitors

The encouraging results from the early studies led to further examination of these checkpoint inhibitors in comparison with the standard of care chemotherapy docetaxel in randomized controlled trials (**Table 2**).

The CheckMate 017 trial was a phase 3 study comparing nivolumab with docetaxel in patients with advanced squamous NSCLC previously treated with platinum-based therapy.[28] A total of 272 patients were randomized to nivolumab at 3 mg/kg every 2 weeks or docetaxel at 75 mg/m^2 every 3 weeks. The primary end point was median OS. Nivolumab was better tolerated than docetaxel and associated with increased ORR (20% vs 9%; $P = .008$), median PFS (3.5 months vs 2.8 months; HR, 0.62; 95% CI, 0.47–0.81; $P <.001$), 1-year PFS (21% vs 6%), median OS (9.2 months vs 6 months; HR, 0.59; 95% CI, 0.44–0.79; $P <.001$), and 1-year OS (42% vs 24%). PD-L1 expression was not prognostic or predictive for nivolumab efficacy compared with docetaxel. These results led to the Food and Drug Administration (FDA) approval of nivolumab in March 2015 for the treatment of patients with advanced squamous NSCLC previously treated with platinum-based chemotherapy.

The Checkmate 057 study compared nivolumab with docetaxel in patients with advanced nonsquamous NSCLC.[29] A total of 582 patients were randomly assigned to nivolumab or docetaxel using the same regimens as in the CheckMate 017 study. Nivolumab was better tolerated and associated with increased ORR compared with docetaxel (19% vs 12%; $P = .02$). The median PFS and 1-year PFS rate were 2.3 months and 19% with nivolumab versus 4.2 months and 8% with docetaxel (HR, 0.92; 95% CI, 0.77–1.1; $P = .39$). Nivolumab was associated with increased median OS (12.2 vs 9.4 months; HR, 0.72; 95% CI, 0.60–0.88; $P <.001$) and 1-year OS (51% vs 39%) compared with docetaxel. Based on the survival benefit and superior toxicity profile, the FDA expanded the approval for nivolumab use to include patients with advanced nonsquamous NSCLC who have progressed on or after platinum-based therapy in October 2015.

The Keynote 010 trial was a phase 2/3 study evaluating the efficacy of pembrolizumab in patients with previously treated advanced NSCLC.[30] Among the 2222 patients whose tumor samples were screened for PD-L1 expression, 1475 (66%) had PD-L1 expression in at least 1% of TCs. Among them, 1034 patients met the eligibility criteria and were randomly assigned in a 1:1:1 fashion to pembrolizumab, 2 mg/kg, pembrolizumab,

Table 2
Randomized clinical trials of checkpoint inhibitors

	CM017[28]	CM057[29]	KN010 (2 mg/kg)[30]	KN010 (10 mg/kg)[30]	POPLAR[31]
Treatment vs doc	Nivolumab	Nivolumab	Pembrolizumab	Pembrolizumab	Atezolizumab
ORR vs Doc	20% vs 9%	19% vs 12%	18% vs 9%	18% vs 9%	15% vs 15%
Median PFS vs Doc	3.5 m vs 2.8 m	2.3 m vs 4.2 m	3.9 m vs 4.0 m	4.0 m vs 4.0 m	2.7 m vs 3.0 m
Median OS vs Doc	9.2 m vs 6.0 m	12.2 m vs 9.4 m	10.4 m vs 8.5 m	12.7 m vs 8.5 m	12.6 m vs 9.7 m
HR for OS (95% CI)	0.59 (0.44–0.79)	0.73 (0.59–0.89)	0.71 (0.58–0.88)	0.61 (0.49–0.75)	0.73 (0.53–0.99)

Abbreviations: CM, CheckMate; Doc, docetaxel; KN, Keynote.

10 mg/kg, or docetaxel, 75 mg/m² every 3 weeks. Adverse events of any grade and grade 3 to 5 for patients treated with pembrolizumab, 2 mg/kg, 10 mg/kg, and docetaxel occurred in 63% and 13%, 66% and 16%, and 81% and 35% of patients, respectively. The most common side effects in patients treated with pembrolizumab were decreased appetite, fatigue, rash, and nausea. For the total population, the ORR for pembrolizumab, 2 mg/kg, pembrolizumab, 10 mg/kg, and docetaxel were 18%, 18% and 9%, respectively. The median PFS and OS for each group were 3.9 months and 10.4 months, 4 months and 12.7 months, and 4 months and 8 months, respectively. Both doses of pembrolizumab improved the median OS compared with docetaxel (pembrolizumab, 2 mg/kg, vs docetaxel: HR, 0.71; 95% CI, 0.58–0.88; P = .0008; pembrolizumab, 10 mg/kg, vs docetaxel: HR, 0.61; 95% CI, 0.49–0.75; P <.0001). The ORR among patients with PD-L1 expression greater than or equal to 50% was 8% in the docetaxel group, 30% in the pembrolizumab, 2 mg/kg, and 29% for pembrolizumab, 10 mg/kg. In this patient population, the median OS for pembrolizumab, 2 mg/kg, 10 mg/kg, and docetaxel were 14.9, 17.3, and 8.2 months (pembrolizumab, 2 mg/kg, vs docetaxel: HR, 0.54; 95% CI, 0.38–0.77; P = .0002; pembrolizumab, 10 mg/kg, vs docetaxel: HR, 0.50; 95% CI, 0.36–0.70; P <.0001). Pembrolizumab was approved by the FDA in October 2015 for patients with previously treated advanced NSCLC and tumor positive for PD-L1 expression.

The POPLAR trial was a phase 2 study comparing atezolizumab with docetaxel in 287 patients with previously treated advanced stage NSCLC.[31] Patients were randomly assigned to receive atezolizumab, 1200 mg, or docetaxel, 75 mg/m², intravenously every 3 weeks. The primary end point was median OS. Neither the PFS (2.7 months vs 3.0 months; HR, 0.94; 95% CI, 0.72–1.23) nor the objective RR (15% vs 15%) were significantly different between the atezolizumab and the docetaxel arms. However, atezolizumab was associated with a significant improvement in median OS compared with docetaxel (12.6 months vs 9.7 months; HR, 0.73; 95% CI, 0.53–0.99; P = .04). The increased median OS improvement from atezolizumab compared with docetaxel was directly related to the PD-L1 expression on TCs, ICs, or both. Among patients with no PD-L1 expression in TCs or ICs, the median OS for atezolizumab and docetaxel was identical at 9.7 months. Grade 3 or 4 treatment-related adverse events occurred in 11% of patients receiving atezolizumab versus 39% in those treated with docetaxel. Fatigue, decreased appetite, nausea, diarrhea, and asthenia were the most common adverse events with atezolizumab.

PREDICTIVE FACTORS OF CHECKPOINT INHIBITORS

Because only a minority of NSCLC patients achieves benefit from single-agent immune checkpoint inhibitors, there has been an intense search for biomarkers.

Programmed Death-ligand 1 Expression

PD-L1, which may be expressed in TCs and its interaction with PD1 is the target for the therapeutic antibodies, is the most commonly evaluated biomarker to predict for benefit from anti-PD1 or anti-PD-L1 checkpoint inhibitors. Nevertheless, despite the strong rationale for the predictive role of PD-L1 expression, the results from clinical trials have not clearly established its role in patient selection. For patients treated with nivolumab, the CheckMate 017 study showed no predictive role for PD-L1 expression on ORR, PFS, or OS.[28] In contrast, the CheckMate 057 showed that improved outcomes for nivolumab compared with docetaxel was observed only in patients with positive PD-L1 expression.[29] Among patients treated with pembrolizumab in the Keynote 001 trial, the ORR was significantly higher in patients with PD-L1 expression of at least 50% compared with those with expression of 1% to 49% and less than 1%.[26] In the Keynote 010, which enrolled only patients with positive PD-L1 expression, the benefit from pembrolizumab compared with docetaxel was higher in patients with PS greater than or equal to 50% than in those with PS 1% to 49%.[30] In the POPLAR study, the benefit from atezolizumab compared with docetaxel was observed only in patients with PD-L1 expression in either TCs or ICs.[31] Nevertheless, although the studies have consistently reported increased ORR, PFS, and OS for checkpoint inhibitors among patients with PD-L1-positive tumors, patients with negative tumors may also benefit from the therapy. In a recent meta-analysis including 1567 patients treated with anti-PD1 or anti-PD-L1 antibodies, there was an increase in ORR among patients with PD-L1 expression tumors compared to those with no PD-L1 expression (29% vs 13%; HR, 2.08; 95% CI, 1.49–2.91; P <.01), although the 1-year OS was similar (28% vs 27%; HR, 0.96; 95% CI, 0.87–1.06; P = .39).[32] Some of the caveats for the use of PD-L1 expression as a biomarker for benefit from immune checkpoint inhibitors include the use of multiple PD-L1 detection antibodies with different staining techniques, cells evaluated, and cutoff points for positive result or scoring system.[33]

Mutation Burden

Rizvi and colleagues[34] examined the impact of mutational landscape on the efficacy of pembrolizumab in NSCLC. In this study, whole-genome sequencing was performed on the tumor samples of two cohorts of patients with NSCLC treated with pembrolizumab. Patients with high somatic nonsynonymous mutation burden (defined as higher than the median burden of the cohort) derived more benefit from treatment with pembrolizumab compared with those with mutation burden lower than median. Seventy-three percent of patients with high mutation burden had durable clinical benefit (defined as partial response (PR) or SD lasting at least 6 months) versus 13% of those with low mutation burden. Patients with high mutation burden also had a higher ORR (63% vs 0%; P = .03) and longer PFS (14.5 months vs 3.7 months; P = .01).

Because patients that are never smokers or harbor *EGFR* activating mutations have lower mutation burden than smokers with wild-type *EGFR*,[35] the OS improvement from nivolumab compared with docetaxel in the CheckMate 057 observed in smokers (0.70; 95% CI, 0.56–0.86) and *EGFR* wild-type (HR, 0.66; 95% CI, 0.51–0.86) but not in never-smokers (HR, 1.02; 95% CI, 0.64–1.61) or *EGFR* mutant (1.18; 95% CI, 0.69–2.00) was expected.[29] Nevertheless, although current or former smokers had increased ORR from pembrolizumab in the Keynote 001 compared with never smokers, when patients were evaluated according to PD-L1 expression, smoking status did not predict for responses.[26] Furthermore, for patients treated with pembrolizumab, self-reported smoking status did not correlate with treatment efficacy, which was instead associated with smoking signature defined as transversion-high tumors.[34]

FIRST LINE IMMUNE CHECKPOINT INHIBITION

With the safety and efficacy of immune checkpoint inhibitors in previously treated patients, recent studies have focused on their use in the first line setting. In the Checkmate 012 trial, 52 patients were treated with nivolumab 3 mg/kg every 2 weeks until tumor progression or unacceptable toxicity.[36] The ORR was 23%, including 9 out of 32 (28%) in patients with PD-L1 positive and 2 out of 14 (14%) with no PD-L1 expression. The median PFS and OS were 3.6 months and 19.4 months respectively. The Keynote-024 randomized 305 patients with PD-L1 expression on at least 50% of tumor cells to receive either pembrolizumab or platinum-based chemotherapy according to investigator's choice.[37] Pembrolizumab was associated with lower fewer adverse effects (73.4% vs 90%), higher ORR (44.8% vs 27.8%) and median PFS

(10.3 vs 6.0 months, HR 0.5; 95% CI 0.37–0.68, P < 0.001). Although the median OS was not reached in either treatment group, the estimated percentage of patients alive at 6 months was higher in the pembrolizumab arm (80.2% vs 72.4%). With the better safety profile and improvement in both PFS and OS compared to chemotherapy, pembrolizumab should be considered a new standard of care for previously untreated patients with tumor PD-L1 staining of at least 50% and no contraindications for immune checkpoint therapy.

SUMMARY

The advancements in immunotherapy have provided a new approach for the management of patients with NSCLC. Although studies with vaccines have not been successful, immune checkpoint inhibitors against the PD-1/PD-L1 pathway are associated with a remarkable benefit in a small percentage of patients. Two anti-PD-1 antibodies, nivolumab and pembrolizumab, have been approved for previously treated patients based on the improved OS and decreased toxicity compared with docetaxel.

REFERENCES

1. Siegel RL, Miller KD, Jemal A. Cancer statistics, 2016. CA Cancer J Clin 2016;66: 7–30.
2. Govindan R, Page N, Morgensztern D, et al. Changing epidemiology of small-cell lung cancer in the United States over the last 30 years: analysis of the surveillance, epidemiologic, and end results database. J Clin Oncol 2006;24:4539–44.
3. Morgensztern D, Ng SH, Gao F, et al. Trends in stage distribution for patients with non-small cell lung cancer: a National Cancer Database survey. J Thorac Oncol 2010;5:29–33.
4. Mok TS, Wu YL, Thongprasert S, et al. Gefitinib or carboplatin-paclitaxel in pulmonary adenocarcinoma. N Engl J Med 2009;361:947–57.
5. Solomon BJ, Mok T, Kim DW, et al. First-line crizotinib versus chemotherapy in ALK-positive lung cancer. N Engl J Med 2014;371:2167–77.
6. Shaw AT, Ou SH, Bang YJ, et al. Crizotinib in ROS1-rearranged non-small-cell lung cancer. N Engl J Med 2014;371:1963–71.
7. Masters GA, Temin S, Azzoli CG, et al. Systemic therapy for stage IV non-small-cell lung cancer: American Society of Clinical Oncology Clinical Practice Guideline Update. J Clin Oncol 2015;33:3488–515.
8. Brahmer JR. Harnessing the immune system for the treatment of non-small-cell lung cancer. J Clin Oncol 2013;31:1021–8.
9. Iyengar P, Gerber DE. Locally advanced lung cancer: an optimal setting for vaccines and other immunotherapies. Cancer j 2013;19:247–62.
10. Vansteenkiste J, Zielinski M, Linder A, et al. Adjuvant MAGE-A3 immunotherapy in resected non-small-cell lung cancer: phase II randomized study results. J Clin Oncol 2013;31:2396–403.
11. Vansteenkiste JF, Cho BC, Vanakesa T, et al. Efficacy of the MAGE-A3 cancer immunotherapeutic as adjuvant therapy in patients with resected MAGE-A3-positive non-small-cell lung cancer (MAGRIT): a randomised, double-blind, placebo-controlled, phase 3 trial. Lancet Oncol 2016;17(6):822–35.
12. Butts C, Maksymiuk A, Goss G, et al. Updated survival analysis in patients with stage IIIB or IV non-small-cell lung cancer receiving BLP25 liposome vaccine (L-BLP25): phase IIB randomized, multicenter, open-label trial. J Cancer Res Clin Oncol 2011;137:1337–42.

13. Butts C, Socinski MA, Mitchell PL, et al. Tecemotide (L-BLP25) versus placebo after chemoradiotherapy for stage III non-small-cell lung cancer (START): a randomised, double-blind, phase 3 trial. Lancet Oncol 2014;15:59–68.

14. Nemunaitis J, Dillman RO, Schwarzenberger PO, et al. Phase II study of belagenpumatucel-L, a transforming growth factor beta-2 antisense gene-modified allogeneic tumor cell vaccine in non-small-cell lung cancer. J Clin Oncol 2006;24:4721–30.

15. Giaccone G, Bazhenova LA, Nemunaitis J, et al. A phase III study of belagenpumatucel-L, an allogeneic tumour cell vaccine, as maintenance therapy for non-small cell lung cancer. Eur J Cancer 2015;51:2321–9.

16. Alfonso S, Valdes-Zayas A, Santiesteban ER, et al. A randomized, multicenter, placebo-controlled clinical trial of racotumomab-alum vaccine as switch maintenance therapy in advanced non-small cell lung cancer patients. Clin Cancer Res 2014;20:3660–71.

17. Kotsakis A, Papadimitraki E, Vetsika EK, et al. A phase II trial evaluating the clinical and immunologic response of HLA-A2(+) non-small cell lung cancer patients vaccinated with an hTERT cryptic peptide. Lung cancer 2014;86:59–66.

18. Limacher JM, Quoix E. TG4010: a therapeutic vaccine against MUC1 expressing tumors. Oncoimmunology 2012;1:791–2.

19. Quoix E, Lena H, Losonczy G, et al. TG4010 immunotherapy and first-line chemotherapy for advanced non-small-cell lung cancer (TIME): results from the phase 2b part of a randomised, double-blind, placebo-controlled, phase 2b/3 trial. Lancet Oncol 2016;17:212–23.

20. Creelan BC, Antonia S, Noyes D, et al. Phase II trial of a GM-CSF-producing and CD40L-expressing bystander cell line combined with an allogeneic tumor cell-based vaccine for refractory lung adenocarcinoma. J Immunother 2013;36:442–50.

21. Nemunaitis J, Jahan T, Ross H, et al. Phase 1/2 trial of autologous tumor mixed with an allogeneic GVAX vaccine in advanced-stage non-small-cell lung cancer. Cancer Gene Ther 2006;13:555–62.

22. Pardoll DM. The blockade of immune checkpoints in cancer immunotherapy. Nat Rev Cancer 2012;12:252–64.

23. Brahmer JR, Drake CG, Wollner I, et al. Phase I study of single-agent anti-programmed death-1 (MDX-1106) in refractory solid tumors: safety, clinical activity, pharmacodynamics, and immunologic correlates. J Clin Oncol 2010;28:3167–75.

24. Topalian SL, Hodi FS, Brahmer JR, et al. Safety, activity, and immune correlates of anti-PD-1 antibody in cancer. N Engl J Med 2012;366:2443–54.

25. Gettinger SN, Horn L, Gandhi L, et al. Overall survival and long-term safety of nivolumab (anti-programmed death 1 antibody, BMS-936558, ONO-4538) in patients with previously treated advanced non-small-cell lung cancer. J Clin Oncol 2015;33:2004–12.

26. Garon EB, Rizvi NA, Hui RN, et al. Pembrolizumab for the treatment of non-small-cell lung cancer. N Engl J Med 2015;372:2018–28.

27. Herbst RS, Soria JC, Kowanetz M, et al. Predictive correlates of response to the anti-PD-L1 antibody MPDL3280A in cancer patients. Nature 2014;515:563–7.

28. Brahmer J, Reckamp KL, Baas P, et al. Nivolumab versus docetaxel in advanced squamous-cell non-small-cell lung cancer. N Engl J Med 2015;373:123–35.

29. Borghaei H, Paz-Ares L, Horn L, et al. Nivolumab versus docetaxel in advanced nonsquamous non-small-cell lung cancer. N Engl J Med 2015;373:1627–39.

30. Herbst RS, Baas P, Kim DW, et al. Pembrolizumab versus docetaxel for previously treated, PD-L1-positive, advanced non-small-cell lung cancer (KEYNOTE-010): a randomised controlled trial. Lancet 2015;387(10027):1540–50.

31. Fehrenbacher L, Spira A, Ballinger M, et al. Atezolizumab versus docetaxel for patients with previously treated non-small-cell lung cancer (POPLAR): a multicentre, open-label, phase 2 randomised controlled trial. Lancet 2016; 387(10030):1837–46.
32. Aguiar PN Jr, Santoro IL, Tadokoro H, et al. The role of PD-L1 expression as a predictive biomarker in advanced non-small-cell lung cancer: a network meta-analysis. Immunotherapy 2016;8:479–88.
33. Shukuya T, Carbone DP. Predictive markers for the efficacy of Anti-PD-1/PD-L1 Antibodies in lung cancer. J Thorac Oncol 2016;11(7):976–88.
34. Rizvi NA, Hellmann MD, Snyder A, et al. Cancer immunology. Mutational landscape determines sensitivity to PD-1 blockade in non-small cell lung cancer. Science 2015;348:124–8.
35. Govindan R, Ding L, Griffith M, et al. Genomic landscape of non-small cell lung cancer in smokers and never-smokers. Cell 2012;150:1121–34.
36. Gettinger S, Rizvi NA, Chow LQ, et al. Nivolumab monotherapy for first-line treatment of advanced non-small cell lung cancer. J Clin Oncol 2016;34:2980–7.
37. Reck M, Rodriguez-Abreu D, Robinson AG, et al. Pembrolizumab versus chemotherapy for PD-L1 positive non-small-cell lung cancer. N Engl J Med (in press).

Advances in Small Cell Lung Cancer

Gregory P. Kalemkerian, MD[a],*, Bryan J. Schneider, MD[b]

KEYWORDS

- Lung cancer • Small cell • Chemotherapy • Radiation therapy • Genomics
- Targeted therapy • Immunotherapy

KEY POINTS

- Small cell lung cancer (SCLC) is a high-grade neuroendocrine tumor with rapid growth, early metastatic spread and initial responsiveness to therapy.
- Limited stage (LS)-SCLC is curable, with long-term survival of 20% to 25% when treated with platinum-based chemotherapy plus thoracic radiation and prophylactic cranial irradiation.
- Extensive stage (ES)-SCLC is incurable, but combination chemotherapy can prolong survival and improve quality of life.
- Although many potential molecular targets have been identified, targeted therapy has not demonstrated consistent clinical activity in SCLC.
- Future advances will depend on therapeutic strategies that target the pathways driving cancer cell survival and immunologic avoidance.

INTRODUCTION

Small cell lung cancer (SCLC) is an aggressive neuroendocrine tumor with clinical and pathologic characteristics distinct from those of non-SCLC. The primary cause of SCLC is tobacco use, with more than 95% of patients being current or former smokers. In the United States, the decreasing prevalence of cigarette smoking has resulted in a decrease in the incidence of SCLC. The frequency of SCLC as a proportion of all lung cancer cases peaked at 17% to 20% in the late 1980s, but is now 13% to 15%.[1,2] Despite the decrease in incidence, SCLC remains the seventh most common cause of cancer-related death in the United States. From 1973 to 2002, the 5-year overall survival rate only increased from 4.3% to 6.3%.[1]

[a] Division of Hematology/Oncology, Department of Internal Medicine, University of Michigan, C350 Med Inn–SPC 5848, 1500 East Medical Center Drive, Ann Arbor, MI 48109-5848, USA;
[b] Division of Hematology/Oncology, Department of Internal Medicine, University of Michigan, C411 Med Inn–SPC 5848, 1500 East Medical Center Drive, Ann Arbor, MI 48109-5848, USA
* Corresponding author.
E-mail address: kalemker@umich.edu

Hematol Oncol Clin N Am 31 (2017) 143–156
http://dx.doi.org/10.1016/j.hoc.2016.08.005
0889-8588/17/© 2016 Elsevier Inc. All rights reserved.

hemonc.theclinics.com

STAGING SYSTEMS

The Veterans' Administration Lung Study Group (VALSG) 2-stage classification has been the standard system for staging SCLC for decades.[3] This system defines limited stage (LS) as disease confined to 1 hemithorax, including contralateral mediastinal and ipsilateral supraclavicular lymph nodes, if all disease can be safely encompassed in a radiation port. Extensive stage (ES) is defined as disease that cannot be classified as limited, including malignant pleural or pericardial effusions and hematogenous metastases. The classification of metastases to contralateral supraclavicular or hilar lymph nodes is debatable, with individualized treatment based on the ability to safely treat all areas of disease with radiotherapy (RT).

It has been suggested that the TNM staging classification should replace the VALSG system for SCLC.[4] This recommendation is based on the finding that the individual tumor (T), node (N), and metastasis (M) classifiers, and the stage I through IV groupings are predictive of overall survival in SCLC.[5] However, the degree of prognostic discrimination with the TNM system is less impressive in SCLC than in non-SCLC. In addition, nearly all of the clinical trials that guide the treatment of patients with SCLC have used the VALSG staging system, so the immediate application of TNM staging may confuse clinical decision making. Nonetheless, TNM staging is useful in the selection of patients for surgical resection (ie, T1-2 N0), and should be incorporated into clinical trial design and tumor registries.

INITIAL ASSESSMENT AND STAGING

LS-SCLC is a curable disease, but ES-SCLC is not, so the primary goal of staging is to look for distant metastases. The initial evaluation of patients with newly diagnosed SCLC is highlighted in **Box 1**. An MRI scan will detect brain metastases in 10% to 15% of newly diagnosed patients without neurologic symptoms.[6] Fewer than 5% of patients will have bone marrow involvement as the only site of metastatic disease, so bone marrow aspiration/biopsy should only be considered in patients with significant hematological abnormalities.

Box 1
Initial evaluation for small cell lung cancer

Complete medical history and physical examination

Pathologic review of biopsy with immunohistochemical analysis

Laboratory studies
    Complete blood count (white blood cells, hemoglobin/hematocrit, platelets)
    Serum electrolytes (Na, K, Cl, HCO_3, Ca)
    Renal function tests (blood urea nitrogen, creatinine)
    Liver function tests (AST, ALT, bilirubin, alkaline phosphatase)
    Serum lactate dehydrogenase (lactate dehydrogenase)
    Nutritional status (total protein, albumin)

CT of the chest and upper abdomen (liver, adrenal glands) with intravenous contrast

^{18}F-fluorodeoxyglucose-PET/CT (whole body)

MRI or CT of brain with intravenous contrast

Bone scan (optional if PET obtained)

Performance status assessment

Abbreviations: ALT, alanine aminotransferase; AST, aspartate aminotransferase; CT, computed tomography; MRI, magnetic resonance imaging; PET, positron emission tomography.

Recently, ^{18}F-fluorodeoxyglucose (FDG)-PET has been incorporated into the staging evaluation of SCLC.[7] If PET is obtained, then bone scan is not necessary because FDG-PET imaging is as sensitive as bone scan for the detection of bone metastases. The sensitivity of FDG-PET imaging is 100% for the detection of SCLC. A systematic review of studies comparing FDG-PET imaging with conventional imaging procedures reported that 16% of patients with LS-SCLC by conventional imaging were upstaged to ES by FDG-PET imaging, whereas 11% of patients with ES-SCLC by conventional imaging were downstaged to LS.[8] A metaanalysis of studies defined the sensitivity and specificity of FDG-PET for the detection of ES-SCLC as 97.5% and 98.2%, respectively.[9] However, FDG-PET is inferior to MRI and CT scanning for the detection of brain metastases. A review of 7 studies found that FDG-PET led to a change in the initial management in 28% of patients, with one-third owing to a change in stage and the rest owing to adjustment of RT fields in patients with LS-SCLC, which may result in better locoregional disease control.[10]

The addition of FDG-PET imaging to conventional imaging studies improves the accuracy of staging and RT planning in patients with SCLC, and is recommended in the initial workup. Owing to the potential for false-positive findings, pathologic confirmation is recommended for any PET-detected lesion that results in a change in treatment.

TREATMENT OF SMALL CELL LUNG CANCER

The management of SCLC is often complicated by the fact that many patients present with debilitating symptoms of disease. The high prevalence of cigarette smoking also results in comorbidities that further impair performance status.

Stage-Specific Therapy

LS-SCLC is a potentially curable disease. Surgical resection followed by adjuvant chemotherapy is indicated for the few patients (<5%) who present with true stage I (T1-2 N0) disease. The standard of care for most patients with LS-SCLC consists of 4 to 6 cycles of cisplatin/carboplatin and etoposide plus early, concurrent thoracic RT. Prophylactic cranial irradiation (PCI) is recommended for patients with good performance status who achieve a robust response to initial therapy. Standard therapy yields an objective tumor response in 90% of patients and a 5-year survival rate of 20% to 25%.

ES-SCLC is an incurable disease in which platinum-based chemotherapy is given with palliative intent. Combination chemotherapy results in an objective response in 60% to 70% of patients. Patients with a good response to chemotherapy and a good performance status should be considered for PCI and/or thoracic RT, which may improve survival. Although chemotherapy improves quality of life and prolongs survival, relapse with relatively chemoresistant disease is inevitable, and fewer than 10% of patients with ES-SCLC remain alive 2 years after diagnosis. The stage-specific treatment of patients with SCLC is outlined in **Box 2**.

Thoracic Radiotherapy in Limited Stage Small Cell Lung Cancer

The expanded use of RT has yielded modest improvements in outcomes for patients with both LS-SCLC and ES-SCLC. In LS-SCLC, metaanalyses demonstrated that the addition of definitive thoracic RT to chemotherapy significantly improved the 2- to 3-year overall survival rate by 5.4%.[11,12] Subsequently, a metaanalysis reported that early thoracic RT (initiated before the third cycle of chemotherapy) resulted in a 5% improvement in 2-year overall survival when compared with late RT.[13] Another metaanalysis of 4 trials reported that patients with a shorter interval between the start of any

---

Box 2
Treatment of small cell lung cancer

Limited stage

Cisplatin/carboplatin + etoposide $\times$ 4 to 6 cycles

Early, concurrent thoracic radiotherapy

Prophylactic cranial irradiation for responders

Surgical resection followed by adjuvant chemotherapy (stage I only)

Extensive stage

Platinum-based chemotherapy (eg, carboplatin + etoposide) $\times$ 4 to 6 cycles

Prophylactic cranial irradiation for responders

Thoracic radiation for responders

Recurrent disease

Single-agent chemotherapy (eg, topotecan, paclitaxel)

Palliative radiotherapy, as needed for symptoms

Clinical trials of investigational therapeutic agents

---

treatment and the end of RT had a better 5-year survival rate (relative risk, 0.62; P = .0003).[14] Based on these findings, early concurrent chemoradiotherapy is the standard approach for patients with LS-SCLC.

The role of hyperfractionated thoracic RT remains controversial. Turrisi and colleagues[15] reported a phase III trial in which 417 patients with LS-SCLC were randomized to receive cisplatin plus etoposide (PE) with 45 Gy of early, concurrent thoracic RT given either once daily or twice daily. Twice-daily RT resulted in a significant improvement in overall survival (5 years, 26% vs 16%; P = .04). However, patients on the once-daily RT arm received a relatively low dose of radiation that was not biologically equivalent to the dose delivered on the twice-daily RT arm. Bonner and colleagues[16] reported another randomized trial of hyperfractionated RT in which 262 patients with LS-SCLC were assigned to receive PE plus either once-daily thoracic RT to 50.4 Gy or twice-daily RT to 48 Gy in a split course. RT was started with the third cycle of chemotherapy in both arms. There were no differences in survival between the arms. The late initiation of RT and the use of a split course of RT in the twice-daily arm are both considered suboptimal therapy. Therefore, the potential benefit of hyperfractionated RT in LS-SCLC remains unclear.

Thoracic Radiotherapy in Extensive Stage Small Cell Lung Cancer

The role of thoracic RT in patients with ES-SCLC is also controversial. Jeremic and colleagues[17] reported a study in which patients who had an excellent response to initial PE were randomized to receive either hyperfractionated thoracic RT (54 Gy) plus concurrent chemotherapy or further PE without RT. Overall survival was significantly better in patients on the RT arm (median, 17 vs 11 months; P = .041). A recent phase III study by Slotman and colleagues[18] randomized 495 patients with ES-SCLC who responded to first-line chemotherapy to either thoracic RT (30 Gy) or no RT. Thoracic RT did not significantly improve the primary endpoint of 1-year overall survival (33% vs 28%; P = .07), but did improve 2-year overall survival (13% vs 3%; P = .004). These trials suggest that patients with ES-SCLC who have responded well to chemotherapy may benefit from RT to residual thoracic disease.

Prophylactic Cranial Irradiation

Approximately 60% of patients with SCLC develop brain metastases. A metaanalysis of randomized trials of PCI in mostly LS-SCLC reported a 25% decrease in the incidence of brain metastases (58% vs 33%; P<.001) and a 5.4% improvement in the 3-year survival rate (15.3% vs 20.7%; P = .01) with PCI.[19] To evaluate the effects of PCI in ES-SCLC, the European Organization for Research and Treatment of Cancer randomized 286 patients with ES-SCLC who had responded to first-line chemotherapy to either PCI or no PCI, and found that PCI decreased the incidence of brain metastases (14.6% vs 40.4%; P<.001) and improved the 1-year survival rate (27.1% vs 13.3%; P = .003).[20] Despite a short-term decline in quality of life, PCI did not have a lasting effect on global quality-of-life scores.[21] However, preliminary data from Japan have cast doubt on these findings, with a randomized trial of PCI versus no PCI in patients with ES-SCLC that demonstrated a trend toward better survival in the no PCI arm (median, 15 vs 10 months; P = .09).[22] Pending the final results of this study, PCI (25 Gy in 10 fractions) is recommended for patients with LS-SCLC or ES-SCLC and good performance status who have had a robust response to initial therapy.

First-Line Chemotherapy

SCLC usually responds well to initial chemotherapy and RT, with relatively rapid improvement in symptoms. Many cytotoxic drugs have activity in SCLC, but the duration of response with single-agents is short (**Box 3**). Alkylator-based regimens, such as cyclophosphamide, doxorubicin, and vincristine, improved response rates to 60% to 80% and median survival to 7 to 10 months.[23] In LS-SCLC, up to 25% of patients remained disease free at 2 years. Subsequently, PE was found to have efficacy similar to that of alkylator-based regimens, with more tolerable toxicity.[24,25] One phase III study comparing PE to cyclophosphamide, epirubicin, and vincristine reported significantly better overall survival with PE (10.2 vs 7.8 months; P = .0004).[26] In addition, metaanalyses reported a modest survival benefit for patients treated with cisplatin-based therapy.[27,28] Therefore, PE became the primary regimen for both ES-SCLC and LS-SCLC.

Many other systemic approaches have been assessed, but none have proven superior to PE. Many studies have evaluated combinations of cisplatin/carboplatin plus a topoisomerase 1 inhibitor (**Table 1**). In Japan, a phase III study randomized 154 patients with previously untreated ES-SCLC to PE or cisplatin plus irinotecan (PI) and

---

Box 3
Active chemotherapy drugs in small cell lung cancer

DNA-intercalating agents: cisplatin, carboplatin

Alkylating agents: cyclophosphamide, ifosfamide, temozolomide, bendamustine

Microtubule inhibitors: vincristine, vinblastine, vinorelbine

Microtubule stabilizers: paclitaxel, docetaxel

Topoisomerase I inhibitors: irinotecan, topotecan

Topoisomerase II inhibitors: etoposide, teniposide

Anthracyclines: doxorubicin, epirubicin, amrubicin

Antimetabolites: methotrexate, gemcitabine

Table 1
Randomized trials of cisplatin/carboplatin plus irinotecan/topotecan in extensive stage small cell lung cancer

Trial	Arm	N	Response Rate		Overall Survival			
			%	P	Median	1 y (%)	2 y (%)	P
Noda et al,[29] 2002	IP	77	84	.02	12.8 mo	58.4	19.5	.002
	EP	77	68		9.4 mo	37.7	5.2	
Hanna et al,[30] 2006	IP	221	48	NS	9.3 mo	35	8	.74
	EP	110	44		10.2 mo	35	8	
Lara et al,[31] 2009	IP	324	60	.56	9.9 mo	41	NR	.71
	EP	327	57		9.1 mo	34	NR	
Zatloukal et al,[32] 2010	IP	202	39	NS	10.2 mo	42	16	.06
	EP	203	47		9.7 mo	39	8	
Hermes et al,[33] 2008	IC	105	17[a]	.02	8.5 mo	NR	NR	.02
	EC	104	7[a]		7.1 mo	NR	NR	
Schmittel et al,[34] 2006	IC	35	67	.24	9.0 mo[b]	27[b]	NR	.03
	EC	35	59		6.0 mo[b]	11[b]	NR	
Eckardt et al,[35] 2006	TP	389	63	NS	9.0 mo	31	NR	.48
	EP	395	69		9.2 mo	31	NR	
Fink et al,[36] 2012	TP	358	56	.01	45 wk	40	NR	.30
	EP	345	46		41 wk	36	NR	

Abbreviations: EC, etoposide + carboplatin; EP, etoposide + cisplatin; IP, irinotecan + cisplatin; IC, irinotecan + carboplatin; NR, not reported; NS, not significant; TP, topotecan + cisplatin.
[a] Complete response rate.
[b] Progression-free survival.

reported that PI significantly improved response rate, progression-free survival, and overall survival.[29] However, randomized trials in Western countries have failed to confirm the superiority of PI over PE with no differences in efficacy outcomes, but less toxicity with PE.[30–32]

In efforts to decrease toxicity, carboplatin plus irinotecan and cisplatin plus topotecan have also been studied in SCLC with mixed results[33–36] (see **Table 1**). Metaanalyses have found a modest improvement in overall survival with combinations of a platinum agent plus irinotecan or topotecan, leaving the question of optimal first-line therapy unresolved.[37,38]

It is unlikely that empiric chemotherapy will further improve outcomes in patients with SCLC. Many chemotherapy-based strategies, including dose intensification, dose-dense regimens, 3-drug regimens, alternating non–cross-resistant regimens, maintenance therapy, consolidation therapy, and even high-dose consolidation with hematologic stem cell support, have failed to yield convincing improvements in survival. Many of these aggressive approaches also resulted in unacceptable toxicity, so cisplatin/carboplatin plus etoposide remains the standard of care for patients with SCLC.

Cisplatin versus carboplatin

In practice, many oncologists substitute carboplatin for cisplatin given its more favorable toxicity profile. The only trial that directly compared PE with carboplatin plus etoposide (CE) in patients with SCLC found no difference in efficacy.[39] The COCIS metaanalysis of 4 trials that compared cisplatin- with carboplatin-based therapy for first-line treatment of both LS-SCLC and ES-SCLC reported no difference in response rate (67% vs 66%, $P = .83$), progression-free survival (median, 5.5 vs 5.3 months, $P = .25$), or overall survival (median, 9.6 vs 9.4 months, $P = .37$).[40] Carboplatin-based regimens caused more grade 3 to 4 myelosuppression, whereas cisplatin resulted in more nausea, neurotoxicity, and nephrotoxicity. These data suggest that carboplatin is as effective as cisplatin in both LS-SCLC and ES-SCLC and that it has a more manageable toxicity profile.

Recurrent disease
Recurrent SCLC is divided into 2 categories: refractory/resistant (progression <3 months from completion of initial therapy) or relapsed/sensitive (progression >3 months). Rates of response to second-line therapy are substantially lower in patients with refractory/resistant disease. The reinitiation of the front-line chemotherapy regimen is recommended if the initial response duration is 6 months or more based on reported response rates of 50% to 60%.[41,42] The benefit of second-line chemotherapy in recurrent SCLC was evaluated in a randomized trial comparing oral topotecan with best supportive care. Although topotecan induced response in only 7% of patients, it did significantly improve overall survival (median, 26 vs 14 weeks; $P = .01$).[43]

Combination regimens usually yield higher response rates than single agents, but overall survival is not improved and their toxicity erodes quality of life. One phase III trial compared single-agent topotecan with cyclophosphamide, doxorubicin, and vincristine in patients with relapsed SCLC and found no difference in response rate (24% vs 18%; $P = .29$) or overall survival (median, 25 vs 25 weeks; $P = .79$).[44] However, hematologic toxicity was significantly greater with cyclophosphamide, doxorubicin, and vincristine. Therefore, single-agent chemotherapy is the standard treatment for patients with relapsed SCLC.

Several other drugs have demonstrated phase II activity in relapsed SCLC, including paclitaxel, docetaxel, oral etoposide, and vinorelbine. The most recently reported active agents are temozolomide (response rates of 20% and 12%, respectively) and bendamustine (response rates of 29% and 26%, respectively).[45–48]

EMERGING THERAPIES
Chemotherapy

Amrubicin has promising activity in patients with SCLC, with a single-agent response rate of 79% in untreated patients.[49] However, a phase III trial comparing cisplatin plus amrubicin with PI in previously untreated patients with ES-SCLC reported similar response rates, but overall survival favoring PI.[50] In relapsed SCLC, a phase III trial randomized patients to receive either amrubicin or topotecan and showed a significant improvement in response rate with amrubicin (31% vs 17%; $P<.001$), but no difference in overall survival (median, 7.5 vs 7.8 months; $P = .17$).[51] Owing to these disappointing results, amrubicin is not available in the United States.

Angiogenesis Inhibitors

SCLC is a highly vascular tumor and most patients have elevated serum levels of vascular endothelial growth factor, a key mediator of angiogenesis. Sunitinib, an inhibitor of vascular endothelial growth factor receptor, was studied as maintenance therapy in ES-SCLC in a trial that randomized 85 patients to receive PE followed by either sunitinib or placebo.[52] Although sunitinib improved progression-free survival (median, 3.8 vs 2.3 months; $P = .037$), there was no difference in overall survival and sunitinib was poorly tolerated.

Table 2
Molecularly targeted agents in clinical development in small cell lung cancer

Mechanism of Action	Agent	Target
Angiogenesis/multikinase inhibition	Bevacizumab	VEGF
	Sunitinib	VEGFR, KIT, FLT3, RET, PDGFR
	Cediranib	VEGFR-1/2/3
	Nintedanib	VEGFR, FGFR, PDGFR, SRC, LCK, FLT3
	Ponatinib	VEGFR, FGFR, ABL, FLT3, TIE2
	Lucitanib	VEGFR, FGFR
Growth factor pathway inhibition	Trametinib	MEK
	Tivantinib	MET
	Rilotumumab	MET
	Everolimus	mTOR
	Sirolimus	mTOR
	Gedatolisib	mTOR, PI3K
	Buparlisib	PI3K
	MK2206	AKT
	Auranofin	JAK/STAT
	Pasireotide	SSTR2
Cell cycle inhibition	Roniciclib	CDK 1/2/4/9
	G1T28	CDK 4/6
	AZD1775	WEE1
Proapoptotic agents	Navitoclax	BCL-2
	LCL161	SMAC
Cancer stem cell pathways	Erismodegib	SMO
	BMS-833923	SMO
	Tarexumab	NOTCH 2/3
HDAC inhibition	Belinostat	HDAC
DNA demethylation	CC-486	DNA methyltransferase
	GSK2879552	LSD1
Microtubule inhibition	Alisertib	Aurora A kinase
DNA repair	Veliparib	PARP
	Olaparib	PARP
	LY2606368	CHK1
	VX-970	ATR kinase
Protein degradation and transport	Ganetespib	HSP 90
	Carfilzomib	Proteasome
	Selinexor	CRM1
Immune checkpoint inhibition	Ipilimumab	Anti–CTLA-4
	Tremelimumab	Anti–CTLA-4
	Pembrolizumab	Anti–PD1
	Nivolumab	Anti–PD1
	Atezolizumab	Anti–PDL1
	Durvalumab	Anti–PDL1
Surface antigens	Lorvotuzumab	CD56-NCAM
	Rovalpituzumab tesirine	DLL3
	SC-002	
	BMS-986012	Fucosyl-GM1
	TF2/Lu^{177}- IMP-288	CEA

Abbreviations: CDK, cyclin-dependent kinase; CEA, carcinoembryonic antigen; CTLA-4, cytotoxic T-lymphocyte antigen 4; FGFR, fibroblast growth factor receptor; HDAC, histone deacetylase; HSP, heat shock protein; mTOR, mammalian target of rapamycin; NCAM, neural cell adhesion molecule; PARP, poly-ADP ribose polymerase; PDGFR, platelet derived growth factor receptor; PI3K, phosphatidylinositol-3-kinase; SMAC, second mitochondria-derived activator of caspases; SMO, smoothened; SSTR2, somatostatin receptor 2; VEGFR, vascular endothelial growth factor receptor.

Targeted Anticancer Therapy

Preclinical studies have led to the identification of many molecular targets for novel therapeutic approaches in SCLC. Many of these biologically rational strategies have been evaluated in clinical trials, but few have demonstrated clinical activity and none have reached routine practice.[53,54] Despite these setbacks, many molecularly targeted therapies are currently being evaluated in clinical trials in SCLC (**Table 2**).

The most promising recent strategy targets DLL3, a Notch ligand that is overexpressed predominantly in SCLC tumor-initiating cells. Rovalpituzumab-tesirine consists of a monoclonal antibody targeting DLL3 linked to a DNA-damaging toxin. In a phase I study, rovalpituzumab-tesirine demonstrated a response rate of 23% in all patients with relapsed SCLC, and 44% in those with high levels of DLL3 expression treated at the recommended phase II dose.[55]

Next-generation molecular techniques, including whole-genome sequencing, have been used to identify genetic derangements that might serve as new therapeutic targets or predictive biomarkers in SCLC. A consistent finding of these studies is the extremely high frequency of protein-altering mutations in SCLC. Other consistent findings are the near ubiquity of alterations in the *p53* and *RB1* tumor suppressor genes and the high frequency of *Myc*-family gene amplification.[56–58] These studies have also identified many new potential targets in SCLC, including histone modifiers (CREBBP, MLL), the PI3K-PTEN pathway, FGFR1, the neural cell migration factor SLIT2, DNA-repair enzymes (PARP1), cell cycle checkpoint regulators (EZH2), and mediators of "stem cell" characteristics (NOTCH, Hedgehog, SOX2).[56–59]

In cancers with high mutational burdens such as SCLC, it is likely that tumor cell heterogeneity and the dysregulation of multiple pathways will limit the activity of any single targeted intervention. Clinical advances in these diseases will require complex combinations of agents targeting several molecular drivers of cell proliferation and survival.

Immunotherapy

Immune checkpoint inhibitors have shown promise in many tumor types, including SCLC. CTLA-4 is an immune checkpoint protein expressed on activated T cells that downregulates T-cell activation. Ipilimumab, an anti–CTLA-4 monoclonal antibody, enhances T-cell activation. A randomized phase II trial treated 164 patients with ES-SCLC with carboplatin and paclitaxel plus either concurrent or phased ipilumumab or placebo, and found that patients receiving phased ipilumumab, given after 2 cycles of chemotherapy, had a higher response rate and overall survival than those receiving placebo.[60]

Activated T cells also express PD-1, another immune checkpoint receptor. Many cancer cells produce PD-L1, the PD-1 ligand, resulting in localized immunosuppression that protects tumors from immune surveillance. In a phase Ib trial, pembrolizumab, an anti-PD1 antibody, yielded a response rate of 35% in patients with PD-L1–positive SCLC.[61] A phase I/II study in relapsed SCLC reported response rates of 18% with nivolumab, another anti-PD1 antibody, and 17% with the combination of nivolumab plus ipilumumab.[62]

SUMMARY

SCLC remains one of the greatest challenges in oncology. Over the past 40 years, clinical advances in the treatment of SCLC have had a relatively modest impact on overall survival (**Table 3**). Although RT is an important component of therapy, SCLC is primarily a systemic disease, so further therapeutic gains will require improvements in

| Table 3
Advances in SCLC	
Era	Advances
1970s	Combination alkylator-based chemotherapy
1980s	Combination platinum-based chemotherapy
Chemotherapy + thoracic RT for LS-SCLC
1990s	Early, concurrent thoracic RT in LS-SCLC
Second-line chemotherapy
PCI for LS-SCLC |
| 2000s | Hyperfractionated thoracic RT for LS-SCLC
Irinotecan + cisplatin in ES-SCLC (Japan)
PCI for ES-SCLC |
| 2010s | Sequential thoracic RT for ES-SCLC
Immunotherapy as second-line therapy |

Abbreviations: ES-SCLC, extensive stage small cell lung cancer; LS-SCLC, limited stage small cell lung cancer; PCI, prophylactic cranial irradiation; RT, radiotherapy; SCLC, small cell lung cancer.

systemic therapy. Future advances will rely on ongoing efforts to identify pathways that drive cancer cell survival, proliferation, invasion and metastasis, and to develop treatments that interfere with these critical targets.

REFERENCES

1. Navada S, Lai P, Schwartz AG, et al. Temporal trends in small cell lung cancer: analysis of the national surveillance, epidemiology, and end-results database. J Clin Oncol 2006;24(18S):384s.
2. Govindan R, Page N, Morgensztern D, et al. Changing epidemiology of small-cell lung cancer in the United States over the last 30 years: analysis of the surveillance, epidemiologic, and end-results database. J Clin Oncol 2006;24:4539–44.
3. Zelen M. Keynote address on biostatistics and data retrieval. Cancer Chemother Rep 3 1973;4:31–42.
4. American Joint Committee on Cancer (AJCC). AJCC Cancer staging handbook. 7th Edition. New York: Springer; 2010. p. 299–323.
5. Shepherd FA, Crowley J, Van Houtte P, et al. The IASLC Lung Cancer Staging Project: proposals regarding the clinical staging of small cell lung cancer in the forthcoming (seventh) edition of the tumor, node, metastasis classification for lung cancer. J Thorac Oncol 2007;2:1067–77.
6. Hochstenbag MMH, Twijinstra A, Wilmink JT, et al. Asymptomatic brain metastases in small cell lung cancer: MR-imaging is useful at initial diagnosis. J Neurooncol 2000;48:243–8.
7. Kalemkerian GP, Loo BW, Akerley W, et al. NCCN clinical practice guidelines in oncology. Small cell lung cancer, version 1.2016. Available at: http://www.nccn.org/professionals/physician_gls/pdf/sclc.pdf. Accessed April 30, 2016.
8. Jett JR, Schild SE, Kesler KA, et al. Treatment of small cell lung cancer. diagnosis and management of lung cancer, 3rd ed: American college of chest physicians evidence-based clinical practice guidelines. Chest 2013;143(5 suppl):e400S–19S.
9. Lu YY, Chen JH, Liang JA, et al. 18FDG PET or PET/CT for detecting extensive disease in small-cell lung cancer: a systematic review and meta-analysis. Nucl Med Commun 2014;35:697–703.

10. van Loon J, De Ruysscher D, Wanders R, et al. Selective nodal irradiation on basis of [18]FDG-PET scans in limited-disease small-cell lung cancer: a prospective study. Int J Radiat Oncol Biol Phys 2010;77:329–36.

11. Warde P, Payne D. Does thoracic irradiation improve survival and local control in limited-stage small-cell carcinoma of the lung? A meta-analysis. J Clin Oncol 1992;10:890–5.

12. Pignon JP, Arriagada R, Ihde DC, et al. A meta-analysis of thoracic radiotherapy for small-cell lung cancer. N Engl J Med 1992;327:1618–24.

13. Fried DB, Morris DE, Poole C, et al. Systematic review evaluating the timing of thoracic radiation therapy in combined modality therapy for limited-stage small cell lung cancer. J Clin Oncol 2004;22:4785–93.

14. De Ruysscher D, Pijls-Johannesma M, Bentzen SM, et al. Time between the first day of chemotherapy and the last day of chest radiation is the most important predictor of survival in limited-disease small-cell lung cancer. J Clin Oncol 2006;24:1057–63.

15. Turrisi AT, Kim K, Blum R, et al. Twice-daily compared with once-daily thoracic radiotherapy in limited small-cell lung cancer treated concurrently with cisplatin and etoposide. N Engl J Med 1999;340:265–71.

16. Bonner JA, Sloan JA, Shanahan TG, et al. Phase III comparison of twice-daily split-course irradiation versus once-daily irradiation for patients with limited-stage small-cell lung carcinoma. J Clin Oncol 1999;17:2681–91.

17. Jeremic B, Shibamoto Y, Nikolic N, et al. Role of radiation therapy in the combined-modality treatment of patients with extensive disease small-cell lung cancer: a randomized study. J Clin Oncol 1999;17:2092–9.

18. Slotman BJ, van Tinteren H, Praag JO, et al. Use of thoracic radiotherapy for extensive stage small-cell lung cancer: a phase 3 randomised controlled trial. Lancet 2015;385:36–42.

19. Auperin A, Arriagada R, Pignon JP, et al. Prophylactic cranial irradiation for patients with small-cell lung cancer in complete remission. Prophylactic cranial irradiation overview collaborative group. N Engl J Med 1999;341:476–84.

20. Slotman B, Faivre-Finn C, Kramer G, et al. Prophylactic cranial irradiation in extensive small-cell lung cancer. N Engl J Med 2007;357:664–72.

21. Slotman BJ, Mauer ME, Bottomley A, et al. Prophylactic cranial irradiation in extensive disease small-cell lung cancer: short-term health-related quality of life and patient reported symptoms: results of an international Phase III randomized controlled trial by the EORTC radiation oncology and lung cancer groups. J Clin Oncol 2009;27:78–84.

22. Seto T, Takahashi T, Yamanaka T, et al. Prophylactic cranial irradiation has a detrimental effect on the overall survival of patients with extensive disease small cell lung cancer: results of a Japanese randomized phase III trial. J Clin Oncol 2014; 32(15S):477s.

23. Lowenbraun S, Bartolucci A, Smalley RV, et al. The superiority of combination chemotherapy over single agent chemotherapy in small cell lung carcinoma. Cancer 1979;44:406–13.

24. Fukuoka M, Furuse K, Saijo N, et al. Randomized trial of cyclophosphamide, doxorubicin, and vincristine versus cisplatin and etoposide versus alternation of these regimens in small-cell lung cancer. J Natl Cancer Inst 1991;83:855–61.

25. Roth BJ, Johnson DH, Einhorn LH, et al. Randomized study of cyclophosphamide, doxorubicin, and vincristine versus etoposide and cisplatin versus alternation of these two regimens in extensive small-cell lung cancer: a phase III trial of the Southeastern cancer study group. J Clin Oncol 1992;10:282–91.

26. Sundstrøm S, Bremnes RM, Kaasa S, et al. Cisplatin and etoposide regimen is superior to cyclophosphamide, epirubicin, and vincristine regimen in small-cell lung cancer: results from a randomized phase III trial with 5 years' follow-up. J Clin Oncol 2002;20:4665–72.
27. Mascaux C, Paesmans M, Breghmans T, et al. A systematic review of the role of etoposide and cisplatin in the chemotherapy of small cell lung cancer with methodology assessment and meta-analysis. Lung Cancer 2000;30:23–36.
28. Mascaux C, Paesmans M, Breghmans T, et al. A systematic review of the role of etoposide and cisplatin in the chemotherapy of small cell lung cancer with methodology assessment and meta-analysis. Lung Cancer 2000;30:23–36.
29. Noda K, Nishiwaki Y, Kawahara M, et al. Irinotecan plus cisplatin compared with etoposide plus cisplatin for extensive small-cell lung cancer. N Engl J Med 2002; 346:85–91.
30. Hanna N, Bunn PA, Langer C, et al. Randomized phase III trial comparing irinotecan/cisplatin with etoposide/cisplatin in patients with previously untreated extensive-stage small-cell lung cancer. J Clin Oncol 2006;24:2038–43.
31. Lara PN, Natale R, Crowley J, et al. Phase III trial of irinotecan/cisplatin compared with etoposide/cisplatin in extensive-stage small-cell lung cancer: clinical and pharmacogenomic results from SWOG S0124. J Clin Oncol 2009;27:2530–5.
32. Zatloukal P, Cardenal F, Szxzesna A, et al. A multicenter international randomized phase III study comparing cisplatin in combination with irinotecan or etoposide in previously untreated small-cell lung cancer patients with extensive disease. Ann Oncol 2010;21:1810–6.
33. Hermes A, Bergman B, Bremmew R, et al. Irinotecan plus carboplatin versus oral etoposide plus carboplatin in extensive small-cell lung cancer: a randomized phase III trial. J Clin Oncol 2008;26:4261–7.
34. Schmittel A, von Weikersthal LF, Sebastian M, et al. A randomized phase II trial of irinotecan plus carboplatin versus etoposide plus carboplatin treatment in patients with extended disease small-cell lung cancer. Ann Oncol 2006;17:663–7.
35. Eckardt JR, von Pawel J, Papai Z, et al. Open-label, multicenter, randomized, phase III study comparing oral topotecan/cisplatin versus etoposide/cisplatin as treatment for chemotherapy-naive patients with extensive-disease small-cell lung cancer. J Clin Oncol 2006;24:2044–51.
36. Fink TH, Huber RM, Heigener DF, et al. Topotecan/cisplatin compared with cisplatin/etoposide as first-line treatment for patients with extensive disease small-cell lung cancer. J Thorac Oncol 2012;7:1432–9.
37. Jiang J, Liang X, Zhou X, et al. A meta-analysis of randomized controlled trials comparing irinotecan/platinum with etoposide/platinum in patients with previously untreated extensive-stage small cell lung cancer. J Thorac Oncol 2010;5:867–73.
38. Lima JP, dos Santos LV, Sasse EC, et al. Camptothecins compared with etoposide in combination with platinum analog in extensive stage small cell lung cancer: systematic review with meta-analysis. J Thorac Oncol 2010;5:1986–93.
39. Sklaros DV, Samantas E, Kosmidis P, et al. Randomized comparison of etoposide-cisplatin vs. etoposide-carboplatin and irradiation in small-cell lung cancer: a Hellenic Cooperative Oncology Group study. Ann Oncol 1994;5:601–7.
40. Rossi A, DiMaio M, Chiodini P, et al. Carboplatin- or cisplatin-based chemotherapy in first-line treatment of small-cell lung cancer: the COCIS meta-analysis of individual patient data. J Clin Oncol 2012;30:1692–8.
41. Postmus PE, Berendsen HH, van Zandwijk N, et al. Retreatment with the induction regimen in small cell lung cancer relapsing after an initial response to short term chemotherapy. Eur J Cancer Clin Oncol 1987;23:1409–11.

42. Giaccone G, Ferrati P, Donadio M, et al. Reinduction chemotherapy in small cell lung cancer. Eur J Cancer Clin Oncol 1987;23:1697–9.

43. O'Brien MER, Ciuleanu TE, Tsekov H, et al. Phase III trial comparing supportive care alone with supportive care with oral topotecan in patients with relapsed small-cell lung cancer. J Clin Oncol 2006;24:5441–7.

44. Von Pawel J, Schiller JH, Shepherd FA, et al. Topotecan versus cyclophosphamide, doxorubicin, and vincristine for the treatment of recurrent small-cell lung cancer. J Clin Oncol 1999;17:658–67.

45. Pietanza MC, Kadota K, Huberman K, et al. Phase II trial of temozolomide in patients with relapsed sensitive or refractory small cell lung cancer, with assessment of methylguanine-DNA methyltransferase as a potential biomarker. Clin Cancer Res 2012;18:1138–45.

46. Zauderer MG, Drilon A, Kadota K, et al. Trial of a 5-day dosing regimen of temozolomide in patients with relapsed small cell lung cancers with assessment of methylguanine-DNA methyltransferase. Lung Cancer 2014;86:237–40.

47. Schmittel A, Knodler M, Hortig P, et al. Phase II trial of second-line bendamustine chemotherapy in relapsed small cell lung cancer patients. Lung Cancer 2007;55:109–13.

48. Lammers PE, Shyr Y, Li CI, et al. Phase II study of bendamustine in relapsed chemotherapy sensitive or resistant small-cell lung cancer. J Thorac Oncol 2014;9:559–62.

49. Yana T, Negoro S, Takada M, et al. Phase II study of amrubicin in previously untreated patients with extensive-disease small cell lung cancer: West Japan thoracic oncology group study. Invest New Drugs 2007;25:253–8.

50. Satouchi M, Kotani Y, Shibata T, et al. Phase III study comparing amrubicin plus cisplatin with irinotecan plus cisplatin in the treatment of extensive-disease small-cell lung cancer: JCOG 0509. J Clin Oncol 2014;32:1262–8.

51. von Pawel J, Jotte R, Spigel DR, et al. Randomized phase III trial of amrubicin versus topotecan as second-line treatment for patients with small cell lung cancer. J Clin Oncol 2014;32:4012–9.

52. Ready NE, Pang HH, Gu L, et al. Chemotherapy with or without maintenance sunitinib for untreated extensive-stage small-cell lung cancer: a randomized, double-blind, placebo-controlled phase II study – CALGB 30504 (Alliance). J Clin Oncol 2015;33:1660–5.

53. Pietanza MC, Byers LA, Minna JD, et al. Small cell lung cancer: will recent progress lead to improved outcomes? Clin Cancer Res 2015;21:2244–54.

54. Schneider BJ, Kalemkerian GP. Personalized therapy of small cell lung cancer. In: Ahmad A, Gadgeel SM, editors. Lung cancer and personalized medicine: novel therapies and clinical management. New York: Springer; 2016. p. 149–74.

55. Pietanza MC, Spigel D, Bauer TM, et al. Safety, activity and response durability assessment of single-agent rovalpituzumab tesirine, a delta-like protein 3 (DLL3)-targeted antibody drug conjugate, in small cell lung cancer. 2015 European Cancer Congress, Vienna, Austria, September 25–29, 2015. Abstract 7LBA.

56. Peifer M, Fernandez-Cuesta L, Sos ML, et al. Integrative genome analyses identify key somatic driver mutations of small-cell lung cancer. Nat Genet 2012;44:1104–10.

57. Rudin CM, Durnick S, Stawiski EW, et al. Comprehensive genomic analysis identifies SOX2 as a frequently amplified gene in small-cell lung cancer. Nat Genet 2012;44:1111–6.

58. George J, Lim JS, Jang SJ, et al. Comprehensive genomic profiles of small cell lung cancer. Nature 2015;524:47–53.

59. Byers LA, Wang J, Nilsson MB, et al. Proteomic profiling identifies dysregulated pathways in small cell lung cancer and novel therapeutic targets including PARP1. Cancer Discov 2012;2:798–811.

60. Reck M, Bondarenko I, Luft A, et al. Ipilimumab in combination with paclitaxel and carboplatin as first-line therapy in extensive-disease-small-cell lung cancer: results from a randomized, double-blind, multicenter phase 2 trial. Ann Oncol 2013;24:75–83.

61. Ott PA, Fernandez MEE, Hiret S, et al. Pembrolizumab (MK-3475) in patients with extensive-stage small cell lung cancer: preliminary safety and efficacy results from KEYNOTE-028. J Clin Oncol 2015;33(15S):400s.

62. Antonia SJ, Lopez-Martin JA, Bendell JC, et al. Nivolumab alone and nivolumab plus ipilumumab in recurrent small cell lung cancer (CheckMate 032): a multicenter, open-label, phase 1/2 trial. Lancet Oncol 2016;17:883–95.

Systemic Treatment of Brain Metastases

Saiama N. Waqar, MBBS, MSCI[a,*], Daniel Morgensztern, MD[a],
Ramaswamy Govindan, MD[b]

KEYWORDS

- Lung cancer • Chemotherapy • Targeted therapy • Immunotherapy
- Brain metastases

KEY POINTS

- Brain metastases are a significant problem in patients with lung cancer, with lung cancer accounting for 50% of brain metastases diagnosed on CT scans.
- For patients with small cell lung cancer (SCLC) and widespread systemic disease along with asymptomatic intracranial brain metastases, it is reasonable to treat upfront with systemic chemotherapy, delaying whole-brain radiation therapy (WBRT) until symptomatic progression of brain metastases.
- Platinum doublet agents are active in the treatment of asymptomatic brain metastases from non–SCLC (NSCLC) but do not replace radiation.
- For selected patients with targetable molecular alterations detected in their tumors, small molecule tyrosine kinase inhibitor (TKI) therapy may be appropriate for treatment of brain metastases.
- The role of immunotherapy in the treatment of brain metastases from lung cancer remains to be established.

INTRODUCTION

Lung cancer continues to be the leading cause of cancer-related death in the United States.[1] Approximately 40% of patients have metastatic disease at presentation and are treated with palliative intent, with the goals of maintaining quality of life and

Disclosure Statement: Dr S.N. Waqar does not have any disclosures to report; Dr D. Morgensztern has a consulting/advisory role with Genentech, Heat Biologics, Celgene, and Bristol-Myers Squibb. He is on the speaker's bureau for Boehringer Ingelheim and Genentech; Dr R. Govindan has consulting/advisory role for GlaxoSmithKline, Boehringer Ingelheim, Clovis Oncology, Helsinn Therapeutics, Genentech/Roche, Abbvie, Celgene, Bayer, and Novartis. He reports receiving honoraria from Boehringer Ingelheim.
[a] Washington University School of Medicine, 660 South Euclid Avenue, Campus Box 8056, St Louis, MO 63110, USA; [b] Section of Medical Oncology, Washington University School of Medicine, 660 South Euclid Avenue, Campus Box 8056, St Louis, MO 63110, USA
* Corresponding author.
E-mail address: saiamawaqar@wustl.edu

improving survival.[2] Brain metastases are a significant problem in patients with lung cancer, which accounts for 50% of brain metastases diagnosed by CT scans.[3] With the advent of improved imaging modalities, such as MRI for staging and detection of subclinical disease, coupled with the modest improvement in survival from therapeutic advances in the systemic treatment of lung cancer, an increase in incidence of brain metastases is expected.

The histologic distribution of metastases from lung cancer is as follows: small cell carcinoma 31%, adenocarcinoma 21%, large cell carcinoma 21%, and squamous cell carcinoma 8%.[4] It is estimated that approximately 8% of patients with NSCLC have brain metastases at presentation, with clinical risk factors, including younger age, female gender, adenocarcinoma or large cell histology, tumor size greater than 3 cm, higher tumor grade, and regional lymph node involvement.[5] A retrospective review of patients with stage III NSCLC treated with combined modality therapy on Southwest Oncology Group protocols reveals a cumulative 24-month estimate for brain metastases of 22% for adenocarcinoma, 8% for squamous NSCLC, and 17% for other histologies.[6]

WBRT has been demonstrated to improve outcome in patients with brain metastases with brain response rate (RR) of 35%, resulting in improvement in headache (82%), lost motor function (61%–74%), and mentation.[7,8] The Radiation Therapy Cooperative Group (RTOG) 0901 and 7361 studies demonstrated that there was no significant difference in survival with different fractionation schedules for palliative WBRT, with reported median overall survival (OS) of 4.1 and 3.4 months in these 2 studies, respectively.[8] Furthermore, the RTOG 7606 found no improvement in survival with a dose of 50 Gy compared with the standard 30-Gy dose.[9] The RTOG 9104 compared 32 Gy twice daily radiation to 30 Gy in 10 fractions and also found no survival advantage for the higher dose of 32 Gy twice daily.[10] Therefore, 30 Gy over 10 fractions is the standard WBRT regimen.

Several prognostic factors in patients with brain metastases have been described. Gaspar and colleagues[11] examined a 1200-patient data set pooled from 3 RTOG trials conducted between 1979 and 1993. They used recursive partitioning analysis, a statistical tool used to create a regression tree according to prognostic indicators, which divided patients into 3 classes. The best survival was noted in patients less than 65 years of age with Karnofsky performance scale score (KPS) of 70 or more and controlled primary tumor with brain as only site of metastases, with median survival of 7.1 months (class I). The worst survival was seen in patients with KPS less than 70, with median survival of 2.3 months (class III), whereas the remaining patients (class II) had a median survival of 4.2 months.

The graded prognostic index is another model developed using 4200 patients from 5 RTOG studies.[12] For patients with lung cancer, 4 variables were included in the model: age, KPS, number of metastases, and presence of extracranial metastases, based on which scores were assigned to each variable. The cumulative scores were used to determine prognosis: a score of 3.5 to 4 was associated with a median survival of 11 months, whereas at the other extreme, a score of 0 to 1 was associated with a median survival of 2.8 months.

For select patients with limited number of metastases, stereotactic brain radiosurgery (SRS) may be used. In the RTOG 9005 study, 156 patients with recurrent brain tumors were treated with SRS.[13] Tumors less than 2 cm were treated to 24 Gy and tumors larger than 2 cm up to 3 cm were treated to 18 Gy whereas tumors between 3.1 cm and 4 cm were treated to 15 Gy. The median survival was 11.4 months. Prognosis varies according to number of lesions, largest lesion volume, age, KPS, and status of systemic disease and a Score Index for Radiosurgery has been developed ranging from 0 to 10. Patients with score 1 to 2 have median survival of 2.9 months whereas those with 8 to 10 have survival of 31.4 months.[14]

SYSTEMIC CHEMOTHERAPY FOR SMALL CELL LUNG CANCER

Brain metastases from SCLC have been conventionally treated with WBRT. Given the frequency of brain metastases from SCLC and poor prognosis associated with them, prophylactic cranial radiation is recommended for patients with limited stage disease. The thought had been that chemotherapeutic agents do not cross the blood-brain barrier in sufficient concentrations to result in an intracranial response. Nevertheless, disruption of the blood-brain barrier by metastases can actually allow intracranial penetration of systemic agents.[15] This is further supported by early reports of intracranial response in patients with SCLC treated with combination systemic chemotherapy.[16]

Front-Line Platinum-based or Cyclophosphamide-Based Regimens

A small prospective study using a regimen of etoposide, cyclophosphamide, doxorubicin, and vincristine in 14 patients with previously untreated SCLC with asymptomatic brain metastases reported an intracranial RR of 82%, with no deterioration of neurologic status (**Table 1**).[17]

The current standard of care for the front-line treatment of SCLC includes a platinum agent with either etoposide or irinotecan. The intracranial RR to single-agent carboplatin is 40% in patients with symptomatic brain metastasis, whereas it is higher for the carboplatin and irinotecan combination at 65%.[18,19] These data suggest that for patients with widespread systemic disease along with asymptomatic intracranial brain metastases, it is reasonable to initiate the treatment with systemic chemotherapy while delaying WBRT until the completion of the initial treatment course or progression of the brain metastases.

Topotecan

Topotecan is the only agent approved in the second-line setting for relapsed SCLC. A phase II study of this agent was conducted in 30 patients with relapsed SCLC with asymptomatic brain metastases and 14 of them had received 1 prior line of chemotherapy, whereas 16 had received at least 2 prior lines of treatment and 8 patients had received prior WBRT.[20] The first 22 patients received the planned dose of topotecan, 1.5 mg/m^2, intravenously as a 30-minute infusion for 5 consecutive days of a 21-day cycle, but due to thrombocytopenia, the last 8 patients were treated with the lower dose of 1.25 mg/m^2. Intracranial response was observed in 33% of the treated patients, which was numerically higher than the systemic RR of 29%.[20] Myelosuppression is a common toxicity of this agent, however, with grade 3 and grade 4 leukopenia observed in 28% and 22% of patients respectively. Grade 3 and grade 4 thrombocytopenia were observed in 17% and 11% of patients, respectively, and 17% of patients had grade 3 infection.

SYSTEMIC CHEMOTHERAPY FOR NON–SMALL CELL LUNG CANCER

Brain metastases are a significant problem in patients with NSCLC, with approximately 8% requiring brain radiotherapy at presentation.[5] Unlike SCLC, PCI has not been shown to improve median survival in patients with stage IIII NSCLC.[21] Several studies have evaluated the role of chemotherapy in patients with brain metastases from NSCLC (**Table 2**).

Table 1
Activity of chemotherapy in patients with brain metastasis from small cell lung cancer

Regimen	N	Study Type	Prior Whole-brain Radiation Therapy	Prior Chemotherapy	Brain Response Rate (%)	Median Survival (mo)	Reference
Cyclophosphamide, doxorubicin, vincristine and etoposide with WBRT	14	Single-arm prospective study, WBRT added at cycle 4	No	No	82	7.8	Lee et al,[17] 1989
Cyclophosphamide, vincristine, etoposide	19	Retrospective analysis of patients with brain metastasis in 610-patient randomized trial	No	No	53	6.5	Twelves et al,[101] 1990
Cyclophosphamide, doxorubicin, and etoposide	24	Prospective single-arm 181-patient study that allowed asymptomatic brain metastases, received WBRT if became symptomatic	No	No	27	8.3	Seute et al,[102] 2006
Cisplatin, teniposide, vincristine, followed by multidrug regimen	21	Prospective study, brain radiation withheld till progression in brain	No	No	85	3.6	Kristjansen et al,[103] 1993
Carboplatin and irinotecan	15	Phase II	Yes, 13/15	Yes, all patients	65	6	Chen et al,[19] 2008
Carboplatin	19	Symptomatic brain metastases			40	3.5	Groen et al,[18] 1993
Topotecan	30	Phase II	Yes, 8/30	Yes, all patients	33	3.6	Korfel et al,[20] 2002
Teniposide with or without WBRT	120	Phase III randomized study	No	No	57 in combination arm, 22 in teniposide-only arm	3.5 vs 3.2	Postmus et al,[104] 2000

Table 2
Activity of first-line platinum doublet chemotherapy in patients with brain metastasis from non–small cell lung cancer

Regimen	N	Study Type	Brain Response Rate (%)	Median Survival (mo)	Reference
Carboplatin and paclitaxel	5	Preliminary data from prospective study	20	—	Lee et al,[22] 1997
Cisplatin and vinorelbine with early vs delayed WBRT	176	Phase III	33 for early WBRT, 27 for delayed	5.1 for early WBRT vs 5.5 for delayed	Robinet et al,[23] 2001
Cisplatin and pemetrexed	43	Phase II	41.9	7.4	Barlesi et al,[25] 2011
Cisplatin and pemetrexed with concurrent WBRT	42	Phase II	68.3	12.6	Dinglin et al,[24] 2013

Platinum Agents

Historically, trials of first-line chemotherapy in NSCLC have excluded patients with brain metastases due to their poor prognosis. Only 1 patient had intracranial response in a preliminary report of 5 patients treated on a clinical trial of carboplatin and paclitaxel, for an intracranial RR of 20%.[22] The phase III Groupe Français de Pneumo-Cencérologie (GFPC) protocol 95-1 compared early versus delayed WBRT with concurrent cisplatin and vinorelbine in 176 patients with inoperable brain metastases.[23] The intracranial RRs were 27% for the delayed radiation (chemotherapy-alone) group and 33% for the chemotherapy with early WBRT. The median survival duration was not significantly different between the 2 groups (24 and 21 weeks respectively, $P = .83$). These results suggested that timing of WBRT did not influence survival of NSCLC with brain metastases when treated with concurrent chemotherapy. Two phase II studies evaluated the activity of cisplatin and pemetrexed in the treatment of brain metastasis.[24,25] The GFPC 07-01 study enrolled chemotherapy-naïve patients with metastatic NSCLC and brain metastases who were ineligible for radiosurgery to up to 6 cycles of cisplatin, 75 mg/m^2, and pemetrexed, 500 mg/m^2, every 3 weeks.[25] Patients received WBRT at the time of chemotherapy completion or at disease progression. The brain metastases RR was 41.9%, whereas extracranial RR was 34.9%. The median survival time in the study was 7.4 months. In a second phase II trial, 42 patients with metastatic NSCLC to the brain were treated with up to 6 cycles of the same regimen of cisplatin and pemetrexed concurrent with WBRT to a dose of 30 Gy in 10 fractions.[24] The RR in the brain and extracranially were 68.3% and 34.1%, respectively, with a median OS of 12.6 months.

Temozolomide

Temozolomide is an alkylating agent approved for the treatment of primary brain tumors, such as glioblastoma.[26] Its intracranial activity led to the study of this agent's activity in tumors that are metastatic to the brain. Two phase II clinical trials evaluated the activity of single-agent temozolomide in heavily pretreated patients with solid tumors, including NSCLC and SCLC, with brain metastases.[27,28] Both studies used a regimen of temozolomide, 150 mg/m^2/d, for 5 days, repeated every 28 days and reported disease control rates (DCRs) of 20.8% to 41% with a median OS of 4.5 to 6.6 months. In the larger of the two studies, which enrolled 41 patients and including 22 with NSCLC, 2 patients (9%) had a partial response (PR).[28] A second study investigated temozolomide in 30 patients with NSCLC with progression of brain metastases after at least 1 line of chemotherapy and WBRT.[29] The dose of temozolomide was escalated to 200 mg/m^2/d with subsequent cycles if no grade 3 or grade 4 hematologic toxicities were observed. Three patients (10%) achieved objective response of brain metastases, with 2 complete responses (CRs). No grade 3 or grade 4 toxicities were observed. Three patients were long-term survivors, having survived beyond a year after the start of temozolomide.

The European Organisation for Research and Treatment of Cancer Lung Cancer Group 08965 study evaluated the activity of single-agent temozolomide, 200 mg/m^2/d for 5 days every 28 days, in chemotherapy-naïve patients with NSCLC.[30] The study included 2 groups of patients, those with brain metastases (n = 12) and patients without brain metastases (n = 13). Treatment was continued until disease progression or unacceptable toxicity, for a maximum of 6 cycles. This study was closed early due to lack of objective responses in either group of patients.

Temozolomide has also been studied in combination with brain radiotherapy. The RTOG 0320 trial was a phase III trial of WBRT at a dose of 37.5 Gy in 15 fractions and SRS alone versus WBRT and SRS with either temozolomide or erlotinib in patients with 1 to 3 brain metastases.[31] The primary endpoint was OS. This study closed prematurely due to poor accrual after enrolling 126 patients. The median survival times for WBRT and SRS–alone group of 13.4 months was numerically higher (although not statistically significant) than WBRT and SRS with temozolomide (6.3 months) or WBRT, SRS, and erlotinib (6.1 months), suggesting a trend toward possible deleterious effect of adding temozolomide or erlotinib to WBRT and SRS.

Antifolate Agents

Pemetrexed is an antifolate chemotherapeutic agent approved for the treatment of nonsquamous NSCLC. In patients with central nervous system (CNS) metastases, pemetrexed distributes from the plasma to the cerebrospinal fluid (CSF) within 1 to 4 hours of dosing, and the resulting CSF concentration of pemetrexed is less than 5% of the plasma concentration.[32] A total of 21 patients with CNS metastases were treated with intravenous pemetrexed at doses of 500 mg/m^2 (n = 3), 750 mg/m^2 (n = 3), 900 mg/m^2 (n = 12), or 1050 mg/m^2 (n = 3) every 3 weeks with restaging neuroimaging performed every 6 weeks in a small study.[32] This study included 4 patients with metastatic lung cancer, 3 of whom had received 1 prior line of chemotherapy, and the fourth patient had received 2 prior lines of chemotherapy. Three of the 4 patients had received prior WBRT. No intracranial responses were observed in patients with lung cancer, although 2 patients had stable disease.

Intrathecal Chemotherapy

Leptomeningeal carcinomatosis is associated with significant morbidity and poor outcome.[33] Intrathecal (IT) chemotherapy, mostly with methotrexate and cytarabine, has been used as a treatment modality in this setting. A randomized controlled trial of IT sustained-release cytarabine (DepoCyt) versus IT methotrexate in 61 patients with solid tumors and positive CNS cytology included 3 patients with NSCLC and 2 patients with SCLC.[34] Patients were randomized to IT DepoCyt (31 patients) or IT methotrexate. The RRs were similar among the DepoCyt group (26%) and methotrexate group (20%), but time to neurologic progression was greater in the DepoCyt arm compared with the methotrexate arm (58 days vs 30 days; log-rank test $P = .007$).

MOLECULARLY TARGETED THERAPY FOR BRAIN METASTASIS

Lung cancer is a genetically complex disease and the study of molecular mechanisms leading to brain metastases in this malignancy has been particularly challenging, because often patients are treated for their brain lesions based on radiographic findings. In select cases, where surgical resection is clinically indicated, tissue suitable for molecular analysis can be obtained. The paired analysis of patient-matched primary and brain metastases, from cancers including lung, has shed some light on the branched evolution of brain metastases relative to the primary tumors, and potential targets for cyclin dependent kinase inhibitors, inhibitors of EGFR, phosphatidyl inositol 3 kinase (PI3K)/AKT/mammalian target of rapamycin (mTOR), and mitogen-activated protein kinase (MAPK) cyclin-dependent kinase (CDK) pathways.[35,36]

The identification of targetable somatic molecular alterations, such as epidermal growth factor receptor (*EGFR*) mutations and anaplastic lymphoma kinase (*ALK*) gene rearrangements, has changed standard of care in select patients.

Epidermal Growth Factor Receptor

EGFR mutations have been reported in 22% of patients with metastatic lung adenocarcinoma enrolled in the Lung Cancer Mutation Consortium study.[37] *EGFR* mutations are seen more commonly in patients who are never-smokers or light smokers, of Asian ethnicity, and are female gender.[38] The first-generation reversible EGFR-TKIs, erlotinib and gefitinib, have demonstrated improved progression-free survival (PFS) compared with front-line chemotherapy in patients with *EGFR*-mutant NSCLC, which led to their approval by the Food and Drug Administration (FDA) for the treatment of patients with metastatic *EGFR*-mutant NSCLC.[39–42] Case reports and case series emerged of impressive intracranial responses in patients treated with EGFR-TKI therapy.[43–45] This led to several retrospective and prospective studies evaluating the intracranial response to EGFR-TKI therapy, either alone or in combination with brain radiotherapy (**Table 3**).[46–53] Intracranial RRs range from 58.3% in Asian patients with unselected adenocarcinoma and asymptomatic brain metastases, which included some *EGFR*-mutant lung cancers, to as high as 88.9% in patients with *EGFR*-mutant NSCLC.[46,49]

The accumulation of erlotinib in the brain metastasis of a patient with *EGFR* exon 19 deletion has been visualized using dynamic PET/CT with [^{11}C]-erlotinib, a novel PET tracer, demonstrating that erlotinib does penetrate into the brain.[54] CSF concentrations of erlotinib and gefitinib, however, are low, reaching only 2.77% and 1.3% of the plasma concentrations, respectively.[55,56] High-dose intermittent erlotinib has been demonstrated to produce more profound and sustained target inhibition in mice carrying *EGFR*-mutant lung cancer xenografts.[57] High-dose erlotinib, however, has not been shown to effectively control extracranial disease progression in patients with advanced *EGFR*-mutant NSCLC with disease progression on standard-dose erlotinib, with RR of 9.1%.[58] This may possibly be due to T790M mutation as the mechanism of resistance.

In contrast, high-dose pulsatile erlotinib, at doses of 1500 mg orally once a week, has been shown to achieve therapeutic concentrations in the CSF.[59] Several case reports and small series have demonstrated the intracranial activity and tolerability of high-dose pulsatile erlotinib in patients with progressive CNS metastases.[59–62] The

Table 3
Activity of epidermal growth factor receptor tyrosine kinase inhibitor's in patients with brain metastasis from non–small cell lung cancer

Classification	Agent	Activating Epidermal Growth Factor Receptor Mutation	Study Type	N	Brain Response Rate (%)	Median Overall Survival (mo)	Reference
First generation	Gefitinib	Yes	Retrospective	9	88.9	—	Li et al,[46] 2011
	Gefitinib	Yes	Phase II clinical trial	41	87.8	21.9	Iuchi et al,[47] 2013
	Erlotinib	Yes	Retrospective	17	82.4	12.9	Porta et al,[48] 2011
	Erlotinib	Asian, adenocarcinoma, included some EGFR-mutant	Phase II clinical trial, asymptomatic brain metastases	48	58.3	18.9	Wu et al,[49] 2013
	Erlotinib plus concurrent WBRT	Unselected	Phase II clinical trial	40	86	11.8	Welsh et al,[50] 2013
	WBRT with or without erlotinib	Unselected	Phase II, if mutation status known, received WBRT with erlotinib, if unknown, received WBRT monotherapy	54; 23 got erlotinib	95.6	10.7	Zhuang et al,[51] 2013
	High-dose pulsatile weekly erlotinib	Yes	Case series	9	67	12	Grommes et al,[60] 2011
	Gefitinib or erlotinib	Yes	Phase II clinical trial	28	83	15.9	Park et al,[52] 2012
	Gefitinib or erlotinib	Asian never-smokers	Retrospective	23	73.9	18.8	Kim et al,[53] 2009
Second generation	Afatinib	Yes	TKI pretreated, as part of compassionate use program	31	35	9.8	Hoffknecht et al,[66] 2015

largest of these studies, a case series of 9 patients, reported an RR of 67% and stable disease in 11%.[60] The median time to CNS progression and median OS were 2.7 months and 12 months, respectively. Molecular analysis of the brain metastases from 4 of these patients did not reveal acquired resistance mutations in the *EGFR* gene. CNS response to high-dose icotinib after standard-dose erlotinib failure has also been reported.[63]

The second-generation EGFR-TKI afatinib was developed as an irreversible inhibitor of EGFR, HER2, and HER4, and, similarly to erlotinib and gefitinib, has been shown to improve PFS compared with front-line chemotherapy for metastatic disease.[64] Afatinib has shown some activity in patients with intracranial metastases with progression on first-generation EGFR-TKI therapy.[65] Intracranial RR of 35% to afatinib have been reported in patients who were TKI pretreated and received afatinib as part of the compassionate use program.[66]

Despite the initial clinical benefit with first-generation and second-generation EGFR-TKIs in *EGFR*-mutant NSCLC, patients eventually experience disease progression. Rebiopsy of progressing lesions showed that *EGFR* 790M is the predominant mechanism of acquired resistance, present in more than 50% of the cases.[67] Osimertinib is a novel small molecule inhibitor of the *EGFR* T790M resistance mutation and recently was granted accelerated approval by the FDA. CNS responses to osimertinib in 2 cases of T790M-positive NSCLC have been described, after progression on first-generation EGFR-TKI therapy.[68] Moreover, CNS response to osimertinib has also been observed in 3 patients with new brain metastases while on treatment with rociletinib, which is another *EGFR* T790M inhibitor.[69] Updated results of the phase I BLOOM study (NCT02228369) osimertinib cohort of patients with leptomeningeal disease from *EGFR*-mutant NSCLC were reported at the 2016 American Society of Clinical Oncology (ASCO) annual meeting.[70] The key inclusion criteria included known sensitizing *EGFR* L858R mutation or exon 19 deletion, prior EGFR-TKI therapy, performance status 0 to 2, stable extracranial disease, and at least 1 leptomeningeal lesion by MRI scan. All 21 patients were Asian and had adenocarcinoma histology, and 11 of 21 had received prior WBRT. Patients received osimertinib, 160 mg orally, once daily. Seven patients (33.3%) had confirmed radiographic response with 2 patients showing confirmed CSF cytology clearance and 5 patients had improvement in neurologic function. Stable disease was observed in 9 (42.8%) of patients.

AZD3759 is a novel EGFR-TKI that has been designed specifically to penetrate the CNS, facilitating the treatment of brain and leptomeningeal metastases in patients with *EGFR*-mutant NSCLC.[71] Preliminary results of the AZD3759 cohort of the BLOOM trial were also reported at the 2016 ASCO annual meeting, which included 21 patients with measurable brain lesions and 5 patients with CSF cytology confirmed leptomeningeal metastases.[72] Drug-related grade 3 or higher adverse events included rash (7%), pruritis (7%), diarrhea (3%), and acne (3%). Two patients treated at the 500-mg twice-daily dose experienced dose-limiting toxicities of grade 3 skin rash and grade 2 intolerable mucositis. The maximum tolerated dose was determined to be 300 mg twice daily, with 200 mg twice daily recommended for the phase II dose, due to tolerability. Tumor shrinkage in the brain target lesions was observed in 11 of 21 patients, with 3 confirmed PR and 3 unconfirmed PR.

Anaplastic Lymphoma Kinase

The echinoderm microtubule-associated protein-like 4 *(EML4)-ALK* gene fusion was first described as an oncogenic driver in lung cancer in 2007, resulting from an inversion within the short arm of chromosome 2.[73] Several other fusion partners of *ALK* have been described, resulting in more than 20 different *ALK* fusion variants, which lead to constitutive activation of the ALK kinase and downstream signaling results in dysregulated cell survival and proliferation.[74] The frequency of *ALK* fusions in NSCLC is approximately 5% and clinical risk factors include light smokers or never-smokers; adenocarcinoma, especially the signet ring subtype; and absence of other oncogenic drivers, such as *EGFR* and *KRAS*.[75,76] Crizotinib, initially designed as a small molecule TKI targeting *c-MET*, was found to also inhibit *ALK* and *ROS1* fusions and became the first ALK inhibitor approved for use in patients with ALK-rearranged NSCLC. The PRO-FILE 1014 was a phase III clinical trial comparing front-line chemotherapy with crizo-tinib in patients with ALK-rearranged NSCLC, which met its primary endpoint of improved PFS in the crizotinib arm (**Table 4**).[77] This study allowed patients with stable treated brain metastases, which comprised 23% of the patients enrolled. Intracranial DCR for patients treated with crizotinib was 85% at 12 weeks and 56% at 24 weeks and the median intracranial time to progression was 15.7 months. The 12-week intra-cranial DCR of crizotinib, based on a pooled retrospective analysis of patients with brain metastases treated on the phase II PROFILE 1005 study and the phase III PRO-FILE 1007 trial comparing crizotinib to second-line chemotherapy, was 56% for pa-tients with previously untreated asymptomatic brain metastases and 62% for patients with previously treated brain metastases.[78]

Approximately half of patients treated with crizotinib experience CNS relapse.[79] This highlights the need for novel ALK inhibitors with intracranial penetration. Both cer-itinib and alectinib are second-generation ALK inhibitors approved for the treatment of *ALK*-positive NSCLCs that seem to have CNS penetration. Ceritinib demonstrated intracranial activity both in ALK inhibitor-naïve patients (brain RR 42.1% and brain DCR of 79%) and ALK inhibitor pretreated patients (brain RR 18.6%, brain DCR 65.3%) in a retrospective analysis of intracranial responses in the ASCEND-1 phase 1 study of ceritinib.[80] The AF-002JG phase 1 trial of alectinib allowed patients with asymptomatic brain metastases, which was present in 45% of the patients, and demonstrated an intracranial DCR of 90% with 52.4% brain RR and 29% CR rate. The median duration of CNS response was 8.2 months for patients with measurable lesions at baseline.[81] The phase II NP28761 study of alectinib also allowed patients with asymptomatic neurologically stable brain metastases and reported an astounding 100% intracranial DCR.[82] The brain RR was reported as 75% overall, with median duration of CNS response of 11.1 months.

Several next-generation ALK inhibitors in development seem to have activity in treating brain metastases. The results of the phase II ALTA trial of brigatinib, in patients with crizotinib refractory ALK-positive NSCLC, were presented at the 2016 ASCO annual meeting.[83] Active brain metastases were defined as lesions with no prior radio-therapy or those with investigator-assessed progression after prior radiotherapy. In patients with measurable active brain metastases at baseline, the intracranial RR was 37% at the 90-mg dose level and 73% at the 180-mg dose level. Median intracra-nial PFS was 15.6 (95% CI, 6.5–15.6 months) in patients treated in the brigatinib, 90-mg daily, cohort and not reached in the brigatinib, 180-mg daily, cohort. An update on the phase I dose escalation study of lorlatinib (NCT01970865) presented at this meeting reported intracranial RR of 31% in 32 patients with baseline brain lesions, treated in the ALK positive cohort.[84]

Preliminary results from the phase I study of X-396, a novel ALK and ROS1 inhibitor, reported an RR of 55% in patient with *ALK*-positive NSCLC, with PR observed in 6 of 11 evaluable patients, which included 2 patients with intracranial responses.[85] Durable complete resolution of brain metastases has also been reported for entrectinib, an in-hibitor of ALK, ROS1 and NTRK1, NTRK2, and NTRK-3.[86]

Other Targetable Molecular Alterations

Both vemurafenib and dabrafenib have been approved by the FDA for the treatment of *BRAF V600E* mutant melanoma; dabrafenib's approval label also extends to *BRAF V600K* mutant melanoma. A phase I study of dabrafenib in patients with BRAF mutant solid tumors included a cohort of patients with *BRAF* mutant melanoma with untreated brain lesions[87]; 9 of 10 patients had reductions in the size of brain lesions. In patients with *BRAF V600E* mutant melanoma brain metastases, larger tumor size, greater number of brain lesions, and progressive extracranial disease were associated with decreased intracranial response to veumrafenib.[88] BRAF mutations are rare in NSCLC, ranging from 1% to 2%; half of these are *BRAF V600E* mutations.[89,90] Dabrafenib has activity in *BRAF* V600E mutant NSCLC, with an investigator-assessed overall RR of 33% (95% CI, 23–45) in a single-arm, phase II study including 84 patients.[91] This study did allow patients with asymptomatic untreated brain metastases smaller than 1 cm to enroll, and 1 such patient was noted to have complete resolution of the brain lesion at the 6-week and 12 week-assessments but then was taken off the study due to nonadherence to protocol. Four patients developed new brain metastases while treated on this study. In addition to this, a single patient case of *BRAF*-mutant NSCLC with metastasis to brain with intracranial response to vemurafenib has been documented.[92]

RET gene rearrangements are seen in 1% to 2% of NSCLCs. Several clinical trials are investigating the activity of RET inhibitors in patients with *RET* fusion-positive NSCLC. Preliminary results from a phase II clinical trial of cabozantinib in this patient population demonstrated responses in 2 of the 3 treated patients; 1 of these patients had bilateral retinal metastases at baseline, which decreased in size on follow-up ophthalmologic examination, with resolution of blurry vision. A third treated patient had stable disease as best response.[93] Intracranial response to the RET inhibitor, vandetinib, in combination with everolimus has also been reported.[94]

Bevacizumab is anti–vascular endothelial growth factor monoclonal antibody approved for use in patients with nonsquamous metastatic NSCLC. The PASSPORT trial was a phase II trial examining the safety of bevacizumab in patients with nonsquamous NSCLC and previously treated brain metastases.[95] Patients receiving treatment in the first-line setting (n = 76) received bevacizumab with platinum doublet or erlotinib at physician's discretion, whereas patients treated in the second-line setting (n = 39) received bevacizumab in combination with single-agent chemotherapy or erlotinib. The median on-study duration was 6.3 months, and patients received a median of 5 cycles of bevacizumab, with no reported episodes of greater than or equal to grade 2 CNS hemorrhage. Two patients did experience grade 5 pulmonary hemorrhage attributed to bevacizumab.

IMMUNOTHERAPY

The immune checkpoints are dysregulated in malignancies such as lung cancer. Recently, the anti–PD-1 agent nivolumab was approved by the FDA for treatment of patients with advanced NSCLC who fail platinum doublet therapy, based on improvement of OS, in comparison to docetaxel.[96,97] Pembrolizumab, another anti–PD-1 antibody, has also been approved for use in patients with refractory advanced NSCLCs whose tumors were PD-L1 positive[98] NCT02085070 is a phase II study of pembrolizumab, 10 mg/kg IV every 2 weeks, in patients with advanced NSCLC or melanoma with at least 1 untreated brain lesion.[99,100] A total of 18 patients were accrued to the NSCLC cohort, with patients to undergo safety evaluation at 4 weeks with brain MRI and response evaluation at 8 weeks. In cases of stable disease (SD) or response,

Table 4
Activity of anaplastic lymphoma kinase inhibitors in patients with brain metastasis from non-small cell lung cancer

Agent	n	Study Type	Eligibility	Brain Response Rate (%)	Duration of Central Nervous System Response	Intracranial Disease Control Rate (%)	Median Progression-free Survival (months)	Median Intracranial TTP (months)	Reference
Crizotinib	79	PROFILE 1014 phase III study compared with pemetrexed and cisplatin/carboplatin	Allowed stable treated brain metastases (23% of patients)	—	—	85 at 12 wk, 56 at 24 wk	9	15.7	Solomon et al,[105] 2016
	275	Pooled retrospective analysis of patients with brain metastases in phase II PROFILE 1005 of crizotinib and phase III PROFILE 1007 (crizotinib vs second-line chemotherapy)	Allowed asymptomatic previously untreated brain metastases (N = 109)	18 for untreated brain metastases, 33 for previously treated	—	56 at 12 wk for untreated brain metastases 62 for previously treated brain metastases	5.9 for untreated and 6 for treated	7 for untreated and 13.2 for previously treated	Costa et al,[78] 2015
Ceritinib	124	Retrospective analysis of intracranial responses in ASCEND-1 phase I study	Allowed asymptomatic untreated brain metastases	42.1 in ALK inhibitor-naïve and 18.6 in ALK inhibitor pretreated patients	Not evaluable for ALK inhibitor-naïve patients, 6.9 mo for ALK inhibitor pretreated patients	79 of ALK inhibitor-naïve patients; 65.3 in ALK inhibitor pretreated patients	6.9	—	Kim et al,[80] 2016

Alectinib	21	AF-002JG phase I portion	Allowed asymptomatic brain metastases (45% of patients)	52.4, 29 CRs	Not evaluable, 8.2 mo for patients with measurable lesions at baseline	90	—	Gadgeel et al,[81] 2014
	52	Phase II NP28761 study	Allowed asymptomatic neurologically stable brain metastases	75 overall; 66.6 in previously untreated (CR rate of 55.5%)	11.1 mo	100	10.3	Shaw et al,[82] 2016
Brigatinib	151	Phase I/II study	Allowed if neurologically stable, leptomeningeal carcinomatosis excluded	37 in the 90-mg cohort, 73 in the 180-mg cohort in patients with measurable active brain metastases	—	88 in the 90-mg cohort, 83 in the 180-mg cohort in patients with measurable brain metastases	15.6 for 90-mg cohort, not reached for 180-mg cohort	Kim et al,[83] 2016
Lorlatinib	32	Phase I/II study	Untreated brain metastases allowed	31, 25 CR rate	—	—	—	Solomon et al,[84] 2016

Abbreviation: TTP, time to progression.

patients continued treatment unit disease progression. At the time of tumor progression, patients were allowed to undergo local therapy for the progressive lesion, with continuation of pembrolizumab if deriving a clinical benefit. The brain metastasis RR was 33% (6 PRs in 18 evaluable patients), which included 4 CRs, and these responses were durable and ongoing in all except 1 patient. The systemic RR was also 33% in the NSCLC cohort. The NCT02696993 is a phase I/II trial of nivolumab plus radiation or nivolumab in combination with radiation and ipilimumab in patients with NSCLC.

SUMMARY

Patients with SCLC with asymptomatic brain metastases and uncontrolled systemic disease can be treated with front-line platinum doublet chemotherapy, whereas the WBRT is delayed until tumor progression or completion of chemotherapy. Platinum doublet agents are active in the treatment of asymptomatic brain metastases from NSCLC but should not replace WBRT. In patients who are not candidates for SRS and have uncontrolled systemic disease, where there is an urgency to treat, it is reasonable to start systemic chemotherapy and follow the brain lesions closely, with salvage WBRT at progression, or after chemotherapy is completed. For selected patients with targetable molecular alterations, small molecule TKI therapy may be appropriate for treatment of brain metastases. The role of immunotherapy for the treatment of brain metastases from NSCLC remains to be established and is currently being addressed in several ongoing studies.

REFERENCES

1. Siegel RL, Miller KD, Jemal A. Cancer statistics, 2016. CA Cancer J Clin 2016; 66:7–30.
2. Morgensztern D, Ng SH, Gao F, et al. Trends in stage distribution for patients with non-small cell lung cancer: a National Cancer Database survey. J Thorac Oncol 2010;5:29–33.
3. Delattre JY, Krol G, Thaler HT, et al. Distribution of brain metastases. Arch Neurol 1988;45:741–4.
4. Ryan GF, Ball DL, Smith JG. Treatment of brain metastases from primary lung cancer. Int J Radiat Oncol Biol Phys 1995;31:273–8.
5. Waqar SN, Waqar SH, Trinkaus K, et al. Brain metastases at presentation in patients with non-small cell lung cancer. Am J Clin Oncol 2015. [Epub ahead of print].
6. Gaspar LE, Chansky K, Albain KS, et al. Time from treatment to subsequent diagnosis of brain metastases in stage III non-small-cell lung cancer: a retrospective review by the Southwest Oncology Group. J Clin Oncol 2005;23:2955–61.
7. El Gantery MM, Abd El Baky HM, El Hossieny HA, et al. Management of brain metastases with stereotactic radiosurgery alone versus whole brain irradiation alone versus both. Radiat Oncol 2014;9:116.
8. Borgelt B, Gelber R, Kramer S, et al. The palliation of brain metastases: final results of the first two studies by the Radiation Therapy Oncology Group. Int J Radiat Oncol Biol Phys 1980;6:1–9.
9. Kurtz JM, Gelber R, Brady LW, et al. The palliation of brain metastases in a favorable patient population: a randomized clinical trial by the Radiation Therapy Oncology Group. Int J Radiat Oncol Biol Phys 1981;7:891–5.
10. Murray KJ, Scott C, Greenberg HM, et al. A randomized phase III study of accelerated hyperfractionation versus standard in patients with unresected brain

metastases: a report of the Radiation Therapy Oncology Group (RTOG) 9104. Int J Radiat Oncol Biol Phys 1997;39:571–4.

11. Gaspar L, Scott C, Rotman M, et al. Recursive partitioning analysis (RPA) of prognostic factors in three Radiation Therapy Oncology Group (RTOG) brain metastases trials. Int J Radiat Oncol Biol Phys 1997;37:745–51.

12. Sperduto PW, Berkey B, Gaspar LE, et al. A new prognostic index and comparison to three other indices for patients with brain metastases: an analysis of 1,960 patients in the RTOG database. Int J Radiat Oncol Biol Phys 2008;70:510–4.

13. Buatti JM, Friedman WA, Meeks SL, et al. RTOG 90-05: the real conclusion. Int J Radiat Oncol Biol Phys 2000;47:269–71.

14. Weltman E, Salvajoli JV, Brandt RA, et al. Radiosurgery for brain metastases: a score index for predicting prognosis. Int J Radiat Oncol Biol Phys 2000;46:1155–61.

15. Stewart DJ. A critique of the role of the blood-brain barrier in the chemotherapy of human brain tumors. J Neurooncol 1994;20:121–39.

16. Kantarjian H, Farha PA, Spitzer G, et al. Systemic combination chemotherapy as primary treatment of brain metastasis from lung cancer. South Med J 1984;77:426–30.

17. Lee JS, Murphy WK, Glisson BS, et al. Primary chemotherapy of brain metastasis in small-cell lung cancer. J Clin Oncol 1989;7:916–22.

18. Groen HJ, Smit EF, Haaxma-Reiche H, et al. Carboplatin as second line treatment for recurrent or progressive brain metastasis from small cell lung cancer. Eur J Cancer 1993;29A:1696–9.

19. Chen G, Huynh M, Chen A, et al. Chemotherapy for brain metastases in small-cell lung cancer. Clin Lung Cancer 2008;9:35–8.

20. Korfel A, Oehm C, von Pawel J, et al. Response to topotecan of symptomatic brain metastases of small-cell lung cancer also after whole-brain irradiation. a multicentre phase II study. Eur J Cancer 2002;38:1724–9.

21. Lester JF, MacBeth FR, Coles B. Prophylactic cranial irradiation for preventing brain metastases in patients undergoing radical treatment for non-small-cell lung cancer: a Cochrane Review. Int J Radiat Oncol Biol Phys 2005;63:690–4.

22. Lee JS, Pisters KM, Komaki R, et al. Paclitaxel/carboplatin chemotherapy as primary treatment of brain metastases in non-small cell lung cancer: a preliminary report. Semin Oncol 1997;24:S12-52–55.

23. Robinet G, Thomas P, Breton JL, et al. Results of a phase III study of early versus delayed whole brain radiotherapy with concurrent cisplatin and vinorelbine combination in inoperable brain metastasis of non-small-cell lung cancer: Groupe Francais de Pneumo-Cancerologie (GFPC) Protocol 95-1. Ann Oncol 2001;12:59–67.

24. Dinglin XX, Huang Y, Liu H, et al. Pemetrexed and cisplatin combination with concurrent whole brain radiotherapy in patients with brain metastases of lung adenocarcinoma: a single-arm phase II clinical trial. J Neurooncol 2013;112:461–6.

25. Barlesi F, Gervais R, Lena H, et al. Pemetrexed and cisplatin as first-line chemotherapy for advanced non-small-cell lung cancer (NSCLC) with asymptomatic inoperable brain metastases: a multicenter phase II trial (GFPC 07-01). Ann Oncol 2011;22:2466–70.

26. Stupp R, Mason WP, van den Bent MJ, et al. Radiotherapy plus concomitant and adjuvant temozolomide for glioblastoma. N Engl J Med 2005;352:987–96.

27. Christodoulou C, Bafaloukos D, Kosmidis P, et al. Phase II study of temozolomide in heavily pretreated cancer patients with brain metastases. Ann Oncol 2001;12:249–54.

28. Abrey LE, Olson JD, Raizer JJ, et al. A phase II trial of temozolomide for patients with recurrent or progressive brain metastases. J Neurooncol 2001;53:259–65.

29. Giorgio CG, Giuffrida D, Pappalardo A, et al. Oral temozolomide in heavily pretreated brain metastases from non-small cell lung cancer: phase II study. Lung Cancer 2005;50:247–54.

30. Dziadziuszko R, Ardizzoni A, Postmus PE, et al. Temozolomide in patients with advanced non-small cell lung cancer with and without brain metastases. a phase II study of the EORTC Lung Cancer Group (08965). Eur J Cancer 2003;39:1271–6.

31. Sperduto PW, Wang M, Robins HI, et al. A phase 3 trial of whole brain radiation therapy and stereotactic radiosurgery alone versus WBRT and SRS with temozolomide or erlotinib for non-small cell lung cancer and 1 to 3 brain metastases: Radiation Therapy Oncology Group 0320. Int J Radiat Oncol Biol Phys 2013;85: 1312–8.

32. Kumthekar P, Grimm SA, Avram MJ, et al. Pharmacokinetics and efficacy of pemetrexed in patients with brain or leptomeningeal metastases. J Neurooncol 2013;112:247–55.

33. Chamberlain MC. Leptomeningeal metastasis. Curr Opin Neurol 2009;22: 665–74.

34. Glantz MJ, Jaeckle KA, Chamberlain MC, et al. A randomized controlled trial comparing intrathecal sustained-release cytarabine (DepoCyt) to intrathecal methotrexate in patients with neoplastic meningitis from solid tumors. Clin Cancer Res 1999;5:3394–402.

35. Brastianos PK, Carter SL, Santagata S, et al. Genomic characterization of brain metastases reveals branched evolution and potential therapeutic targets. Cancer Discov 2015;5:1164–77.

36. Paik PK, Shen R, Won H, et al. Next-generation sequencing of stage IV squamous cell lung cancers reveals an association of PI3K aberrations and evidence of clonal heterogeneity in patients with brain metastases. Cancer Discov 2015;5: 610–21.

37. Sholl LM, Aisner DL, Varella-Garcia M, et al. Multi-institutional oncogenic driver mutation analysis in lung adenocarcinoma: the lung cancer mutation consortium experience. J Thorac Oncol 2015;10:768–77.

38. Rosell R, Moran T, Queralt C, et al. Screening for epidermal growth factor receptor mutations in lung cancer. N Engl J Med 2009;361:958–67.

39. Zhou C, Wu YL, Chen G, et al. Erlotinib versus chemotherapy as first-line treatment for patients with advanced EGFR mutation-positive non-small-cell lung cancer (OPTIMAL, CTONG-0802): a multicentre, open-label, randomised, phase 3 study. Lancet Oncol 2011;12:735–42.

40. Rosell R, Carcereny E, Gervais R, et al. Erlotinib versus standard chemotherapy as first-line treatment for European patients with advanced EGFR mutation-positive non-small-cell lung cancer (EURTAC): a multicentre, open-label, randomised phase 3 trial. Lancet Oncol 2012;13:239–46.

41. Mitsudomi T, Morita S, Yatabe Y, et al. Gefitinib versus cisplatin plus docetaxel in patients with non-small-cell lung cancer harbouring mutations of the epidermal growth factor receptor (WJTOG3405): an open label, randomised phase 3 trial. Lancet Oncol 2010;11:121–8.

42. Inoue A, Kobayashi K, Maemondo M, et al. Updated overall survival results from a randomized phase III trial comparing gefitinib with carboplatin-paclitaxel for chemo-naive non-small cell lung cancer with sensitive EGFR gene mutations (NEJ002). Ann Oncol 2013;24:54–9.

43. Cappuzzo F, Ardizzoni A, Soto-Parra H, et al. Epidermal growth factor receptor targeted therapy by ZD 1839 (Iressa) in patients with brain metastases from non-small cell lung cancer (NSCLC). Lung Cancer 2003;41:227–31.

44. Cappuzzo F, Calandri C, Bartolini S, et al. ZD 1839 in patients with brain metastases from non-small-cell lung cancer (NSCLC): report of four cases. Br J Cancer 2003;89:246–7.

45. Lai CS, Boshoff C, Falzon M, et al. Complete response to erlotinib treatment in brain metastases from recurrent NSCLC. Thorax 2006;61:91.

46. Li Z, Lu J, Zhao Y, et al. The retrospective analysis of the frequency of EGFR mutations and the efficacy of gefitinib in NSCLC patients with brain metastasis. ASCO Meeting Abstracts 2011;29:e18065.

47. Iuchi T, Shingyoji M, Sakaida T, et al. Phase II trial of gefitinib alone without radiation therapy for Japanese patients with brain metastases from EGFR-mutant lung adenocarcinoma. Lung Cancer 2013;82:282–7.

48. Porta R, Sanchez-Torres JM, Paz-Ares L, et al. Brain metastases from lung cancer responding to erlotinib: the importance of EGFR mutation. Eur Respir J 2011;37:624–31.

49. Wu YL, Zhou C, Cheng Y, et al. Erlotinib as second-line treatment in patients with advanced non-small-cell lung cancer and asymptomatic brain metastases: a phase II study (CTONG-0803). Ann Oncol 2013;24:993–9.

50. Welsh JW, Komaki R, Amini A, et al. Phase II trial of erlotinib plus concurrent whole-brain radiation therapy for patients with brain metastases from non-small-cell lung cancer. J Clin Oncol 2013;31:895–902.

51. Zhuang H, Yuan Z, Wang J, et al. Phase II study of whole brain radiotherapy with or without erlotinib in patients with multiple brain metastases from lung adenocarcinoma. Drug Des Devel Ther 2013;7:1179–86.

52. Park SJ, Kim HT, Lee DH, et al. Efficacy of epidermal growth factor receptor tyrosine kinase inhibitors for brain metastasis in non-small cell lung cancer patients harboring either exon 19 or 21 mutation. Lung Cancer 2012;77:556–60.

53. Kim JE, Lee DH, Choi Y, et al. Epidermal growth factor receptor tyrosine kinase inhibitors as a first-line therapy for never-smokers with adenocarcinoma of the lung having asymptomatic synchronous brain metastasis. Lung Cancer 2009;65:351–4.

54. Weber B, Winterdahl M, Memon A, et al. Erlotinib accumulation in brain metastases from non-small cell lung cancer: visualization by positron emission tomography in a patient harboring a mutation in the epidermal growth factor receptor. J Thorac Oncol 2011;6:1287–9.

55. Togashi Y, Masago K, Masuda S, et al. Cerebrospinal fluid concentration of gefitinib and erlotinib in patients with non-small cell lung cancer. Cancer Chemother Pharmacol 2012;70:399–405.

56. Zhao J, Chen M, Zhong W, et al. Cerebrospinal fluid concentrations of gefitinib in patients with lung adenocarcinoma. Clin Lung Cancer 2013;14:188–93.

57. Schottle J, Chatterjee S, Volz C, et al. Intermittent high-dose treatment with erlotinib enhances therapeutic efficacy in EGFR-mutant lung cancer. Oncotarget 2015;6:38458–68.

58. Kuiper JL, Heideman DA, Thunnissen E, et al. High-dose, weekly erlotinib is not an effective treatment in EGFR-mutated non-small cell lung cancer-patients with

acquired extracranial progressive disease on standard dose erlotinib. Eur J Cancer 2014;50:1399–401.

59. Clarke JL, Pao W, Wu N, et al. High dose weekly erlotinib achieves therapeutic concentrations in CSF and is effective in leptomeningeal metastases from epidermal growth factor receptor mutant lung cancer. J Neurooncol 2010;99: 283–6.

60. Grommes C, Oxnard GR, Kris MG, et al. Pulsatile high-dose weekly erlotinib for CNS metastases from EGFR mutant non-small cell lung cancer. Neuro Oncol 2011;13:1364–9.

61. Kuiper JL, Smit EF. High-dose, pulsatile erlotinib in two NSCLC patients with leptomeningeal metastases–one with a remarkable thoracic response as well. Lung Cancer 2013;80:102–5.

62. Dhruva N, Socinski MA. Carcinomatous meningitis in non-small-cell lung cancer: response to high-dose erlotinib. J Clin Oncol 2009;27:e31–2.

63. Guan Y, Zhao H, Meng J, et al. Dramatic response to high-dose icotinib in a lung adenocarcinoma patient after erlotinib failure. Lung Cancer 2014;83:305–7.

64. Sequist LV, Yang JC, Yamamoto N, et al. Phase III study of afatinib or cisplatin plus pemetrexed in patients with metastatic lung adenocarcinoma with EGFR mutations. J Clin Oncol 2013;31:3327–34.

65. Hata A, Katakami N. Afatinib for erlotinib refractory brain metastases in a patient with EGFR-mutant non-small-cell lung cancer: can high-affinity TKI substitute for high-dose TKI? J Thorac Oncol 2015;10:e65–6.

66. Hoffknecht P, Tufman A, Wehler T, et al. Efficacy of the irreversible ErbB family blocker afatinib in epidermal growth factor receptor (EGFR) tyrosine kinase inhibitor (TKI)-pretreated non-small-cell lung cancer patients with brain metastases or leptomeningeal disease. J Thorac Oncol 2015;10:156–63.

67. Camidge DR, Pao W, Sequist LV. Acquired resistance to TKIs in solid tumours: learning from lung cancer. Nat Rev Clin Oncol 2014;11:473–81.

68. Ricciuti B, Chiari R, Chiarini P, et al. Osimertinib (AZD9291) and CNS response in two radiotherapy-naive patients with EGFR-mutant and T790M-positive advanced non-small cell lung cancer. Clin Drug Investig 2016;36(8):683–6.

69. Sequist LV, Piotrowska Z, Niederst MJ, et al. Osimertinib responses after disease progression in patients who had been receiving rociletinib. JAMA Oncol 2016;2:541–3.

70. Yang JCH, Kim DW, Kim SW, et al. Osimertinib activity in patients (pts) with leptomeningeal (LM) disease from non-small cell lung cancer (NSCLC): Updated results from BLOOM, a phase I study. ASCO Meeting Abstracts 2016;34:9002.

71. Kim DW, Yang JCH, Chen K, et al. AZD3759, an EGFR inhibitor with blood brain barrier (BBB) penetration for the treatment of non-small cell lung cancer (NSCLC) with brain metastasis (BM): preclinical evidence and clinical cases. ASCO Meeting Abstracts 2015;33:8016.

72. Ahn MJ, Kim DW, Kim TM, et al. Phase I study of AZD3759, a CNS penetrable EGFR inhibitor, for the treatment of non-small-cell lung cancer (NSCLC) with brain metastasis (BM) and leptomeningeal metastasis (LM). ASCO Meeting Abstracts 2016;34:9003.

73. Soda M, Choi YL, Enomoto M, et al. Identification of the transforming EML4-ALK fusion gene in non-small-cell lung cancer. Nature 2007;448:561–6.

74. Shaw AT, Engelman JA. ALK in lung cancer: past, present, and future. J Clin Oncol 2013;31:1105–11.

75. Shaw AT, Yeap BY, Mino-Kenudson M, et al. Clinical features and outcome of patients with non-small-cell lung cancer who harbor EML4-ALK. J Clin Oncol 2009; 27:4247–53.
76. Wong DW, Leung EL, So KK, et al. The EML4-ALK fusion gene is involved in various histologic types of lung cancers from nonsmokers with wild-type EGFR and KRAS. Cancer 2009;115:1723–33.
77. Solomon BJ, Mok T, Kim DW, et al. First-line crizotinib versus chemotherapy in ALK-positive lung cancer. N Engl J Med 2014;371:2167–77.
78. Costa DB, Shaw AT, Ou SHI, et al. Clinical experience with crizotinib in patients with advanced ALK-rearranged non–small-cell lung cancer and brain metastases. J Clin Oncol 2015;33:1881–8.
79. Ou SH, Janne PA, Bartlett CH, et al. Clinical benefit of continuing ALK inhibition with crizotinib beyond initial disease progression in patients with advanced ALK-positive NSCLC. Ann Oncol 2014;25:415–22.
80. Kim DW, Mehra R, Tan DS, et al. Activity and safety of ceritinib in patients with ALK-rearranged non-small-cell lung cancer (ASCEND-1): updated results from the multicentre, open-label, phase 1 trial. Lancet Oncol 2016;17(4):452–63.
81. Gadgeel SM, Gandhi L, Riely GJ, et al. Safety and activity of alectinib against systemic disease and brain metastases in patients with crizotinib-resistant ALK-rearranged non-small-cell lung cancer (AF-002JG): results from the dose-finding portion of a phase 1/2 study. Lancet Oncol 2014;15:1119–28.
82. Shaw AT, Gandhi L, Gadgeel S, et al. Alectinib in ALK-positive, crizotinib-resistant, non-small-cell lung cancer: a single-group, multicentre, phase 2 trial. Lancet Oncol 2016;17:234–42.
83. Kim DW, Tiseo M, Ahn MJ, et al. Brigatinib (BRG) in patients (pts) with crizotinib (CRZ)-refractory ALK+ non-small cell lung cancer (NSCLC): first report of efficacy and safety from a pivotal randomized phase (ph) 2 trial (ALTA). ASCO Meeting Abstracts 2016;34:9007.
84. Solomon BJ, Bauer TM, Felip E, et al. Safety and efficacy of lorlatinib (PF-06463922) from the dose-escalation component of a study in patients with advanced ALK+ or ROS1+ non-small cell lung cancer (NSCLC). ASCO Meeting Abstracts 2016;34:9009.
85. Horn L, Infante JR, Blumenschein GR, et al. A phase I trial of X-396, a novel ALK inhibitor, in patients with advanced solid tumors. ASCO Meeting Abstracts 2014; 32:8030.
86. Farago AF, Le LP, Zheng Z, et al. Durable clinical response to entrectinib in NTRK1-rearranged non-small cell lung cancer. J Thorac Oncol 2015;10:1670–4.
87. Falchook GS, Long GV, Kurzrock R, et al. Dabrafenib in patients with melanoma, untreated brain metastases, and other solid tumours: a phase 1 dose-escalation trial. Lancet 2012;379:1893–901.
88. Gibney GT, Gauthier G, Ayas C, et al. Treatment patterns and outcomes in BRAF V600E-mutant melanoma patients with brain metastases receiving vemurafenib in the real-world setting. Cancer Med 2015;4:1205–13.
89. Kinno T, Tsuta K, Shiraishi K, et al. Clinicopathological features of nonsmall cell lung carcinomas with BRAF mutations. Ann Oncol 2014;25:138–42.
90. Brustugun OT, Khattak AM, Tromborg AK, et al. BRAF-mutations in non-small cell lung cancer. Lung Cancer 2014;84:36–8.
91. Planchard D, Kim TM, Mazieres J, et al. Dabrafenib in patients with BRAF-positive advanced non-small-cell lung cancer: a single-arm, multicentre, open-label, phase 2 trial. Lancet Oncol 2016;17(5):642–50.

92. Robinson SD, O'Shaughnessy JA, Cowey CL, et al. BRAF V600E-mutated lung adenocarcinoma with metastases to the brain responding to treatment with vemurafenib. Lung Cancer 2014;85:326–30.

93. Drilon A, Wang L, Hasanovic A, et al. Response to cabozantinib in patients with RET fusion-positive lung adenocarcinomas. Cancer Discov 2013;3:630–5.

94. Subbiah V, Berry J, Roxas M, et al. Systemic and CNS activity of the RET inhibitor vandetanib combined with the mTOR inhibitor everolimus in KIF5B-RET rearranged non-small cell lung cancer with brain metastases. Lung Cancer 2015;89:76–9.

95. Socinski MA, Langer CJ, Huang JE, et al. Safety of bevacizumab in patients with non-small-cell lung cancer and brain metastases. J Clin Oncol 2009;27: 5255–61.

96. Brahmer J, Reckamp KL, Baas P, et al. Nivolumab versus docetaxel in advanced squamous-cell non-small-cell lung cancer. N Engl J Med 2015;373: 123–35.

97. Borghaei H, Paz-Ares L, Horn L, et al. Nivolumab versus docetaxel in advanced nonsquamous non-small-cell lung cancer. N Engl J Med 2015;373:1627–39.

98. Garon EB, Rizvi NA, Hui R, et al. Pembrolizumab for the treatment of non-small-cell lung cancer. N Engl J Med 2015;372:2018–28.

99. Kluger HM, Goldberg SB, Sznol M, et al. Safety and activity of pembrolizumab in melanoma patients with untreated brain metastases. ASCO Meeting Abstracts 2015;33:9009.

100. Goldberg SB, Gettinger SN, Mahajan A, et al. Pembrolizumab for patients with melanoma or non-small-cell lung cancer and untreated brain metastases: early analysis of a non-randomised, open-label, phase 2 trial. Lancet Oncol 2016; 17(7):976–83.

101. Twelves CJ, Souhami RL, Harper PG, et al. The response of cerebral metastases in small cell lung cancer to systemic chemotherapy. Br J Cancer 1990;61: 147–50.

102. Seute T, Leffers P, Wilmink JT, et al. Response of asymptomatic brain metastases from small-cell lung cancer to systemic first-line chemotherapy. J Clin Oncol 2006;24:2079–83.

103. Kristjansen PE, Soelberg Sorensen P, Skov Hansen M, et al. Prospective evaluation of the effect on initial brain metastases from small cell lung cancer of platinum-etoposide based induction chemotherapy followed by an alternating multidrug regimen. Ann Oncol 1993;4:579–83.

104. Postmus PE, Haaxma-Reiche H, Smit EF, et al. Treatment of brain metastases of small-cell lung cancer: comparing teniposide and teniposide with whole-brain radiotherapy–a phase III study of the European Organization for the Research and Treatment of Cancer Lung Cancer Cooperative Group. J Clin Oncol 2000; 18:3400–8.

105. Solomon BJ, Cappuzzo F, Felip E, et al. Intracranial efficacy of crizotinib versus chemotherapy in patients with advanced ALK-positive non–small-cell lung cancer: results from PROFILE 1014. J Clin Oncol 2016;34(24):2858–65.

Index

Note: Page numbers of article titles are in **boldface** type.

A

Adjuvant chemotherapy, for NSCLC, 32–34
    for anaplastic lymphoma kinase-positive NSCLC, 106–107
    choice of agent, 33–34
    in elderly patients, 34
Alatinib, for EGFR mutated advanced NSCLC, 85–88
Alectinib, for anaplastic lymphoma kinase-positive NSCLC, 104–105
    resistance to, 105
Anaplastic lymphoma kinase (ALK), 17–18
  in targeted therapy for brain metastases of lung cancer, 163–164
Anaplastic lymphoma kinase (ALK) tyrosine kinase inhibitors, potential role of, 106
Anaplastic lymphoma kinase (ALK)-positive NSCLC, diagnosis and treatment, **101–111**
    patient evaluation, 102
    pharmacologic treatment options, 102–107
        ceritinib and alectinib, 104–105
        crizotinib, 102–104
        optimal sequence of therapy, 106
        in patients with CNS disease, 105–106
        potential role of adjuvant treatment, 106
        role of chemotherapy and immunotherapy, 107
        role of nonpharmacologic therapy, 107
Angiogenesis inhibition, in first-line therapy of NSCLC, 61–64
  for SCLC, 147–148
Antifolate agents, for brain metastases from NSCLC, 160

B

Biologic agents, added to platinum combinations in first-line therapy for NSCLC, 61–65
    angiogenesis inhibition, 61–64
    epidermal growth factor receptor inhibition, 64–65
Biomarkers, chemotherapy, 35
  of lung cancer, **13–29**
    genomic, 14–22
        anaplastic lymphoma kinase, 17–18
        B-RAF proto-oncogene, serine/threonine kinase, 20–21
        discoidin domain receptor tyrosine kinase 2, 22
        epidermal growth factor receptor, 16–17
        fibroblast growth factor receptor, 21–22
        human epidermal growth factor receptor 2, 19
        Kirsten rat sarcoma (KRAS) viral oncogene homolog, 18
        MET proto-oncogene, 20
        neurotrophic receptor tyrosine kinase 1, 21

Hematol Oncol Clin N Am 31 (2017) 177–187
http://dx.doi.org/10.1016/S0889-8588(16)30156-3
0889-8588/17

Biomarkers (*continued*)
       phosphatidylinositol-4,5-bisphosphonate 3-kinase catalytic subunit alpha, 21
       RET proto-oncogene, 19–20
       ROS proto-oncogene 1, receptor tyrosine kinase, 18–19
    histologic subtyping, 14
    immunotherapy markers, 22–23
       cytotoxic T-lymphocyte-associated antigen 4, 23
       programmed death-ligand 1 receptor, 23
BRAF proto-oncogene serine/threonine kinase, 20–21
  in lung adenocarcinoma, 120–121
Brain metastases, of lung cancer, systemic treatment of, **155–174**
    antifolate agents, 160
    immunotherapy, 165–168
    intrathecal chemotherapy, 160–161
    molecularly targeted therapy for, 161–165
       anaplastic lymphoma kinase, 163–164
       epidermal growth factor receptor, 161–163
       other targeted alterations, 165
    systemic chemotherapy for NSCLC, 157–160
       platinum agents, 159
       temozolomide, 159–160
    systemic chemotherapy for SCLC, 157
       front-line platinum- or cyclophosphamide-based regimens, 157
       topotecan, 157

C

c-MET, amplification and mutation in, 119–120
Ceritinib, for anaplastic lymphoma kinase-positive NSCLC, 104–105
    resistance to, 105
Chemoradiation, for unresectable stage III NSCLC, 48–52
    radiation dose and fractionation, 51
    radiation techniques, 51–52
    role of induction, consolidation, and maintenance therapy, 49–51
    selection of chemotherapy regimen, 49
    timing of, 48–49
Chemotherapy, adjuvant, for NSCLC, 32–34
    choice of agent, 33–34
    in elderly patients, 34
  for anaplastic lymphoma kinase-positive NSCLC, 107
  for brain metastases of NSCLC, 157–160
    platinum agents, 159
    temozolomide, 159–160
  for brain metastases of SCLC, 157
    front-line platinum- or cyclophosphamide-based regimens, 157
    topotecan, 157
  first-line, for NSCLC, **59–70,** 71
    addition of biologic agents to platinum combinations, 61–65
    maintenance therapy, 65–68
    patient evaluation, 59–60
    with platinum combinations, 60–61

first-line, for SCLC, 145–147
   cisplatin vs carboplatin, 146–147
   emerging agents, 147
intrathecal, for brain metastases from lung cancer, 160–161
neoadjuvant, for NSCLC, 34–35
second-line, for NSCLC, **71–81**
   docetaxel, 73–75
   epidermal growth factor receptor TKIs, 76–77
   first-line treatment, 71
   maintenance therapy, 72
   pemetrexed, 75–76
   single-agent vs combination regimens, 72–73
for unresectable stage III NSCLC, 48–49
   role of induction, consolidation and maintenance therapy, 49–51
   selection of regimen, 49
   timing, 48–49
Chromosomal rearrangements, in lung cancer, 4–5
Clonal heterogeneity, in lung cancer, implications for therapy, 6–8
Copy number alterations, in lung cancer, 3–4
Cranial irradiation, prophylactic, in SCLC, 145
Crizotinib, for anaplastic lymphoma kinase-positive NSCLC, 102–104
   resistance to, 103–104
Cyclophosphamide-based regimens, for brain metastases from SCLC, 157
Cytotoxic T-lymphocyte-associated antigen 4 (CTLA-4), 23

D

Discoidin domain receptor tyrosine kinase 2 (DDR2), 22
Docetaxel, in second-line chemotherapy for NSCLC, 73–75

E

Elderly patients, adjuvant chemotherapy for NSCLC in, 34
Epidermal growth factor receptor (EGFR), 16–17
   inhibition of in first-line therapy of NSCLC, 64–65
   in targeted therapy for brain metastases of lung cancer, 161–163
Epidermal growth factor receptor (EGFR) mutated advanced NSCLC, **83–99**
   acquired resistance mechanisms and predictive biomarkers, 88–89
   characteristics of mutated subsets, 84–85
   comparison of EGFR TKIs, 86–88
   EGFR TKI monotherapy as first-line therapy, 85–86
   management of acquired resistance, 89–92
Epidermal growth factor receptor (EGFR) tyrosine kinase inhibitors (TKIs), for advanced
   EGFR mutated NSCLC, 85–88
      comparison of, 86–88
      monotherapy with, 85–86
   in second-line therapy for NSCLC, 76–77
Ertolinib, for EGFR mutated advanced NSCLC, 85–88

F

Fibroblast growth factor receptor, 21–22
First-line systemic therapy, for NSCLC, **59–70,** 71
    addition of biologic agents to platinum combinations, 61–65
      angiogenesis inhibition, 61–64
      epidermal growth factor receptor inhibition, 64–65
    maintenance therapy, 65–68
    patient evaluation overview, 59–60
    with platinum combinations, 60–61

G

Gefitinib, for EGFR mutated advanced NSCLC, 85–88
Genomic biomarkers, in NSCLC, 14–22
    anaplastic lymphoma kinase, 17–18
    B-RAF proto-oncogene, serine/threonine kinase, 20–21
    discoidin domain receptor tyrosine kinase 2, 22
    epidermal growth factor receptor, 16–17
    fibroblast growth factor receptor, 21–22
    human epidermal growth factor receptor 2, 19
    Kirsten rat sarcoma (KRAS) viral oncogene homolog, 18
    MET proto-oncogene, 20
    neurotrophic receptor tyrosine kinase 1, 21
    phosphatidylinositol-4,5-bisphosphonate 3-kinase catalytic subunit alpha, 21
    RET proto-oncogene, 19–20
    ROS proto-oncogene 1, receptor tyrosine kinase, 18–19

H

Histologic subtyping, of NSCLC, 14
Human epidermal growth factor receptor 2 (HER2), 19

I

Immune checkpoint inhibitors, in NSCLC, 134–138
    early phase clinical studies with, 135–136
    mutation burden, 138
    predictive factors of, 137–138
      mutation burden, 138
      PD-L1 expression, 137–138
    randomized clinical trials with, 136–137
Immune-based therapy, next-generation sequencing and, for lung cancer, 8
Immunotherapy, for brain metastases of lung cancer, 165–168
    in NSCLC, **131–140**
    adjuvant settings, 132–133
    for anaplastic lymphoma kinase-positive, 107
    checkpoint inhibitors, 134–138
    first-line therapy, 134
    immune checkpoint inhibitors, early phase clinical studies with, 135–136
      mutation burden, 138

predictive factors of, 137–138
randomized clinical trials with, 136–137
maintenance therapy, 133–134
previously treated patients, 134
vaccines, 131–132
for SCLC, 149
Immunotherapy markers, in lung cancer, 22–23
cytotoxic T-lymphocyte-associated antigen 4, 23
programmed death-ligand 1 receptor, 23
Intrathecal chemotherapy, for brain metastases from lung cancer, 160–161

K

Kirsten rat sarcoma (KRAS) viral oncogene homolog, 18, 121–123
KRAS viral oncogene homolog, 18, 121–123

L

Locally advanced non-small cell lung cancer, treatment of, **45–57**
patient evaluation, 45–47
resectable stage III, 47–48
surveillance, 53
treatment complications, 52–53
unresectable stage III, 48–52
radiation dose and fractionation, 51
radiation techniques, 51–52
role of induction, consolidation, and maintenance systemic therapy, 49–51
selection of chemotherapy regimen, 49
timing of chemotherapy and radiotherapy, 48–49
Lung cancer, brain metastases, systemic treatment of, **155–174**
antifolate agents, 160
immunotherapy, 165–168
intrathecal chemotherapy, 160–161
molecularly targeted therapy for, 161–165
systemic chemotherapy for NSCLC, 157–160
systemic chemotherapy for small cell lung cancer, 157
next-generation sequencing of, **1–12**
chromosomal rearrangements, 4–5
clonal heterogeneity, 6–8
copy number alterations, 3–4
future directions, 8–9
immune-based therapies, 8
somatic mutations, 2–3
splicing alterations, 6
non-small cell, anaplastic lymphoma kinase-positive, **101–111**
patient evaluation, 102
pharmacologic treatment options, 102–107
role of nonpharmacologic therapy, 107
biomarkers, **13–29**
genomic, 14–22
histologic subtyping, 14

Lung (*continued*)
  immunotherapy markers, 22–23
  epidermal growth factor receptor (EGFR) mutated advanced, **83–99**
    acquired resistance mechanisms and predictive biomarkers, 88–89
    characteristics of mutated subsets, 84–85
    comparison of EGFR TKIs, 86–88
    EGFR TKI monotherapy as first-line therapy, 85–86
    management of acquired resistance, 89–92
  first-line systemic therapy for, **59–70**
    addition of biologic agents to platinum combinations, 61–65
    maintenance therapy, 65–68
    patient evaluation overview, 59–60
    with platinum combinations, 60–61
  immunotherapy in, **131–140**
    adjuvant settings, 132–133
    checkpoint inhibitors, 134–138
    first-line therapy, 134
    maintenance therapy, 133–134
    previously treated patients, 134
    vaccines, 131–132
  locally advanced, treatment of, **45–57**
    patient evaluation, 45–47
    resectable stage III, 47–48
    surveillance, 53
    treatment complications, 52–53
    unresectable stage III, 48–52
  neoadjuvant and adjuvant therapy for, **31–44**
    adjuvant chemotherapy, 32–34
    background, 31–32
    chemotherapy biomarkers, 35
    molecularly targeted therapy, 35–39
    neoadjuvant chemotherapy, 34–35
    radiation therapy, 39
  new targets in, **113–129**
    amplification and mutation in c-MET, 119–120
    BRAF mutations in lung adenocarcinoma, 120–121
    KRAS, 121–123
    oncogenic NTRK1 fusion, 114–116
    oncogenic RET fusion, 116–117
    oncogenic ROS1 fusion, 114–118
  second-line chemotherapy and beyond for, **71–81**
    docetaxel, 73–75
    epidermal growth factor receptor tyrosine kinase inhibitors, 76–77
    first-line treatment, 71
    maintenance therapy, 72
    pemetrexed, 75–76
    single-agent vs combination regimens, 72–73
  small cell, advances in, **141–154**
    initial assessment and staging, 142–143
    staging systems, 142
    treatment, 143–149

emerging therapies, 147–149
first-line chemotherapy, 145–147
prophylactic cranial irradiation, 145
stage-specific therapy, 143
thoracic radiography in extensive stage, 144
thoracic radiography in limited stage, 143–144

M

MET proto-oncogene, 20
Metastases, of lung cancer to the brain, systemic treatment of, **155–174**
   antifolate agents, 160
   immunotherapy, 165–168
   intrathecal chemotherapy, 160–161
   molecularly targeted therapy for, 161–165
      anaplastic lymphoma kinase, 163–164
      epidermal growth factor receptor, 161–163
      other targeted alterations, 165
   systemic chemotherapy for NSCLC, 157–160
      platinum agents, 159
      temozolomide, 159–160
   systemic chemotherapy for SCLC, 157
      front-line platinum- or cyclophosphamide-based regimens, 157
      topotecan, 157
Molecularly targeted therapy. *See* Targeted therapy.

N

Neoadjuvant chemotherapy, for NSCLC, 34–35
Non-small cell lung cancer (NSCLC), anaplastic lymphoma kinase-positive, **101–111**
   patient evaluation, 102
   pharmacologic treatment options, 102–107
      ceritinib and alectinib, 104–105
      crizotinib, 102–104
      optimal sequence of therapy, 106
      in patients with CNS disease, 105–106
      potential role of adjuvant treatment, 106
      role of chemotherapy and immunotherapy, 107
   role of nonpharmacologic therapy, 107
   biomarkers, **13–29**
      genomic, 14–22
         anaplastic lymphoma kinase, 17–18
         B-RAF proto-oncogene, serine/threonine kinase, 20–21
         discoidin domain receptor tyrosine kinase 2, 22
         epidermal growth factor receptor, 16–17
         fibroblast growth factor receptor, 21–22
         human epidermal growth factor receptor 2, 19
         Kirsten rat sarcoma (KRAS) viral oncogene homolog, 18
         MET proto-oncogene, 20
         neurotrophic receptor ttyrosine kinase 1, 21
         phosphatidylinositol-4,5-bisphosphonate 3-kinase catalytic subunit alpha, 21

Non-small (*continued*)
        RET proto-oncogene, 19–20
        ROS proto-oncogene 1, receptor tyrosine kinase, 18–19
    histologic subtyping, 14
    immunotherapy markers, 22–23
        cytotoxic T-lymphocyte-associated antigen 4, 23
        programmed death-ligand 1 receptor, 23
  epidermal growth factor receptor (EGFR) mutated advanced, **83–99**
    acquired resistance mechanisms and predictive biomarkers, 88–89
    characteristics of mutated subsets, 84–85
    comparison of EGFR TKIs, 86–88
    EGFR TKI monotherapy as first-line therapy, 85–86
    management of acquired resistance, 89–92
  epidermal growth factor reeptor mutated advanced, **83–99**
  first-line systemic therapy for, **59–70**
    addition of biologic agents to platinum combinations, 61–65
        angiogenesis inhibition, 61–64
        epidermal growth factor receptor inhibition, 64–65
    maintenance therapy, 65–68
    patient evaluation overview, 59–60
    with platinum combinations, 60–61
  immunotherapy in, **131–140**
    adjuvant settings, 132–133
    checkpoint inhibitors, 134–138
    first-line therapy, 134
    immune checkpoint inhibitros, early phase clinical studies with, 135–136
        mutation burden, 138
        predictive factors of, 137–138
        randomized clinical trials with, 136–137
    maintenance therapy, 133–134
    previously treated patients, 134
    vaccines, 131–132
  locally advanced, treatment of, **45–57**
    patient evaluation, 45–47
    resectable stage III, 47–48
    surveillance, 53
    treatement complications, 52–53
    unresectable stage III, 48–52
        delection of chemotherapy regimen, 49
        radiation dose and fractionation, 51
        radiation techniques, 51–52
        role of induction, consolidation, and maintenance systemic therapy, 49–51
        timing of chemotherapy and radiotherapy, 48–49
  neoadjuvant and adjuvant therapy for, **31–44**
    adjuvant chemotherapy, 32–34
    background, 31–32
    chemotherapy biomarkers, 35
    molecularly targeted therapy, 35–39
    neoadjuvant chemotherapy, 34–35
    radiation therapy, 39
  new targets in, **113–129**

amplification and mutation in c-MET, 119–120
BRAF mutations in lung adenocarcinoma, 120–121
KRAS, 121–123
oncogenic NTRK1 fusion, 114–116
oncogenic RET fusion, 116–117
oncogenic ROS1 fusion, 114–118
second-line chemotherapy and beyond for, **71–81**
docetaxel, 73–75
epidermal growth factor receptor tyrosine kinase inhibitors, 76–77
first-line treatment, 71
maintenance therapy, 72
other therapeutic agents, 77
pemetrexed, 75–76
single-agent vs combination regimens, 72–73
NTRK1, 21, 117–119

O

Osimertinib, for EGFR mutated advanced NSCLC, 85–88

P

PD-L1 receptor, 23
immune checkpoint inhibitor and expression in NSCLC, 137–138
Pemetrexed, in second-line therapy for NCSCL, 75–76
Phosphatidylinositol-4,5-bisphosphonate 3-kinase catalytic subunit alpha (PI3KCA), 21
Platinum-based chemotherapy, first-line, for NSCLC, 60–65
with biologic agents, 61–65
platinum combinations, 60–61
for brain metastases from NSCLC, 159
for brain metastases from small cell lung cancer, 157
Programmed death-ligand 1 (PD-L1) receptor, 23
immune checkpoint inhibitor and expression in NSCLC, 137–138
Prophylactic therapy, cranial irradiation in small cell lung cancer, 145

R

Radiation therapy, adjuvant, for NSCLC, 39
prophylactic cranial irradiation in SCLC, 145
for unresectable stage III NSCLC, 48–52
dose and fractionation, 51
techniques, 51–52
timing, 48–49
Radiography, thoracic, in SCLC, 143–144
extensive stage, 144
limited stage, 143–144
RET proto-oncogene receptor tyrosine kinase, 19–20, 116–117
ROS proto-oncogene 1 receptor tyrosine kinase, 18–19, 114–116

S

Second-line chemotherapy, for NSCLC, **71–81**
    docetaxel, 73–75
    epidermal growth factor receptor tyrosine kinase inhibitors, 76–77
    first-line treatment, 71
    maintenance therapy, 72
    pemetrexed, 75–76
    single-agent vs combination regimens, 72–73
Sequencing, next-generation, of lung cancer, **1–12**
    chromosomal rearrangements, 4–5
    clonal heterogeneity, 6–8
    copy number alterations, 3–4
    future directions, 8–9
    immune-based therapies, 8
    somatic mutations, 2–3
    splicing alterations, 6
Small cell lung cancer (SCLC), **141–154**
    initial assessment and staging, 142–143
    staging systems, 142
    treatment, 143–149
        emerging therapies, 147–149
            angiogenesis inhibitors, 147
            chemotherapy, 147
            immunotherapy, 149
            targeted therapy, 149
        first-line chemotherapy, 145–147
            cisplatin vs carboplatin, 146–147
            recurrent disease, 147
        prophylactic cranial irradiation, 145
        stage-specific therapy, 143
        thoracic radiography, 143–144
            in extensive stage, 144
            in limited stage, 143–144
Somatic mutations, in lung cancer, 2–3
Splicing alterations, in lung cancer, 6
Staging systems, for small cell lung cancer, 142
Systemic therapy. *See also* Chemotherapy.
    first-line, for NSCLC, **59–70,** 71
        addition of biologic agents to platinum combinations, 61–65
            angiogenesis inhibition, 61–64
            epidermal growth factor receptor inhibition, 64–65
        maintenance therapy, 65–68
        patient evaluation overview, 59–60
        with platinum combinations, 60–61

T

Targeted therapy, for brain metastases of lung cancer, 161–165
    anaplastic lymphoma kinase, 163–164
    epidermal growth factor receptor, 161–163

other targeted alterations, 165
new targets in, **113–129**
   amplification and mutation in c-MET, 119–120
   BRAF mutations in lung adenocarcinoma, 120–121
   KRAS, 121–123
   oncogenic NTRK1 fusion, 114–116
   oncogenic RET fusion, 116–117
   oncogenic ROS1 fusion, 114–118
for NSCLC, 35–39
ongoing trials, 36–39
for SCLC, 144
Temozolomide, for brain metastases from NSCLC, 159–160
Thoracic radiography, in SCLC, 143–144
   extensive stage, 144
   limited stage, 143–144
Topotecan, for brain metastases from SCLC, 157
Tyrosine kinase inhibitors (TKIs), anaplasmic lymphoma kinase (ALK), 106
epidermal growth factor receptor (EGFR), 76–77, 85–88
   for advanced EGFR mutated NSCLC, 85–88
      comparison of, 86–88
      monotherapy with, 85–86
   in second-line therapy for NCSCL, 76–77
new target in NSCLC, **113–129**

Moving?

Make sure your subscription moves with you!

To notify us of your new address, find your **Clinics Account Number** (located on your mailing label above your name), and contact customer service at:

Email: journalscustomerservice-usa@elsevier.com

800-654-2452 (subscribers in the U.S. & Canada)
314-447-8871 (subscribers outside of the U.S. & Canada)

Fax number: 314-447-8029

Elsevier Health Sciences Division
Subscription Customer Service
3251 Riverport Lane
Maryland Heights, MO 63043

*To ensure uninterrupted delivery of your subscription, please notify us at least 4 weeks in advance of move.